I0147647

DEPLOYED

DEPLOYED

*A Physician on the Front Lines
of Global Health*

Kevin M. De Cock,
MD, FRCP (UK), DTM&H

JOHNS HOPKINS UNIVERSITY PRESS | BALTIMORE

© 2025 Johns Hopkins University Press
All rights reserved. Published 2025
Printed in the United States of America on acid- free paper
9 8 7 6 5 4 3 2 1

Johns Hopkins University Press
2715 North Charles Street
Baltimore, Maryland 21218
www.press.jhu.edu

Library of Congress Cataloging-in-Publication Data

Names: De Cock, Kevin author
Title: Deployed : a physician on the front lines of global health /
    Kevin M. De Cock.
Description: Baltimore : Johns Hopkins University Press, 2025. |
    Includes bibliographical references and index. | Summary: "In this
    book, Dr. De Cock recounts his career tackling global infectious disease
    crises. It offers an insider's perspective on the challenges of public
    health leadership, scientific discovery, and pandemic response in an
    interconnected world"—Provided by publisher.
Identifiers: LCCN 2025011278 (print) | LCCN 2025011279 (ebook) |
    ISBN 9781421453064 hardcover | ISBN 9781421453071 ebook
Subjects: LCSH: De Cock, Kevin | MESH: Infectious Disease Medicine |
    Communicable Disease Control | Global Health | Public Health
    Practice | Personal Narrative
Classification: LCC RA643 .D4335 2025 (print) | LCC RA643 (ebook) |
    NLM WZ 100
LC record available at https://lccn.loc.gov/2025011278
LC ebook record available at https://lccn.loc.gov/2025011279

A catalog record for this book is available from the British Library.

*Special discounts are available for bulk purchases of this book. For more
information, please contact Special Sales at specialsales@jh.edu.*

EU GPSR Authorized Representative
LOGOS EUROPE, 9 rue Nicolas Poussin,
17000, La Rochelle, France
E-mail: Contact@logoseurope.eu

To my family,
with love and gratitude

CONTENTS

PART III BUREAUCRAT

ILLUSTRATIONS

PROLOGUE

The story of global health is an optimistic one. Like advances in science, progress in global health is not linear, it lurches unevenly, but movement has been inexorably towards safer, longer, and healthier lives everywhere.[1] Such generalization does not minimize the persistent burden of preventable disease and death, the unequal access to modern medicine and public health services, or the ravages from conflict, displacement, and natural disasters. Pessimism can act as a guardrail against injudicious enthusiasm, but it cannot deny what careful measurement has shown—that despite its troubles, the world is healthier than it was.

This book details some personal journeys through medicine and global health over decades that have seen emergence of new pathogens, severe epidemics and several pandemics, and astonishing scientific progress. Some of the lessons learned might have been helpful before initiating travel. Much of the experience was gained working for the US Centers for Disease Control and Prevention (CDC), the world's leading public health agency.

The journeys described could not have been planned prospectively. I have written about them as much to draw meaning for myself from work in global health as to share experiences and conclusions others might find relevant. Examination of one's own career requires controlled self-examination. Balance is required between meek introspection and boastful justification of events that should have been handled better. Criticism of others is best tempered with personal humility.

Life Plans and Infectious Diseases

Kierkegaard's dictum that history is written backwards, but that life must be lived forwards highlights the limits of planning, the importance of serendipity, and the need to seize unpredictable opportunities.[2] While I knew from childhood that I hoped to be a doctor, I had no insight into what such a future might hold. Those outside the profession understand little of what medicine entails, and medical students enter their training with little notion of the careers on which they are embarking.

When I started medical school in the United Kingdom in 1969 and then trained in internal medicine, the world seemed oblivious to pandemic threats. Infectious diseases were considered no longer to pose a challenge. Exotic viruses such as Lassa,[3] Marburg,[4] and Ebola[5] emerged in other parts of the world, but they seemed irrelevant to the practice of modern Western medicine. Classic killers such as tuberculosis or childhood infections were deemed vanquished by vaccines and antimicrobial drugs. The tropical world still faced its burden of malaria, schistosomiasis, and other parasitic diseases, but these were little considered by mainstream medicine. Time spent outside of Western medical centers was judged detrimental to an academic future.

Yet for me, unexpectedly, infectious diseases and Africa came to dominate my subsequent career. Social and political changes over the last half century have come to affect medicine as much as society in general. The changes in global health over my time as a physician have been extraordinary—and this fact alone is worthy of discussion.

It was the AIDS epidemic more than any other phenomenon that highlighted our misjudgment relating to communicable diseases.[6] Apparently out of nowhere, a new infectious disease erupted, spread quickly and widely, and generated fear. It was soon understood that AIDS was but the advanced manifestation of a much more widespread condition of immune deficiency. This was captured in the famous "iceberg slide" from the CDC (Figure P.1). The clinical features of the syndrome aroused fascination and gave the disease a unique mystique, notable for its relentless progression to death, the risk groups affected, and the initially obscure connection with Haiti and Africa. Stigma and discrimination also followed, not lightened by the discovery of HIV as the causative agent.

More than four decades have passed since AIDS was first described, and the intervening years have witnessed large outbreaks of newly recognized as well as old infectious diseases.[7] Most recent and devastating, of course, has been the pandemic of COVID-19. While its long-term consequences remain to be

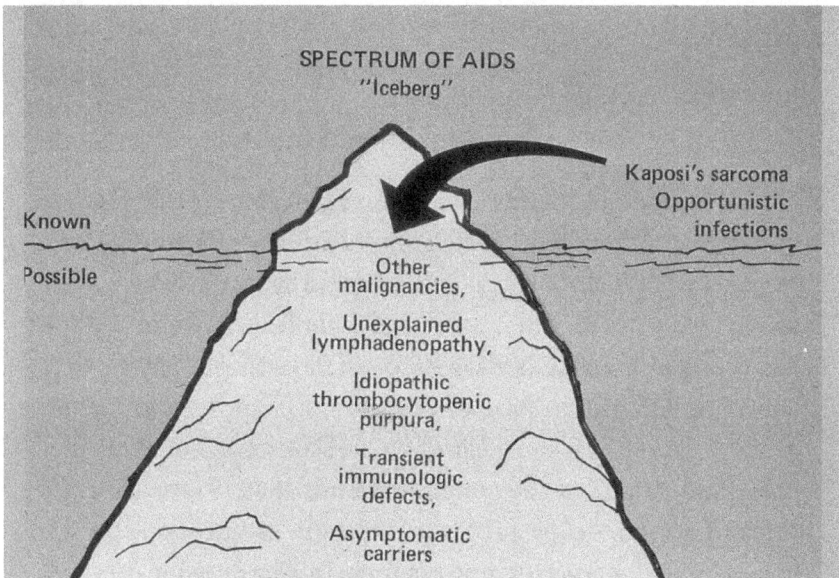

SPECTRUM OF AIDS
"Iceberg"

Kaposi's sarcoma
Opportunistic
infections

Known

Possible

Other
malignancies,

Unexplained
lymphadenopathy,

Idiopathic
thrombocytopenic
purpura,

Transient
immunologic
defects,

Asymptomatic
carriers

Prologue 1 Even before the causative agent (HIV) was discovered, clinicians and epidemiologists suspected AIDS was the severe, end-stage of a syndrome of immunodeficiency with a broad constellation of clinical manifestations.

(Centers for Disease Control and Prevention, "Spectrum of AIDS 'Iceberg,'" slide, circa 1980s. Public domain)

elucidated, COVID-19 should not minimize the significance of these other modern and diverse epidemics.

Severe acute respiratory syndrome (SARS) and Middle East respiratory syndrome (MERS); arboviruses like dengue, Chikungunya, Zika, and yellow fever; and Marburg and Ebola—all have caused important outbreaks. In the poorest parts of the Global South, enteric infections such as cholera and typhoid spread intermittently in epidemic fashion. Antimicrobial resistance has increased.[8] Sexually transmitted infections (STIs), including that ancient disease syphilis, stubbornly resist control. We now have a better understanding of infectious disease emergence, its associated sociopolitical and economic factors, and the consequences of disrupting the balance within our ecosystem. Earlier dismissal of the threat from infectious diseases, it is now evident, was misplaced.

Medicine and Public Health

One of my earliest memories in life is of an etching that hung in my surgeon father's office in Belgium and that now is mine. Drawn in grief by the Austrian artist Ivo Saliger in 1920, the work was inspired by the death of his 22-year-old sister from leukemia.[9] A naked young woman has her arms around the neck of a physician in whites, as death in the form of a kneeling skeleton tries to pull her away, with the physician pushing on the skeleton's skull. Both macabre and poignant, the etching reminds that, no matter one's title or position, the basis of work in health is that of one person in danger or distress reaching out for help. The drawing captures the uncertainty of outcomes in medicine, despite the physician's resolve to do right.

Section I of this book describes my early education and clinical experience. Although I later left clinical medicine for research and public health, what I saw and learned in those earlier years became the core of a professional identity and proved invaluable throughout my personal and working life. And therein, perhaps, is the first lesson: never to forget that medicine and public health concern individuals.

The CDC of the United States is the archetype of a national public health institute.[10] It has had enormous influence and reach since it was established in 1946.[11] Over the years, the CDC has turned to all areas of public health, and its collaborations and networks extend to all parts of the globe. Despite the breadth of its work, the CDC is best known for infectious disease surveillance, and the investigation and control of outbreaks. These topics are central to training in the CDC's Epidemic Intelligence Service (EIS) (a cadre of "disease detectives") and EIS's international offshoots, the Field Epidemiology Training Programs (FETPs).[12] Having embarked on EIS training in 1986, I found the rest of my career revolving around CDC.

Section II of this book describes experiences with African field work. The CDC's work in the West African Ebola epidemic was of historical importance—to the agency itself as well as in the overall chronicle of global health. The final chapter of this section considers early observations on the COVID-19 pandemic from my vantage point as a CDC insider stationed outside the United States (and retired from the agency since the end of 2020). The CDC stumbled during this crisis that should have allowed it to excel. It will take time for the meaning and broad consequences of COVID-19 to become fully understood. The world has become more dangerous, and the need for a strong CDC has increased rather than diminished.

Leadership, Administration, Retirement

Although acute emergencies capture the limelight in clinical medicine and public health, lives are dominated by more day-to-day and long-term considerations. Age and experience lead inexorably to positions of seniority and broader responsibility. One's direct impact seems less obvious when compared with the frenetic activity of the emergency room or the field, and life too easily comes to feel mundane, less exciting. Yet this professional advancement is essential for exerting influence, driving change, and ultimately having broader impact.

Section III of the book deals with experiences in research and public health that required longer-term commitments and engagement in bureaucracy. One chapter considers tuberculosis. Like syphilis and cholera, it is an old disease that is as much a social phenomenon as it is a biological one, epitomizing the social determinants of health and the challenge of health equity.

One lesson from any career is the importance of mistakes. Impact in medicine—lives saved, and mistakes made—are more obvious in clinical work focused on individuals than when dealing with populations. There is truth in the jibe that one murder leads to prison, 100 murders to an institution, and thousands of murders to political exile. Clinical mistakes are more often pursued than public health errors, although the latter may cause far more deaths. The road not travelled can be especially important in population health, where acts of omission, not taking action or intervening, may have even greater consequences than active mistakes.

As COVID-19 illustrated, the stakes for public health are high. We have a duty to learn from our mistakes—and mistakes are inevitable because health practitioners are human. I have commented on some of my own failures. Where I cite missteps of others, it is not for criticism but to encourage thought on what might have been done differently.

Wither Global Health?

Global health as understood today evolved from the disciplines of tropical medicine and international health.[13] Tropical medicine is a term now rarely used, though it continues to feature in the titles of august, predominantly European institutions. I was privileged to study at one such institute, the Liverpool School of Tropical Medicine, and to teach at two others, in London and Antwerp.

There has been increased debate in recent years about the colonial origins and evolution of tropical medicine and its institutions, the influence of tropical medicine on today's global health, and how to democratize promotion of health in the world.[14] These unfinished discussions have been made more acute by geopolitical events and funding decisions in 2025. The epilogue offers some reflections on the meaning and current state of global health. The populations with which global health is concerned will be best served by the thoughtful analysis of a past we cannot change and a definition of a future that is ours to deliver.

2025

"There are decades when nothing happens; and there are weeks when decades happen"—those words ascribed to Vladimir Ilyich Lenin could apply to early 2025 when this book was being finalized. The world now seems more dangerous and unpredictable. An event enhancing uncertainty was the change of administration in the United States.

Following his inauguration in January 2025, President Donald Trump issued an executive order withdrawing the US from the World Health Organization (WHO), reinstituting the order he had issued during the COVID-19 pandemic. Almost all foreign aid has been frozen, and the US Agency for International Development is to be dissolved. Development assistance for health has not been spared, with major interruptions to programs such as the President's Emergency Plan for AIDS Relief (PEPFAR) and the President's Malaria Initiative (PMI), pillars of President George W. Bush's legacy. The consequences in faraway places have been extensive.[15]

In the name of efficiency, Robert F. Kennedy Jr., the new Secretary of Health and Human Services (HHS), moved to reduce HHS staffing by some twenty thousand employees. Reductions of 20–25% of the workforce have occurred at the CDC, the National Institutes of Health (NIH), and the Food and Drug Administration (FDA). At the CDC, extensive cuts have been made to diverse programs and technical groups, including ones that I worked with, such as those addressing HIV/AIDS and global health.

After almost a quarter century of generous funding and notable health impact on scourges like malaria, tuberculosis, and HIV/AIDS, uncertainty has arisen about global health and its future. The unexpected events of early 2025 do not erase experiences or lessons discussed in this book but raise urgent questions about how the world will respond and adapt.

Conclusions

Former CDC Director William ("Bill") Foege taught that epidemiology was the basic science of public health, while its philosophic basis was social justice. Years ago, I asked public health lawyer Lawrence ("Larry") Gostin to define social justice for me: "a fair distribution of the benefits and burdens of society," was his suggestion.[16] Simple frameworks for what we do to assure conditions for people to be healthy—respect for human rights, social justice, evidence-based decision-making—should transcend politics, religion, or ideology.

One of the cultural battles enjoined concerns diversity, equity, and inclusion (DEI).[17] The CDC and other agency websites have been scrubbed, research papers pulled back, and whole areas of scientific investigation defunded or eliminated. The term "equity" has been used frequently in this book because it is critical as a public health goal and should not be viewed as a political or cultural red flag. Equity here does not mean equality but refers to elimination of health disparities, floating all boats. Applied to both health overall and health security, equity means the same outcomes irrespective of different investments required.

Kierkegaard's quote conveys that a priori destinations are never evident, and meaning must be drawn retrospectively from travels undertaken. It is for younger professionals from all over the world to shape the future of global health. They must embark on their own journeys through a discipline in continuous evolution, in need of clearer definition, and inevitably buffeted by events in the broader world. Politicians, academic departments, and institutions rise and fall, but the arc of history is long. The quest is noble and the prize great—health equity in an interconnected world.

DEPLOYED

PART I

CLINICIAN

Although I aspired to be a doctor from early childhood, I had no specific specialty in mind. My reasons for pursuing medicine were typically vague and immature. They mirrored the interview responses most students gave when asked about their motivation— an interest in science and biology, wanting to contribute, working with people, and so forth. Social awareness and an interest in problems of the Global South were enhanced during my gap year and contributed to a focus on infectious and tropical diseases from early on.

The great divide in my clinical training was between the worlds of medicine (referred to in the United States as internal medicine) and surgery. It was evident from my earliest clinical days that I had neither aptitude for nor interest in surgery, and medicine became increasingly obvious as the path to pursue. The surgeons with whom I worked were only too pleased to have as an intern ("houseman" in the United Kingdom), someone interested and committed to the medical welfare of their patients. Although I never regretted my choice of internal medicine as a specialty, it was later that I realized how many other avenues existed that I had little notion of, from forensic psychiatry to medical journalism. I have come to advise students that it is more important to determine what one does not want to do than to strive for certainty about the perfect niche.

Fundamental to the practice of medicine are the science and art of diagnosis. I found much later that the analytic thinking and approaches required in clinical medicine share features with the discipline of epidemiology. It is for that reason that my later transition from clinical work, to which I had been so committed, to public health did not seem like a betrayal. But I am ever conscious of the need to link the welfare of the individual to the needs of the many, and I have missed the interaction with patients.

If I had not been a doctor, I might have been an investigative journalist, another career that requires clear and sequential thinking and deduction. As it is, I am forever grateful for clinical experience and the identity of a physician. Section I of this book deals with my early journey through medicine, to Africa, and the unexpected route through clinical medicine to the US Centers for Disease Control and Prevention.

CHAPTER 1

Why Medicine, Not Politics?

Africa—so much of my life was unexpectedly determined by Africa. Africa, exploited yet overindulged, so often underestimated, misunderstood. Africa, so heterogeneous, yet perceived by the outside world as one large village where everyone lives under the same conditions of underdevelopment. Africa that will influence the world so much more than it has until now, if only because of demography—few recognize that by the end of this century, more than four-fifths of youth in the world will be African.

I do not know why it has dominated my life so, and it was not simply because I later married an African or have African children. To some extent, it was early interest in the plight of countries that were poor, and later, interest and professional opportunities in the health challenges of what today is called the Global South. But much came down to chance.

During my childhood in Flanders in the 1950s, almost every village had someone working in "the Congo," today the Democratic Republic of the Congo. My first awareness of Africa came from hearing my father discussing the quest for Congolese independence at the time of the 1958 Brussels World Fair. A feature at the exhibition, unacceptable today, was a Congolese village with real people, for the viewing interest of Western visitors.

Later, in my English boarding school in the early 1960s, class-mates and I were temporarily inspired at a retreat directed by two White Fathers, Catholic missionaries serving in far-away Africa.[1] And no Belgian child grew up without reading about Tintin and his international adventures, including in Africa,[2] before his political correctness or sexual identity was questioned. Serendip-ity and occasional luck played their role in my journeys in and out of Africa, but it probably all started with a social awakening during a year between school and university.

Flanders: January 1969

Influenza H3N2, so-called Hong Kong flu, caused a pandemic in the late 1960s that sickened millions across the world, including my American mother in the village of Gijzegem in northern Bel-gium. It was late January 1969, and she was confined to the bed-room she had shared with my father until his death 3 years earlier, a death too soon for a 64-year-old surgeon but perhaps too late for a proud man incapacitated over several years by cerebrovascular disease. It was certainly a death too soon for me, his 13-year-old, youngest child.

My parents' bedroom on the ground floor overlooked the lake surrounding the house, a weeping willow prominent on the oppo-site bank to which two herons returned every summer. The early winter morning was characteristically Flemish, cold and grey, when I entered to say goodbye. I was about to hitchhike to Swit-zerland at the beginning of a 9-month gap before entering uni-versity. Three weeks short of my seventeenth birthday, I was impatient with my mother's worry, dismissive of her concern that one hundred dollars in my pocket might be insufficient for safety and survival over the coming month.

My excitement and bravado were tempered by anxiety and self-doubt. I later thought of Laurie Lee's *As I Walked Out One*

Midsummer Morning,[3] reflecting that not only did he express more self-confidence in that earlier tale of coming of age but that he also set off at a kinder time of year. Long after my mother's passing, I remember these and other moments of youthful unkindness with regret and some shame. "And Mary stood at the foot of the cross" was a frequent quote of hers when hearing of any mother's pain or worry about children. Fortunately, my gap year proved eventful, educational, and safe.

Lourdes, France: 1939

Lourdes in southwest France is a site of pilgrimage for Roman Catholics, and especially for the chronically infirm hoping and praying for a cure.[4] A young girl, Bernadette Soubirous, reported seeing the Virgin Mary in 18 separate appearances in the mid-19th century. Water from the local grotto was said to have healed illnesses thought incurable, and an ensuing industry of pilgrimages to Lourdes and its waters continues to this day. In the quest for miracles, up to five million people visit this little town annually, whose indigenous population is barely twenty thousand. Because Lourdes is where my parents met, my siblings and I joke that we have proof of at least one miracle.

Romain De Cock, my father, was born to a small contractor and his wife in the village of Wetteren in East Flanders in 1901. He studied medicine at the nearby University of Ghent, worked for some years as a general practitioner to earn money, and then trained in general surgery. Ghent is in the north of Belgium and Dutch-speaking, but at that time, French was the language of the higher social and educational classes, including for the university teaching of medicine. German, which my father also spoke, was the dominant language of European science, and Latin and Greek were considered an essential basis for medicine.

My mother, Mary Magan, visited Europe with a group of other young and privileged New Yorkers in the fall of 1939, and Lourdes was a required stop on the itinerary of good Catholics such as these. It was while volunteering with the sick, unable to comprehend a disabled Belgian man whom she was attempting to feed, that my father stepped in to assist. He was there as the medical officer accompanying the Flemish pilgrimage. This chance meeting proved the beginning of my mother's subsequent life that took her from a comfortable New York City existence to Belgium for the rest of her days.

I do not know what form courtship took in the late 1930s, but I was surprised at the rapidity of events. Having seen each other so briefly after this initial encounter, my parents agreed to meet in Paris before my mother's return to the United States. My father then did something so out of character that only a *coup de foudre* (lightning strike) could have compelled him to act in this way. He absconded from being on call for the hospital in Aalst, Belgium, and took the train to Paris to meet his date. She declined his offer of champagne at dinner, afraid of becoming drunk, and later recounted how impressed she was that he drank the whole bottle himself. He asked her to marry him and, despite having met only a few times over her short stay in Europe, she agreed. He was 38 years old and she was 25 (Figure 1.1).

John Magan, my maternal grandfather, was a lawyer for the Catholic Archdiocese of New York. So dismayed was he by the news his only daughter brought back from Europe that he retired to his bed for a month. He demanded a reference from the local bishop concerning this potential foreign son-in-law. As luck would have it, my father and the bishop of Ghent were friends who used to meet regularly to converse in Latin. The bishop duly sent a letter of recommendation, but by sea rather than air, and the epistle took weeks to reach New York, enhancing my grandfather's skepticism.

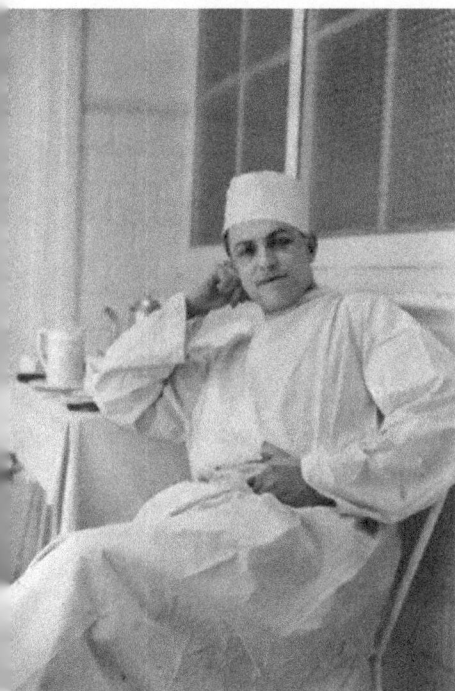

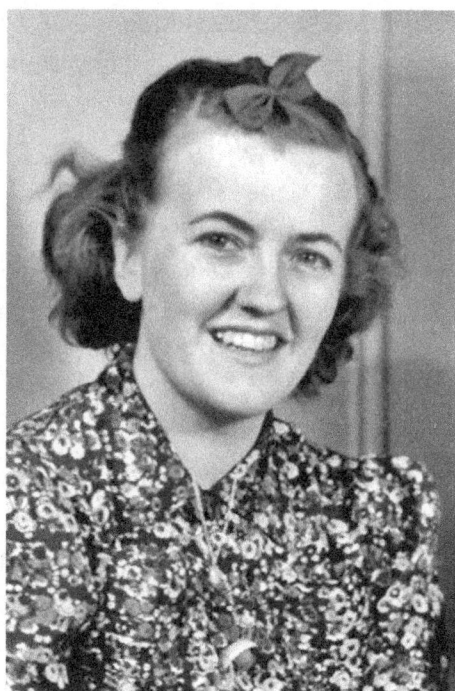

Figure 1.1 *Left*: My father, Romain De Cock, surgeon; *Right*: my mother, Mary Magan, circa 1940s.
(Kevin De Cock, personal collection)

The positive reference eventually arrived, and my parents were married in New York City in January 1940, as Europe was descending into war. When my parents left the church, my father cried, a regular event in moments of emotion but always to the consternation of others unused to such an authoritative figure weeping. My mother consoled him, thinking he was crying from happiness, but he responded that he had never felt so alone in his whole life.

The newlyweds left New York on the last passenger ship departing the United States to Europe early in the war, crossing to Genoa, Italy. Because parts of Western Europe were under German occupation, my American mother needed special transit papers, which the Belgian consulate in Genoa promised but proved unable to provide. Weeks of uncertain waiting took their toll. My father's Flemish melancholy emerged, and he spent days sleeping, pronouncing "happy are the dead" as he chose the arms of Morpheus over those of my mother. Eventually, she took the initiative to contact the American consulate, which delivered the necessary papers, and they were allowed to travel to Belgium. Stories such as these buoyed my mother's lifelong patriotism and belief in the special character and leadership of the United States in the world.

The war years were hard, privileged as my parents were. Patients with limited money would pay for my father's medical services with agricultural produce, so food was never in short supply. The family house in Aalst was next to the railway station, a potential target for bombing by the Allies, so my mother went to stay with friends, owners of a family brewery in the nearby village of Wieze. Caught between German and Allied fighting, Belgium's precarious situation was captured by the Bishop of Ghent, who prayed for "liberation from our 'protectors'" (as the Germans described themselves), and "protection from our 'liberators'" (the Allies).

My siblings and I marvel at our mother's grit as she survived and overcame the challenges of these war years, including being a societal oddity, family hostility to this foreigner, learning new languages and customs, brief detention by the Gestapo, and a late miscarriage. Happier days saw the birth of my sister Jacqui and the liberation, when dozens of American, Canadian, and British troops passed through my parents' house. Their nationalities were less important than the fact that they were English speaking. The euphoria was well captured by a female friend, reputed to have been generous with her affections to the anglophones, who some years later said to my mother "Mary, we don't need another war, what we need is another liberation."

Belgian Childhood

Surgery dominated my father's life, so decisions about education of the four children, two girls and two boys,* were largely made by my mother. Flemish seriousness pervaded life in our multilingual household in which Dutch (the formal version of Flemish), French, and English were readily interchanged by the adults. My anglophone mother had focused on learning French upon arrival in Belgium, and her Flemish was a trilingual mixture quite unique to her. I spoke only Dutch in these early years.

Life was about study and work, which, if not taken seriously, led to shame and family disdain. Paternal approval weighed heavily, with academic success praised and unnecessary financial expenditure criticized. To this day I recall, at the age of six, showing my father a pair of newly bought swimming goggles costing 40 US cents and being rebuked with the curt comment in Flemish: "Wasting money."

Yet, the Flemish work ethic was balanced by Belgian appreciation of life's pleasures and controlled *joie de vivre*. Good food and wine were enjoyed, soccer was followed with enthusiasm no matter how badly the local team fared, and a healthy skepticism was shown toward authority. The Church was respected as a part of weekly life but kept at a distance, despite affection for the nuns who ran the hospitals where my father worked and priests who were family friends. My surgeon father became materially comfortable and locally prominent, but he retained simplicity and the common touch. When asked at a rather aristocratic weekend lunch, "Doctor, do you hunt?" his reported conversation-stopping reply was "No, I kill enough during the week."

---

* Jacqui, born in 1941; Miriam ("Mieken"), born in 1947, deceased in 1975; Romain, born in 1948; Kevin, born in 1952)

My earliest memories, curiously, concern illness—severe measles with fever, vomiting, and the characteristic itchy, blotchy rash; and, earlier, presumed meningitis with a typical post-lumbar puncture headache relieved only by lying flat. For many Belgian children, the comic strip characters of Tintin and his friends were important companions, and they stay with you for life. Tintin defies that joke that there are no famous Belgians (so does the singer Jacques Brel). The intrepid reporter with his little white dog travelled the world and defended the forces of good over evil. Tintin in Africa was a favorite but the comic strip later became criticized for how Africans were depicted in colonial attitudes of the time. Nonetheless, he remains a national icon; more than 60 years later, I found posters depicting Tintin's adventures around the world decorating the walls of the Belgian consulate in Geneva.

Every Flemish village had families with one member who had gone to work in the Belgian Congo, returning home every few years, sometimes if only to die. The brother of a neighbor visited during home leave and gave me a "tam tam," a Congolese drum that I have to this day. Congo was granted independence in 1960 but without investment in its human capacity. Its subsequent history, including its renaming as Zaire and later the Democratic Republic of the Congo, has been turbulent, wasteful, and tragic. Belgium has had difficulty acknowledging the abuses of its early colonial system, and the quest for a balanced historical analysis continues. A turning point in national dialogue, and a cause of shock, was the publication of Adam Hochschild's *King Leopold's Ghost*, depicting the atrocities of King Leopold II's administration of the Congo Free State, then his private property, in the late 19th and early 20th centuries.[5]

The world of adults was an incomprehensible mixture of professional colleagues, friends, and distant relatives. My father was close to a female cousin in Wetteren, the village of his birth and location of a small hospital where he went once weekly to operate. Rachel and my father would drink champagne after his hospital work, and they discussed financial transactions such as the sale of Persian carpets. We children were dragged to old-style, seven-course lunches lasting late into the evening for events such as New Year or a cousin's First Communion. Children were exposed early to wine—a far cry from conditions I experienced later in English boarding schools.

Professionally, my father was a big man in a small environment, in an era when the authority of medical professionals went unchallenged. He was active as a leader in international hospital associations and made a telling comment on a visit to San Francisco that pricked my ears even as a 9-year-old child. He contrasted the impressive medical facilities in the United States with the poorer infrastructure in Belgium, observing there was no comparison when many in our Flemish village still had an outhouse for a toilet. But he commented that a hospital is ultimately only a building, and that good medicine is possible despite adverse conditions, a theme that has stayed with me over the years.

England: 1959–1968

To this day I do not fully understand what made our mother send us to boarding school in England, but send us she did. In 1955 my parents took my brother Romain, just 3 months past his seventh birthday, to Ladycross School* in Seaford,[6] a small town on the Sussex coast. Seaford hosted eight or so boarding schools, of which ours was notorious because we were "the Catholics."

With his usual emotion, my father burst into tears when saying goodbye to his son. Mr. Feeney, the Oxford-educated, English headmaster, was horrified. "Doctor," he said, "pull yourself together. You're setting a bad example to the boy." Only later did I

---

* The school was established in 1891 and closed in 1977.

understand the deep significance of these words. The motto of the school, in Latin, was "The voice of the voice sounds, but the voice of example thunders." "Set a good example" and "do your duty" were the exhortations dominating early school days in England. Although I dismissed them as a child, in later life, when stripped of class and colonial attitudes, they have seemed meaningful.

I joined the same school as my brother in 1959, also at the age of seven and speaking only Flemish. Lumpy porridge and milk, other appalling food, no coffee, compulsory cold showers every morning—the whole experience was redolent of Dickens. Corporal punishment, which I mostly escaped, included being beaten on the behind with a horse crop, leaving linear marks on pale buttocks reminiscent of grilled bread. The English author Graham Greene earlier captured the despair that homesickness inflicted: "Unhappiness in a child," he wrote, "accumulates because he sees no end to the dark tunnel. The thirteen weeks of a term might just as well be thirteen years."[7]

The abrupt separation from parents, home, and all that was familiar made me cry nightly for a month. At the end of the first week, I resolved that this anguish had to stop and that I should return to Belgium to the local day school. I crafted a letter to my parents making what I thought were convincing arguments. So awful did I feel and so persuaded by the merits of my case that I was surprised and devastated when my request was ignored.

That letter came back into my possession four decades later while going through my mother's papers after her death. I reluctantly accepted that this penciled note in bad handwriting was not as persuasive as I had recalled, poignant and tearstained though it was. I now have it framed in my office, an occasional visitor enquiring about the significance of this unusual wall hanging.

The distance between England and Belgium is fixed in miles but has waxed and waned psychologically over the years, again increasing recently because of Brexit. In the late 1950s and early

1960s, these countries were worlds apart. The boat from Ostend to Dover took 3½ hours to cross the English Channel, longer in bad weather. England had not recovered from World War II, which remained a constant reference in adult conversations, just as Brexit does today. The country seemed drab, stiff, old-fashioned, and rather poor.

Apart from the peculiarity of driving on the left side of the road, other observations made impressions on a foreign boy. Cars were antiquated, square, and almost all black. People's clothes were sober and uniform. The beaches were pebbled rather than sandy, and the white cliffs of Dover and rolling South Downs of Sussex seemed like mountains after *le plat pays* (the flat land) of Flanders that was hauntingly captured later in a *chanson* by Jacques Brel.[8]

My time in this first boarding school had its share of friendships, bullying, and peculiar, memorable events. Sharing the only two-person room in the school for a term with an older boy, I was forced to sleep next to an open window that let in rain and regularly left me drenched. Aged eleven, I was refused permission to receive a gift subscription to *Time Magazine* provided by my American brother-in-law, indicative of the restrictive environment that questioned things foreign. The conservative *Daily Telegraph*, however, was available to older boys. Stale bread in the dining room was recycled after being softened with water. An outbreak of food poisoning from a meat and potato pie felled half the school, with boys rushing off sports fields and from classrooms to the unsanitary toilets. A friend and I wrote a report on the outbreak, which we were prevented from disseminating. This education induced a certain resilience, but at cost. It certainly changed our characters and futures.

My American mother was a fervent supporter of President John Kennedy. I read with keen interest about race relations in the United States, President Kennedy's assassination in 1963, and the evolving civil rights struggle. I visited my sister Jacqui and her husband in Chicago in the summer of 1964 and was profoundly affected by deprived Black neighborhoods, seeing poverty I had never witnessed in Europe. In a supermarket I bought the book *Black Like Me* by John Howard Griffin,[9] a white man who darkened his skin and wrote of his experience travelling through the American South as a Black man. My brother-in-law stayed up all night reading it.

I was among a small group of students selected for intense tutoring during the final 2 years of my preparatory school, with a strong emphasis on Latin and Greek. No greater success could be envisaged by the headmaster than his pupils later studying classics at Oxford or Cambridge. I wrote an essay in my scholarship exam for secondary school about my visit to the United States and my thoughts about race relations, wondering later whether my award was related to results in Greek or this manifestation of an awakening social conscience.

I moved to full-time education by the Jesuits ("Give me a child until he is seven and I will show you the man" is the quote frequently attributed to the founder of the Society of Jesus, Ignatius of Loyola) at the famous Stonyhurst College in the north of England.[10] The Jesuits had started educational efforts almost 400 hundred years previously in what is today's France and Belgium and only were allowed to move to the school's English home in 1794. The Jesuits' reputation for providing rigorous education was encapsulated for me in a much later interview given by Anthony ("Tony") Fauci, formerly of the US National Institutes of Health and 11 years older than I. Fauci was educated by the Jesuits in New York City and said that they tried to instill in him "clarity of thought and economy of expression."

I finished school when I was sixteen and applied to medical school with just-adequate academic results. Memorable events were sitting hunched over my small transistor radio in the school dining room listening to reports of the assassinations of Martin

Luther King Jr., and Robert Kennedy in 1968, and negotiating by telephone with students occupying Bristol University Senate House (the occupation was in protest against British support for Nigeria in the Biafran war) about how to attend my university admission interview. I failed to get into Oxford but obtained a place at Bristol University and headed into my gap year.

Looking back, I find it hard to judge this early education, the quality of which my parents took solely on trust. Boarding schools were an integral part of the Great Britain of yesterday, supportive of the country's rigid class system and the needs of tens of thousands or more families serving the Empire or its businesses overseas, all needing to educate their children. The rituals, eccentricities, and traditions of this education were taken as part of the package that would prepare students for the rigors of service and life. Even nomenclature was odd, in that so-called public schools are, in fact, private and fee paying.

Despite loss of the colonies and escalating costs of boarding, the independent school sector in Britain has remained strong, although a substantial proportion of today's boarders are foreign students, many from Asia, and especially China.[11] Similar schools were established in other countries of the Commonwealth, modeled on establishments in Britain, and many persist to this day, educating a more diverse elite and international clientele.

Several recent books provide exhaustive descriptions of experience as well as suffering at British boarding schools.[12, 13] They poignantly capture the pain and longing of young children who face parental and family separation. Their very titles, such as *Stiff Upper Lip*,[12] *Sad Little Boys*,[13] and *The Old Boys*,[14] give insight into some of the history and evolution of these uniquely British institutions. Charles Spencer, the ninth Earl Spencer and brother of the late Princess Diana, wrote a devastating memoir, *A Very Private School*, in which he described abuse and persisting trauma from his early boarding school education in the 1970s.[15] These testimonies all discuss sexual abuse, which, in my own experience, was joked about but never witnessed. Nevertheless, the Jesuits also were later incriminated in abuses that have plagued other sectors of the Catholic church.[16]

To the extent that this "sink or swim" education led me to a medical degree, I remain grateful but also perplexed about whether it all might have been easier. Control of emotion was the expected approach to life's challenges, an attitude that may have promoted resilience but also detachment. "Everyone understands English, but nobody understands the English," said Jean-Claude Juncker, the Luxembourgian former president of the European Commission, exasperated with Brexit. I often think of this quote as I reminisce on these schoolboy experiences.

Between School and University: 1969

I had an undeveloped idea of wanting to do volunteer work during my gap year and discovered the organization Service Civil International (SCI), founded in 1920 by a Swiss pacifist.[17,18] With audacious, perhaps naive, idealism, SCI aimed for reconciliation in Europe after World War I through an emphasis on service, physical work, and nonviolence, captured in its motto *"paix, pelle, et pioche"* (peace, spade, and pickaxe). Its first work camp focused on reconstruction in a village near Verdun in northeastern France, bringing together young people of diverse nationalities, including Swiss, German, and French.

SCI could legitimately claim to have been the progenitor of later, much better known and financed organizations such as the British Voluntary Service Overseas or US Peace Corps. SCI grew into an international organization with branches in several dozen countries that organized 2- to 4-week work camps, as well as medium- and long-term service. By the time I discovered its office in

Brussels, SCI still retained some of its alternative thinking and skepticism of conventional politics.

My first work camp was in Ticino in the Italian-speaking region of Switzerland working on a construction site for a rest home for the elderly. It was for this destination that I came to be hitchhiking south from Belgium on a cold day late in January 1969. Over the next 7 months I did further stints in francophone Switzerland, Belgium, Holland, and Sweden, mostly involving manual labor for socially oriented projects.

This year between school and university offered experiences that complemented my formal education and showed its lacunae. I was exposed to political and social discussions rarely held at school, such as the existence and causes of poverty, the reality of rich and poor countries, and the historical impact of colonialism. I learned about inequality in the world and that it was not just due to chance. I grew intellectually and socially, abetted by falling in love, but began to question the role of medicine in the world. Politics and economics seemed more relevant, and I came to doubt my choice of medicine as a university course and career.

SCI work camps brought together people from varied backgrounds, and many were politically motivated. Intense discussions were held in bars. Late one night in a tavern in Ostend, I was shocked to see two men entwined in a passionate kiss, something I had never seen despite the innuendos about male-to-male sex in English schools. I remember, painfully, the arrogance of youth, as on other occasions we lectured older people drawn into our idealistic discussions.

Hitchhiking is not as safe today as it was in my student days. On a good day you could travel well more than 500 kilometers, especially if picked up by a long-distance truck driver. It was easiest to travel alone; two men hitchhiking had it most difficult, whereas a man and a woman were more trusted. "Travel fast, travel alone; travel far, travel with others" is an oft-quoted

African proverb that applied well to these experiences. My mother started picking up hitchhikers out of a sense of duty. I benefited from the generosity of strangers who sometimes offered food and shelter.

On the first day of my first trip, I covered close to 1,000 kilometers. I was offered a bed by a young couple living on the French side of the border between France and Switzerland, the man in hiding to avoid compulsory service in the Swiss army. To my surprise, the most difficult countries in which to hitchhike were Holland and Sweden; in the latter I had to abandon my efforts and spend my meager funds on a train ticket for the long journey from Malmo to Stockholm.

Adverse events were rare. A French truck driver tried to persuade me to negotiate a sex worker for him in a Belgian village. I declined, dismounted, and trudged off to sleep in a nearby forest. A man driving from Sweden to Germany intentionally left on view the pornography he had bought and appeared to masturbate as he drove, all of which I frostily ignored. A ramshackle car in Sweden, on a long and fast ride, contained four men intent on avoiding police along the way. A ride out of Brussels appeared to take a different direction than stated, but the car's two occupants allowed me to disembark without trouble. In retrospect, several drivers may have picked me up hoping for more than just company, including an older, distinguished-looking man who invited me to tea in his very expensive Brussels apartment. Perhaps I was naive, but I never felt threatened. Today, I advise young people to invest in a rail pass.

Looking Back

Two coincident events profoundly influenced me, perhaps over my whole life, before I left school: my father's terminal illness and the criticism he endured at the end of his career. Accusations of surgical malpractice were leveled against him, and formal investigations were undertaken, including the exhumation of patients who had died postoperatively. He was officially exonerated of wrongdoing or blame, but he was pained by the experience. In a letter to my godfather, he accepted the burden of criticism with the memorable words "tall trees catch the wind."

One school vacation in 1963, I was told my father was ill and had stopped working. He had noticed a breast lump, which he biopsied himself, aided by his trainee surgeons. His deterioration over the following 2½ years was not, despite my mother's insistence, related to proven breast cancer but to cerebrovascular disease. It was sobering to see this giant figure weakened by disease, suffering symptoms and signs that my later medical training enabled me to interpret retrospectively.

His speech became slightly slurred ("dysarthria"), he had difficulties expressing himself ("dysphasia"), was emotionally labile, and wept even more easily than in active life. A major stroke while visiting California to see his first grandchild signaled the end. He died in late January 1966, when I was still 13.

I have wondered ever since what his opinions and comments would have been concerning my career choices. He became a general surgeon in the pre-antibiotic era, before the advent of drugs for tuberculosis, a time when general surgeons did everything. I joke that he likely would have accepted, grudgingly, my choice of internal medicine, but would not have understood my journey into public health. Although he lived through the great influenza pandemic of 1918, he surely would have been surprised by the epidemics of AIDS, Ebola, and coronavirus infections that have characterized recent decades.

The loneliness of boarding schools and absence of a father figure contributed to feelings of solitude, uncertainty, and worry I had about financial security. The internationalism of our background and education promoted flexibility, adaptability, and independence, but also resulted in feelings of rootlessness and not belonging. I generally felt different from others—more privileged than children in our Flemish village; a Belgian in England; an anglophone in Belgium; and foreign-born in the United States. I later joked that Africa thinks all white people look the same, and it was easy to adapt there, amidst refreshing anonymity.

It is now more than half a century since I took my hesitant steps into medical training. My dominant recollection of the last few days before setting off from Belgium to Bristol University was time with my brother, 4 years older, who coincidentally took up medicine later and became an ophthalmologist. Memories include drinking beer with him; a dangerous ride on the back of his motorcycle after seeing the movie *Easy Rider*; thinking a 5-year medical course was impossibly long; the nagging belief that only politics and economics could bring change to the world; and unease that I was embarking on the wrong degree. I am forever grateful that, despite initial hesitancy, I adhered to medicine.

CHAPTER 2

Medicine

You See Only What You Look for
and Recognize Only What You Know

One never knows a chosen profession until deep into it, by which time so much may have been invested that it is difficult to turn back. My doubts about medicine, fortunately, were early rather than late. The fresh-faced students who gathered in Bristol in September 1969 to begin 5 years of medical school had little insight into the nature of their future work. Two years of preclinical studies preceded the final 3 years of clinical engagement, exposure to patients, and qualifying exams. Five years seemed an eternity, and when I arrived in Bristol aged 17 years, the youngest person in my class of about 120 students, I could not imagine ever finishing. In fact, a decade of training in the South West of England would precede international work, and I now marvel at what a leap into the unknown these early years represented.

Anatomy, cell biology, biochemistry, histology, and behavioral science filled the first year. The second year comprised anatomy, physiology, pathology, microbiology, and pharmacology, inching us closer to real patients and their problems. The course was traditional in organization, contrasting with today's promotion of a more holistic and integrated curriculum that bridges the theoretical and clinical worlds.

Our teachers included famous scientists as well as oddballs. A biochemistry professor noted for his brilliance was a womanizing, recovering alcoholic. Our behavioral science teacher was a radical Trotskyite often seen leading demonstrations in the streets of Bristol. Some friends and I asked him to lead a study group on politics and psychology, but the articles he selected for discussion were impenetrable. He repeatedly attempted to manipulate us into participation in protests, arguing that action was the only path to understanding. An aging pathology lecturer, a direct descendant of a historically important British figure, dressed as if still a student. It was not just the young who had their issues.

Anthony ("Tony") Epstein (later Sir Michael Anthony), our dapper professor of pathology, was codiscoverer of the Epstein-Barr virus that bears his name and was first isolated from Burkitt's lymphoma cells.[1] Burkitt's lymphoma was named after the English missionary surgeon Denis Burkitt, who described this form of cancer in Uganda in 1958.[2] This tumor of lymphoid tissue most commonly affects the jaw in children and is especially prevalent in parts of East Africa. The Ugandan connection was thought to be related to malaria altering the immune response, promoting the cancer-inducing potential of the virus. Epstein-Barr virus was also later incriminated as the cause of infectious mononucleosis ("glandular fever")[3] and linked to nasopharyngeal cancer and possibly other lymphoproliferative conditions, including, much later, in patients with AIDS.[4,5]

The naming of diseases or infectious agents is often unfair. Bert Achong was the electron microscopy specialist collaborating with Epstein and was a coauthor of the Lancet paper describing the virus in 1964. However, the contributions of this quiet, unassuming, gay pathologist of Trinidadian origin have been relegated to history by nomenclature. He also discovered the human foamy virus, the first recognized retrovirus infection in man.[6]

Epstein was somewhat of a showman. From his first lecture on our first day, he repeatedly cited work on cellular pathology by the scientist George Palade at the Rockefeller Institute in New York. Such august institutions seemed remote and of another world to the new students. A collective groan was let out some lectures later when Epstein casually said "when I was having lunch last week in New York with George Palade," and we had the first of many insights into the insecurities and other psychologic traits of professionals who, to us, had achieved great success. I was to hear of Palade again—some 15 years later, back in Bristol for my higher-degree ceremony*: I heard Epstein give the oration for the honorary doctorate conferred on George Palade.

Medical students had fuller timetables than other students, and the work required to keep up was intense. My doubts about whether I had chosen the right path persisted, and I wavered between continuing or transferring to study politics and economics. The dean of preclinical studies kindly invited me to his house when he saw my distress, persuaded me that medicine offered broader choices in life than most subjects, gave examples of doctors who became politicians or writers, and pushed me to focus and work. It proved an inspiring and lasting lesson, for in the discipline of application and working harder I found renewed motivation and reward, and my doubts lifted. It was an early example for me of the importance of mentorship and a reminder, only recognized later, to thank those individuals who help us on our journeys.

Medical school years continued the transition from adolescence to adulthood and had their share of insecurities and uncertainty. Once accepted to university, the British system expects

---

* Medicine in the United Kingdom is an undergraduate degree (Bachelor of Medicine, Bachelor of Surgery). The higher Doctor of Medicine (MD) degree is analogous to a Doctor of Philosophy (PhD) degree in medicine.

and facilitates all students to pass, yet a few still fell by the wayside from lack of work or other reasons. Drug use was relatively common—mostly soft drugs—and a few students, less in medicine than in other disciplines, lost their way in the counterculture of the 1960s and '70s.

Patterns for later life were laid down. One classmate left at the end of the course without graduating and died in an alcoholic stupor 2 years later. It was known that she drank excessively and had unsuitable relationships, but I now wonder what support she received and whether she could have been helped more. Another completed exacting training and became an eminent surgeon, but his longstanding alcohol use led to incapacity, early resignation from a high-profile position, and premature death. I was fortunate in discovering exercise as a source of discipline and relief of stress.

Individual vignettes remain of youthful misjudgments, behavior by male teachers toward female students that would be considered unacceptable today, and daily tragedies. Anatomy teaching consisted of lectures as well as demonstration on cadavers by trainee surgeons studying for the Fellowship of the Royal College of Surgeons. Our small group's anatomy demonstrator learned of his wife's late miscarriage of their first child just before one teaching session, and I still see him repeatedly stabbing the orbit of our cadaver's right eye with his scalpel as he struggled to refrain from sobbing.

Beginning work in the hospital made this life choice seem more real, despite our short white coats that communicated the limits of our knowledge and authority. Basic tasks were learned, such as collecting blood samples. The school had the sensitivity to insist students practice on each other, painfully, before we undertook the early-morning ritual of specimen collection from patients. The best way to learn to sew up wounds was to volunteer in the Accident and Emergency Department on Saturday nights, when numerous patients with head wounds were seen, incapacitated as well as anesthetized by drink.

The first hospital year exposed us to internal medicine and general surgery, with an emphasis on medical history taking and physical examinations. The hospital was organized into "firms" consisting of a "consultant" (attending physician) and his (always "his" at that time, now no longer) specialist trainees. Small groups of students were attached to each firm for 8 weeks, allowing continuity with individual patients and teaching. A divide existed between staff employed by the University and those by the hospital, although all worked for the National Health Service (NHS) and saw the same patient population. Only NHS consultants could see private patients, though this occurred in outside facilities.

Consultants were powerful, idiosyncratic figures. Joe Cates was a dominant internist at the Bristol Royal Infirmary with subspecialist interest in endocrinology and diabetes. He was respected for his diagnostic skills and, in earlier years, stopped people in the street if they displayed some manifestation of disease such as a goiter, ordering them to attend his clinic. White spots on black shoes of aging men could indicate sugar in the urine or the urinary indignities of enlarged prostates. The hospital was enthralled when he correctly, and belatedly, made a diagnosis of typhoid in a young woman with fever of unknown origin and a characteristic rash ("rose spots"), indicative of how rare infectious diseases had become.

The student experience offered remarkable insight into patients' lives at a remarkably young age. I was 20 when I completed our obstetrics requirement of delivering 12 babies and dealing with associated minor complications. I was humbled later by young colleagues in Africa who had been trained to perform a cesarean section, something I would be unable to do. My interest in social and political issues and challenges of low-income countries remained, and I chose assignments relevant to these interests.

I received high marks for a presentation on the relative protective effect of sickle cell disease and other abnormalities of hemoglobin against malaria. I noted how some diseases lent themselves to individual patient care as well as public health approaches and epidemiologic study.

I attempted to keep an open mind to subjects deemed outside of the mainstream, such as psychiatry. Again, individual clinical tableaux were imprinted on memory. A woman was brought to the clinic shaking uncontrollably, unable to speak, the victim of severe and recurrent depression that responded only to electroconvulsive therapy. A personal experience of depression lasting 2 to 3 months some years later gave me insight into its mental as well as physical manifestations, a useful lesson for a physician. The sense of hopelessness and despair engendered, the early morning wakening, and weight loss all conveyed how easily it could lead to self-harm.

I saw two female patients with dementia next to each other in a long-term care facility, locked in their inner worlds, one continuously sobbing and the other laughing uproariously, who were to remain in these contrasting positions for the rest of their lives. The long-term care of the mentally and physically disabled was and remains chronically underfunded. A group of medical students organized regular support and visits to an aged facility for patients with mental disability, a place of relative neglect and despair. Closure of large institutions for the mentally and physically disabled was relatively recent, driven by idealism that care in the community was better all round. The promise of improvement was not matched by funding and today's persistent burden of mental illness among the homeless and incarcerated was not anticipated.

Final Year

In our final year we were sent to peripheral hospitals in the South West of England for practical experience, and we also had a 2-month elective period allowing us to follow our own interests. I wanted to see medicine in a low-income country and sought advice from our professor of radiology, Sir Howard Middlemiss. A large, rotund man with a goatee beard, Middlemiss was an internationalist with extensive experience establishing radiology departments in Africa and the Caribbean. He sent trainees to teach in the faculties of Africa's new universities and attracted their graduates to his own department in Bristol. "Go to Kenya," he said to me when I asked where I could go for 2 months. He wrote to the dean in Nairobi and I escaped the 1973 British winter, spending a month at Nairobi's Kenyatta National Hospital and a month upcountry in Kapenguria's District Hospital.

Africa was alien. My knowledge of medicine was inadequate to contribute usefully, and I was bewildered by what I saw. Professor Michael Floyer from the London Hospital Medical School had taken the position of professor of Medicine in Nairobi and was committed to building an African faculty. He took me under his wing, medically as well as socially. He organized an expedition to climb Mount Kenya, which we did on the tenth anniversary of Kenyan independence, seeing fireworks launched from the mountain's other, higher peak by specialist climbers who had reached the summit.

Philip Rees, a British physician long resident in Kenya and working at Kenyatta Hospital, sent me to a rural attachment in Kapenguria by simply writing a short letter to Peter Cox, the missionary District Medical Officer. I took the overnight bus to western Kenya with considerable trepidation. Aware of the danger of losing my money to thieves, I hid my currency in my underwear. Getting off the bus in Kitale, bank notes fell down my leg and out of the bottom of my trousers and I looked ridiculous, scrambling on the ground with a large pack on my back, gathering up my money under the gaze of a bemused crowd.

Cox was hospitable and not taken aback at all by my simply turning up (Rees's letter had never arrived) and expecting to stay for a month—that was how it went in the bush. Kapenguria was famous as the site where Jomo Kenyatta, Kenya's founding president, was imprisoned by the British in the early 1950s. A remote rural area near the Uganda border and Mount Elgon, Kapenguria's people, the Pokot, frequently engaged in battles with their neighbors over cattle theft. Fighting that in early years involved spears was later taken over by gunfights. Cox inspired me because despite his heavy work burden literally doing everything—surgery, medicine, obstetrics, public health—he had written and successfully defended a doctoral dissertation on the local burden of disease.

Small incidents as a student loomed large. I went out with the nurses on a rural preventive medicine visit and was confronted with an extremely ill, breathless, febrile young woman. My diagnosis was pneumonia, based on clinical examination and use of my stethoscope. I had learned the symptoms and signs in theory, but this was my first practical exposure to the syndrome. Extensive negotiation with her nomadic clan was required to transport her to the hospital on the back of our truck, and I was relieved when Cox supported my diagnosis and prescription of penicillin. It was the first life I saved.

We evacuated a young boy with intractable nose bleeding and a peripheral blood film filled with abnormal white cells to Nairobi, undoubtedly to die of acute leukemia. In Nairobi, I sat for hours one night compressing the bleeding penis of a boy with hemophilia who had been subjected to traditional circumcision, against medical advice. Such early clinical experiences are long remembered. Before leaving Kenya, a colleague and I hitchhiked to the coast and met up with other medical school friends who had worked in different mission hospitals, all with clinical tales to recount, recognizing our medical school years were ending.

I learned more medicine in the early months of 1974 than I had over almost all the rest of my course. In medicine, everything relates to everything else, so initial knowledge of a particular subject has no context, and its relevance is difficult to grasp. Intense study began to make things fall into place. Two weeks as a locum house physician in Plymouth, replacing a qualified doctor taking leave, gave me uniquely valuable initiation in practical patient care. It was a revelation in this pre-internet era to learn how to prescribe medicines, where to look up practical information for immediate use, how to order intravenous fluids, or determine how much blood to transfuse.

An extremely competent and hard-working senior resident from Australia, worn down by his hospital as well as family duties, supervised me. My inexperience was evident, and he insisted on being briefed on every admission, no matter what the time of day. I admitted a young woman who had taken a small overdose of sleeping pills, a frequent cause of hospitalization that usually led to referral to the psychiatrists and rapid discharge. As was common, she now felt sheepish and remorseful, and was as unsure of herself as I was. We both laughed uproariously as I tapped her knees and elicited a knee-jerk reflex in ritualistic examination of her central nervous system at two o'clock in the morning.

Final exams were largely practical, involving short and long cases. A child with a hole in the heart, a man with stenosis of his aortic heart valve, and a pregnant woman were among the short cases. My long case involved assessing a young man with bipolar disorder, currently in a manic phase. He flitted from one topic to another as he told his story, characteristic of "flight of ideas." I raced around the hospital after him as he paced impulsively in different directions. The examiners were kind and, for most of us, the exams were an uneventful rite of passage. I crossed the street separating the two sides of the Bristol Royal Infirmary and experienced a sudden feeling of elation and awe as I realized I was now a doctor.

Medical and Surgical Internship

From my earliest days in medical school, I knew I could not be a surgeon. I had never been practical and found anatomy difficult to learn. One of the medical disciplines that has changed the most over my career is radiology. The advent of ultrasound, computerized tomography (CT), magnetic resonance imaging (MRI), and angiography (canulating blood vessels for diagnosis or delivery of interventions such as a stent) has vastly expanded the armamentarium of the radiologists but not lessened their need for deep understanding of anatomy. I have collaborated closely with radiologists over the years but realized theirs also was a discipline for which I was not best suited.

Early in training, emphasis was placed on the great divide: the difference between the medical and the surgical worlds. It was not obvious to many of us that other disciplines might be worthy of consideration, such as oto-rhino-laryngology (ear, nose, and throat) or ophthalmology, let alone forensic pathology, adolescent or forensic psychiatry, medicolegal work, or medical journalism. Jokes were ingrained about medical stereotypes—surgeons do everything but know nothing, physicians (internists) know everything and do nothing, and pathologists know everything and do everything, but only when it is too late. Anesthetists were the half asleep watching the half-awake being half murdered by the half-witted, a jibe, obviously, at surgeons.

Although collaboration generally was good and mutual respect adequate, the hierarchy of medicine and the role of social class in British medicine were not to be underestimated. Graduates of London hospitals, for example, really did feel they were superior. In the United Kingdom at that time, public health was considered a poor career choice, and the subspecialty of sexually transmitted infections (still referred to as venereal disease) was considered a backwater for those who could not succeed in the mainstream.

Internal medicine suited me. It provided a basis for looking across all disciplines, required logic and deduction, needed knowledge but also experience, and, above all, depended on synthesis of information and good judgment. It was a subject that required reasoning rather than manual intervention that characterizes surgery. An overriding emphasis was placed on diagnosis, perhaps the most essential service our profession could deliver to the patient. Although I learned my share of practical procedures over the ensuing years, such as placing emergency pacemakers or starting peritoneal dialysis, these were not my favorite aspects of medicine.

With time I also came to realize that not all surgeons are the same and some truly are "physicians who operate." One such person was my friend Paul Finan, who later became professor of Colorectal Surgery in Leeds. I teased him for his decision to pursue surgery, a life-long memory between us being my taunt that his greatest challenge in this unwise career choice would be deciding what color thread to use. Thoughtful and knowledgeable surgeons challenge their internist colleagues, as I have seen with the best heart surgeons who also are diagnostic cardiologists, or the outstanding liver and biliary tract surgeons with whom I later worked in Los Angeles, CA.

We had to complete 6 months internship in both medicine and surgery, being resident in the hospital every second or third night and weekend. In this way, there were weeks when we worked more than 100 hours, something no longer allowed. Stress and tiredness took their toll. Finan and I laugh in reminiscence at how, despite our friendship, he subjected me to aggressive questioning when I referred a medical patient with intestinal obstruction to his surgical team. Simple discussion made the diagnosis evident, and he apologized profusely for exhaustion-induced impatience.

My own experience as a house surgeon passed uneventfully, my surgical seniors being only too pleased to allow me to look after the medical rather than surgical needs of our patients. Individual stories stick in the mind, such as the months spent on our ward by a courageous young woman with Crohn's disease and its complications of abscesses and fistulae. Overseeing her intravenous nutrition on an open ward was my heavy responsibility, and though we kept her biochemically stable, she succumbed to an infection of her heart valves, like that sometimes seen in people who inject drugs. The senior surgical resident said to me months earlier, somewhat matter-of-factly it seemed to me, "of course she's going to die." In retrospect, it made me understand that, at the time, I still did not have the judgment concerning disease that only comes with experience.

Much of the surgical work was rewarding, including dealing with the urological emergency of urinary retention in men, mostly due to enlargement of the prostate. The simple act of passing a catheter, thus allowing urine to flow and the painful expansion of the bladder to decompress, provided instant, visible, and audible relief. Few patients were so immediately grateful. Some situations were less straightforward. A man assumed to have routine retention turned out to have not prostatic hypertrophy but a severe phimosis, tightening of the foreskin of the penis. As I leaned over trying to catheterize the patient, his functional obstruction suddenly lifted and I received a face full of urine, to his simultaneous relief and embarrassment. I washed my face, containing my disgust by rationalizing that I had only been doused in water containing some electrolytes.

Medicine and surgery are trades as much as academic subjects, and experience cannot be replaced by theory. Put simply, the more one sees and does, the better one gets at a discipline. Working hours today are restricted—a good thing because fatigue leads to mistakes—but one also must wonder whether the physicians and surgeons exiting today's training programs are as prepared as earlier generations for what medical life will throw at them.

Alan Read, the professor of Medicine under whom I trained, was a short, overweight man with an unusually large head. He was an outstanding bedside teacher and lecturer, and wrote some well-received textbooks on clinical methods, general medicine, and liver disease. He was more feared than liked but generated respect and was effective in promoting his department's stature and enhancing the discipline of gastroenterology in Bristol.

When patients are unable to absorb their food, a condition known as malabsorption, steatorrhea results, a condition that produces fatty stools characteristically described as "pale, bulky, and offensive." It was my friend Tim Ewer, who applied this latter moniker to our professor. In fact, Read was kind to me, and I owe him gratitude for support over quite some years. I was both pleased and proud to have him supervise examination of my doctoral dissertation years later. He died of a brain tumor within 18 months of retiring at the age of 65, a warning not to take anything for granted in late careers or aspirations for retirement.

Internship was, at times, an emotional experience. Internists in those earlier days, more in the United Kingdom than in the United States, treated most diseases themselves rather than referring patients to subspecialists. We interns gained broad experience looking after patients with diverse ailments referred to the great professor or consultant, but I wondered whether this lack of referral was the best for all.

Mrs. N was a young woman who was on our wards for months with Hodgkin's disease. Today, this malignant illness is often curable; in those days it was less so. She suffered medicine's awful complications, including a fungal infection of her bloodstream, undoubtedly acquired in the hospital, and then deafness from the antibiotic gentamycin she received in high doses for bacterial infections.

One night, the ward sister (i.e., the senior nurse in charge), an extraordinarily powerful figure, asked me to speak to Mrs. N's husband, who had turned up outside of visiting hours and intoxicated, demanding to see Professor Read. When informed that only I was available, he replied that he was not interested in talking "to some 17 year old." I drew myself up to my full 22-year-old height and said it was me or no one, but his anguish and words were memorable.

Professor Read did see him later, lecturing him that his wife would be cured, an injudicious promise that, alas, was not in the Professor's power to keep, and Mrs. N later died. It was a teaching moment, a reminder never to overpromise: in medicine, hope is a good companion but a poor guide.

Because Read was a hepatologist, we received a disproportionate number of patients with liver disease. A doctor for only about 6 weeks, I was on call when things started to go terribly wrong for a special patient, another professor of medicine who had come from far away with end-stage liver disease. It was emphasized this was not alcoholic cirrhosis—presumably, professors of medicine were immune to this condition—and with today's knowledge, his cirrhosis was likely due to hepatitis C. He had worked for a long time in Egypt, which we now know has some of the highest rates of hepatitis C infection in the world. A complication of liver cirrhosis is portal hypertension, elevated blood pressure in the circulation through the liver before flow back to the heart. Collateral vessels develop to bypass this obstruction, some in the stomach and esophagus, and these can rupture and bleed, sometimes massively. This was now happening to the professor.

How hard to struggle and when to accept defeat always require fine judgment. A senior decision had been made to transfuse 12 units of blood but no more if bleeding had not stopped, and surgery to stem the bleeding was out of the question. I spent all night with this frightened, intelligent man who understood very clearly what was happening, as did his wife hovering by the bedside. He died in the early morning, and as I entered the hospital dining room for breakfast, curious colleagues crowded around and asked for details of the night's events. I broke down and wept.

Specializing in Internal Medicine

Having decided to pursue internal medicine, I had to secure a place in a training program and obtain the essential postgraduate degree, the Membership of the Royal College of Physicians. Bristol had a renal medicine unit that offered dialysis and kidney transplantation, run by a larger-than-life physician called Campbell Mackenzie. Working in this specialized area of medicine gave me an opportunity to study (essential preparation for the first part of the Membership) for a written exam, which I passed on the first attempt.

Training was remarkably unstructured—one just did different jobs and gained experience, thus working up the career ladder and hoping to eventually become a hospital consultant. For those aspiring to academia and positions in teaching institutions, research was a requirement along with a doctoral thesis. I obtained a position on a so-called rotation organized through Professor Read's unit, a series of linked positions in different hospitals and subspecialties over 3 years and including a year in a peripheral hospital in Torquay in the South West of England. My interview for this rotation was memorable because, having just finished the first part of the Membership exam, I was due to leave on holiday in the Seychelles, where a girlfriend had friends who ran a hotel. I had to ask to be interviewed first and then immediately depart for the airport from where I would telephone to hear the outcome. I was fortunate to have Professor Read's support.

"You see only what you look for and recognize only what you know" was an aphorism passed on to me by a family friend in

Belgium from her own physician. It is an insightful observation with special significance in internal medicine. It emphasizes that medicine requires experience. A patient with apparent heart failure caused concern because of his increasing abdominal discomfort and lack of response to treatment. I made several observations and went on my way. He continued to deteriorate and was seen by Professor Read, who made no different recommendations. A young cardiologist finally put the patient's symptoms and signs together and made the correct diagnosis—a pericardial effusion with cardiac tamponade (fluid in the sac around the heart that prevents it from pumping). Drainage of the fluid saved the patient's life.

I had made the pertinent observations but failed to aggregate them, not recognizing a syndrome that I knew in theory but with which I was unfamiliar. Some years later in Nairobi, I was able to save another life in a different cultural context but similar clinical circumstances, that time seeing what I specifically looked for and recognizing it for what it was.

The second part of the exam for Membership of the Royal College of Physicians was practical, involving interpretation of clinical photos, laboratory results, electrocardiograms, imaging, and, later, clinical short and long cases. It was intimidating to be in the Royal College in London, impressed by the weight of centuries of medical history in the building. Up to six attempts to pass part 2 of the exam were allowed, and the failure rate was high. I never understood whether this was to keep standards up or generate income for the College—the exam fees were stiff.

The clinical part of the exam was held in different London hospitals. I failed my first attempt at the degree. I realized I had not done well and knew immediately from the thin envelope that arrived in the post the following week that I had failed—a pass was known to be communicated in a thick envelope containing all kinds of information and requests for money from the College.

Failure, especially after studying so hard, was unfamiliar and de-
pressing to me, but a good life lesson.

My second attempt to pass the Membership in June 1977 was
more auspicious. My long case, a West Indian woman with non-
Hodgkin's lymphoma, had an unusual physical finding, lymph
nodes around the elbow, along with other manifestations of her
disease. The examiner was impressed because he was not aware
of this physical finding. The eminent hepatologist Sheila Sherlock,
an intimidating figure, examined me for short cases, all of which
I diagnosed correctly. I knew I had succeeded when I heard her
"well done" floating through the air as she walked off to the next
candidate.

It was during this early training that I attempted my first medical writing, describing unusual patient presentations or
outcomes.[7-9] Case reports describing individual patients are often
dismissed as simply anecdotal. Nonetheless, they provide writing
experience and sometimes are important—the AIDS epidemic
was brought to the world's attention with a report of five homosexual men with *Pneumocystis* pneumonia.[10] Former CDC director
Bill Foege often quoted the aphorism that the plural of anecdote is
data. I was also exposed to academic competitiveness when Professor Read, my former and later boss, called me to request the
clinical history of a surgical patient with an unusual form of peritonitis caused by a cardiac drug, practolol.[11] The patient featured
in a published case series, but I do not recall my surgical boss being involved.

I returned to Bristol from Torquay in the fall of 1978, having
been offered an extension of a year as a locum senior registrar, a
high position for my current age of 26, on the cardiology unit
where I had worked previously. My early suspicions that this was
the wrong place to be only strengthened with the weeks. The experience taught me to trust instinct more than intellect in professional and other decisions.

As a Belgian, I still had to fulfill my military service obligation, but I had settled on the alternative of serving in a low-income country for 2 years. I decided that now was the time to commit to this requirement, enrolled for the Diploma in Tropical Medicine and Hygiene at the University of Liverpool, and, in early December 1978, informed my employers that I was leaving. It would be another 15 years before I worked in England again, by which time I would have spent time in Africa and the United States.

CHAPTER 3

Tropical Medicine

Tropical Medicine in Liverpool

Alan Read, professor of medicine in Bristol, asked me why I needed a diploma in tropical medicine, since I was knowledgeable in infectious diseases. I suspected his question emanated more from concern at having to find a replacement for me than from esteem for my medical expertise. Because I was funding my own studies, I had enrolled in the 3-month-long course at the Liverpool School of Tropical Medicine; the diploma at the London School of Hygiene and Tropical Medicine then took 6 months of study. A healthy rivalry existed between the schools, with Liverpool reminding the world that it was the first ever such institution, founded in 1898.

I left Bristol on New Year's Day, 1979, concerned about the weather. Walking near Brunel's iconic Clifton Suspension Bridge in the morning, I witnessed a car lose control and crash into parked vehicles on the icy roads. The route to Liverpool became progressively unpleasant and dangerous as I drove north, snow obscuring my vision. I was relieved to arrive in Merseyside, of Beatles fame, where I was to stay for the duration of my course with the mother of my surgeon friend Paul Finan.

The incongruity of studying tropical medicine in England was accentuated by the initial closure of the school because of

flooding from frozen and burst water pipes. The European institutions teaching tropical medicine had been established to
serve the needs of the colonial empires and their servants. I often thought over subsequent years how much more appropriate
and effective it would be if such teaching was conducted in the
Global South.

Arrogant in my knowledge of internal medicine, I was shocked
at the work required to keep up. The teaching was outstanding, except for public health, then still referred to as community medicine. That teaching was so poor that the student body organized
a debate to protest and suggest alternatives, but the dean, the patrician Herbert Gilles, stepped in to prevent this expression of student power. There was a missed opportunity to educate clinically
oriented students like me in epidemiology or imbue them with an
interest in public health. Major political shifts were happening in
health, such as the primary health care movement motivated by
the previous year's famous Alma-Ata Declaration aspiring to
health for all.[1]

We studied practical parasitology and entomology, learning to
examine stool and insect specimens to make specific diagnoses
and identifications. Despite my initial skepticism, this turned
out to be supremely useful later when I had to hold my own
while teaching students in Kenya who had learned some of these
practical skills.

Before leaving Bristol, I had applied and been interviewed for
a post of lecturer in internal medicine at the University of Ife (now
Obafemi Awolowo University) in Ile-Ife, Nigeria. Today, Nigeria
evokes thoughts of corruption and mismanagement, despite being Africa's largest economy. In the 1960s and '70s, it stood out
for the quality of its universities and their literature, arts, and science programs. Institutions like the University of Ibadan were
world-renowned, new universities were springing up, and the
future was full of hope. Ife sounded particularly interesting

because of the connections it had with Bristol. A senior lecturer in radiology whom I knew had worked there, sent by the influential professor of Radiology at the University of Bristol, Howard Middlemiss, and enthused about his experience there.

My interview was held in the imposing Nigeria High Commission on Trafalgar Square in London. I answered the questions, was asked to wait outside, and, when called back in, was offered the position on the spot. I returned to Bristol secure in my decision to resign, but after starting in Liverpool, I heard no more. I became increasingly concerned; I was burning through my savings and still had no contract for work. I scoured the employment pages of the *British Medical Journal* and applied for a position as lecturer in Medicine at the University of Nairobi in Kenya. I received an offer by mail within a short time, accepted the offer, and completed my course. Many months later in Nairobi I received a letter from Ife saying they remained interested in my joining, but I politely replied that time had moved on.

I left the United Kingdom for Kenya in mid-May 1979. I felt anxious and conflicted about stepping into the unknown, an inner voice asking why I was leaving friends, attachments, and the security of the United Kingdom where I had studied and worked for 20 years. An expression I heard years later at the CDC well conveyed my inner turmoil: "Many people want to work in Africa, but far fewer get on the plane."

Nairobi

I was one of the last white expatriates hired by the University of Nairobi. I was met at the airport by the chairman of the Department of Medicine, Professor Walter Gitau, a UK-trained, Kenyan endocrinologist. I was eager to start work as soon as possible but was advised to take time to settle and was temporarily housed at the Fairview Hotel while waiting for university accommodation.

I had come with just one suitcase of clothes and some books, so there was little settling to do. A kilometer from the city center, the Fairview was a charming, colonial-style hotel with a beautiful garden. It was simpler than the larger hotels and was frequented by missionaries, aid workers, and travelers on lower budgets but not quite in the backpack set. Somewhat more developed today, it retains its old-world charm.

I was still at the Fairview when I experienced a warning about my new environment. The Association of Physicians of East and Central Africa was holding its annual meeting at another hotel nearby. Although advised not to walk after dark, I declined the offer of a lift by car to the evening reception. I changed into smart clothes and set off on foot at dusk.

As I walked toward the main road, three young men were coming toward me, one of whom clearly said something about me to the others. I felt fear but ignored my instinct to run back or shout. As they passed, I was grabbed, forced to the ground, and had my wallet with its meager cash taken. They casually sauntered away, and with the sudden bravado from realizing I was not seriously hurt, I asked them to drop the papers that the wallet contained, which they did. My hand was cut, and my pale jacket was now stained with blood. I was halfway to the reception and decided I might as well continue. Causing a stir upon arrival, I drank a strong gin and was taken to the private Nairobi Hospital to have my hand stitched up.

Being mugged within 2 weeks of arrival in Kenya was an inauspicious beginning. I realized I was luckier than many, and the fear this experience instilled was perhaps useful in avoiding future risk. Many others have similar stories, some far worse, and insecurity and crime are threats in many African cities. Stories of muggings and theft were common among Kenyan staff at Kenyatta National Hospital. Nairobi has maintained its unfortunate reputation, sometimes facetiously referred to as "Nairobbery." A joke is that a third of the city is employed protecting another third against the final third; provision of security services has become big business. Security specialists always advise to follow one's instincts about danger and to give up possessions without a fight. Material goods are replaceable, life and limb are not.

Medicine at Kenyatta National Hospital

It had been 6 years since I had been at Kenyatta National Hospital on my student elective and in the intervening period I had qualified as a doctor, trained as a specialist in internal medicine, and obtained a tropical medicine degree. I threw myself into the work, eager to experience what medicine had to offer in this poor, African environment.

The Department of Medicine had about twenty lecturers and senior lecturers, one-third non-Kenyan, including Europeans and Indians (Figure 3.1). Philip Rees, the tropical medicine expert, became a mentor, though distant and slightly aloof in British fashion. I focused on tropical medicine, gastroenterology, and liver disease. A longstanding collaboration had existed between the University of Amsterdam and Nairobi, and a Dutch physician, Piet Kager, later professor of tropical medicine in Amsterdam, worked closely with Rees and became a lifelong friend. The Dutch had a longstanding presence in public health in Kenya, although this was now being wound down. Within a few years it was invisible apart from a building on the hospital campus, referred to ever since as "the Dutch building."

Kenyatta National Hospital was a sprawling complex whose history dated back to the early twentieth century. Its earlier name, still enshrined on plaques in unexpected corners, King George VI Memorial Hospital, indicated its colonial past. The tuberculosis control program had a building on the campus and had conducted important therapeutic trials over the years, supported by the

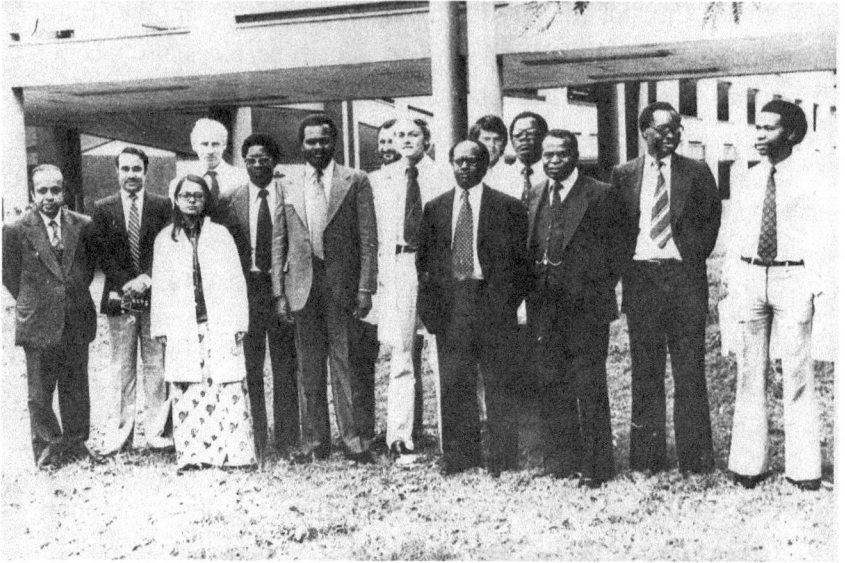

Figure 3.1   University of Nairobi, Department of Medicine, circa. 1981.
(Kevin De Cock, personal collection)

United Kingdom's Medical Research Council. The Wellcome Trust supported a baboon colony for research work on the immunology of schistosomiasis nearby, and a beautiful, if dilapidated, colonial building housed the extensive Wellcome library.

One day, a baboon died unexpectedly and, on autopsy, was found to have tuberculosis (S.B. Lucas, personal communication). Panic ensued, there being concern the infection had spread from the adjacent tuberculosis laboratory, raising anxiety about worker safety as well as the implications for years of immunology research results. An unfortunate PhD student who oversaw the baboons was then discovered to have tuberculosis and was the suspected source of infection.

Kenyatta Hospital acted as primary care center for the underserved population of Nairobi but also as district and provincial hospital and national referral center, all at the same time. It was crowded, busy, and noisy. Typical of such a large national hospital, it consumed about 20% of the national health budget, and was a constant source of criticism. Its numerous medical staff worked either for the university or the Ministry of Health, with some tension between the two groups. Expatriates living in Nairobi were disdainful of the hospital; they sought their own care in the city's well-established private facilities.

I was considered an oddity by the Europeans with whom I played tennis, my dominant leisure activity outside of medicine. They were intrigued by my occupation, place of work, and that I was on a local salary with no expatriate benefits. The pay was so poor that the Belgian authorities eventually recognized me as a volunteer and facilitated a small stipend given to volunteer teachers at the end of their overseas tours.

Expatriates fell into distinct groups. The missionaries, however opinionated and rigid, stayed long term in difficult places in the interior where few others would serve, and they had to be admired for their dedication. The diplomats, development workers, and United Nations crowd lived in a bubble of constant communication and professional entertaining, to which I was occasionally invited. The business community interacted the most with the regular Kenyan population.

Kenyan society itself was rigidly divided among Africans, Asians, and "KCs," Kenyan-born white people referred to as Kenya Cowboys. Kenyans had strong tribal affiliations and divisions. I maneuvered through this social mixture by maintaining my own identity and focusing on medicine, teaching, and research. The eclectic academic staff housed in the apartment complex where I lived were of different nationalities and disciplines, and strong friendships developed. Commitment to medicine and the hospital, good relations with colleagues and students, and my modest lifestyle helped my integration into the Kenyan world.

Piet Kager and Philip Rees had a research interest in leishmaniasis, a parasitic infection spread by sandflies in dry, harsh parts of the country. Wanting to concentrate on his research, Kager was more than pleased for me to take over his supervision of the Adult Observation Ward (AOW), the acute medical admission unit where patients were admitted for evaluation before discharge or transfer to the main wards. Because the hospital was so crowded, the AOW functioned like a ward itself, and patients sometimes stayed there for many days.

The pressure on the AOW was enormous: dozens of patients could be admitted in one day, and overcrowding was normal. Patients often shared beds, lying head to toe, or occupied mattresses on the floor and in the corridors. The facility had a characteristic, unpleasant odor that crept into one's hair and clothes. It was conditions like these that gave the hospital its poor reputation to outsiders, but what quickly struck me was that good medicine could be practiced, even under such adverse conditions. I reminded people that you did not die from sharing a bed or lying on the floor, but you could from medical neglect or mismanagement.

The lingering British influence on the hospital was shown by an interaction with the Kenyan clinical dean, Ambrose Wasunna, the British-trained professor of surgery. He accosted me in the corridor one day, pulled me into a closet, and asked why I did not wear a tie at work. I replied that work on the AOW entailed kneeling on the floor to examine patients and that a tie was impractical. His strange response was that the professor of obstetrics and gynecology also had a hard job, yet he wore a tie every day. I duly complied with his request, noting later that a Swiss colleague who ignored a similar instruction won a small battle but lost relationships.

I quickly realized that the classic tropical diseases I had studied in Liverpool occupied a small and restricted niche in medicine overall. We saw three broad patterns of disease. Most common were the infectious diseases of poverty that accounted for most admissions to the AOW: pneumonia, tuberculosis, diarrheal diseases, and assorted conditions. The second group comprised the diseases that occupy internists everywhere in the world: the common noncommunicable diseases such as hypertension, diabetes, cancer, and less common conditions such as rheumatologic diseases. Finally, there were the classic tropical diseases such as malaria and schistosomiasis, whose distribution in the country were geographically restricted and determined by ecology and climate. I found this categorization useful and accurate, and described it in an article in the *British Medical Journal* after I left Kenya.[2]

The breadth of medicine at Kenyatta National Hospital was extraordinary. I often commented that although I was the teacher, I was receiving a priceless education. One day, my unit admitted eleven patients with meningococcal meningitis, a condition many practitioners in the Global North may not see in their whole professional life. The diagnosis is confirmed by microscopic examination of cerebrospinal fluid obtained by lumbar puncture. One patient's cerebrospinal fluid was under such pressure from the associated brain swelling that the fluid shot out through the needle and into my face. One just accepted these things happened. Seeing so many cases over a 24-hour period clearly indicated a meningitis outbreak in Nairobi. Collaboration between clinicians and the public health authorities was limited, and I was not aware of any further action or investigation being taken.

Tetanus was a frequent diagnosis, again no longer seen in the industrialized world. In another case, when members of a single family were admitted with nausea and vomiting, complaining of seeing double, and we learned that another relative was on the intensive care unit, we diagnosed botulism, a disease from microbial production of a toxin that can contaminate food and cause muscle paralysis, including the respiratory muscles and muscles of the eye. Insects stored in a plastic bag many days earlier and sent down as a delicacy by bus from the interior to Nairobi were the culprit. My training in Bristol had not prepared me for such events.

Some diseases were not themselves infectious, such as primary cancer of the liver or cancer of the cervix. These are, respectively, among the commonest cancers in Kenyan men and women, and we now know that these are long-term consequences of viral infections, hepatitis B and human papillomavirus, respectively. Both are preventable by vaccination.

I shared my departmental office with a suave, sophisticated Ugandan neurologist named Mata Bahemuka. He had trained at Queen's Square in London, the Mecca for neurology, and was proud of that association. We had deep as well as humorous conversations as he puffed on his pipe, and I respected his intellect and clinical acumen. He documented the previously unrecognized high burden of strokes in relatively young Africans, often the consequence of high blood pressure. The *East African Medical Journal* is not widely read internationally but had considerable influence in the region and was a journal where he and I published much of our clinical research.[3-5]

I was saddened to hear some years later that Bahemuka had been killed in Uganda, shot at a gasoline station in Kampala, possibly a robbery or a targeted assassination related to the murky politics evolving in that country. The despot Idi Amin had been ousted by Tanzanian forces the month before my arrival in Nairobi, but Uganda remained unstable until Yoweri Museveni took over in 1986. He remains in power to this day, a complex figure whose early ideals gave way, as seen so often, to brutal determination to remain in charge.

Interesting research on hypertension was being supported by the Wellcome Trust, implemented by Neil Poulter and colleagues from London. The group was tracking migrants from the Nyanza region around Lake Victoria to Nairobi and seeing how their lifestyles and health changed with this move. The migrants' salt intake increased, and their blood pressure increased by about 10 points, an elegant demonstration of some of the consequences of evolving lifestyles on health so much more evident today.[6–11] To my knowledge, Bahemuka and Poulter did not know each other. Yet, Bahemuka's early descriptions of the clinical consequences of hypertension in young Africans were the "why" justifying some of Poulter's work examining the environmental and social factors driving high blood pressure. Today, hypertension is recognized as perhaps the biggest killer in the world, and large-scale efforts address the public health challenge it represents.[12]

I did not see a single heart attack during my 3 years in Nairobi, but decades later, coronary artery disease, obesity, and type 2 diabetes are common. A frequent cause of severe cardiac dysfunction was rheumatic heart disease, the result of earlier rheumatic fever, which can damage the valves of the heart. This remains an underaddressed problem in global health that results in more than 300,000 deaths annually.[13]

I came to realize what a terrible disease diabetes is for people who are poor. For those requiring insulin injections, a condition that usually starts when one is young, assuring supply of the drug and appropriate cool storage can pose overwhelming challenges. It occurred to me that one reason we did not see more patients with insulin-dependent (type 1) diabetes was simply because they had died. I was gratified to help a laboratory technician who supported me in clinical and research work. He sought me out to tell me of new symptoms he could not understand; he was always thirsty, drank more water, passed more urine, felt tired, and was losing weight. We admitted him and rapidly controlled his diabetes with insulin.

Groundbreaking work was done in Tanzania by the British physician Donald McLarty and Tanzanian colleagues assessing the burden of diabetes in the population and describing its impact, as well as advising on its management, all at a time when public health interest in noncommunicable diseases was not in vogue.[14] McClarty committed his career to Tanzania. I heard him present his work at East African medical conferences and was sorry when I learned of his premature death due to melanoma.

I was interested in evaluating new or simplified diagnostic measures and assessing their utility and appropriateness in this low-income, tropical environment, and had productive collaborations assessing ultrasound imaging, endoscopy, and other interventions.[15-20] Ultrasound scanning was simple, though reading the images needed sophisticated training, and it was adaptable to harsh conditions by rendering equipment portable in four-wheel-drive vehicles. It was useful for diagnosing hydatid disease, a parasitic condition causing cysts in different parts of the body and an important public health problem in the remote Turkana region of northern Kenya.

Although I was proud of our clinical work,[21-27] I also developed concerns that have stayed with me over the years in Africa. Things taken for granted are instantly noticed when absent, and two essentials I missed were consistently good nursing care and the sense of urgency that medicine requires. In the public sector of many African countries I have visited, the quality of nursing has been variable. That it is better in the private sector shows that a decent living wage and supportive supervision encourage performance.

Later, when AIDS emerged, stigma and discrimination worsened an already adverse situation of staff all too often blaming patients for their illness. Corruption adds fuel to this fire, and it is well known that, in some places, staff had to be paid if they were to provide any care. Indifference to human suffering is sometimes seen everywhere, but it always surprises me in its contrast to the emphasis on support, generosity, and loyalty to family over individualism that is so strong in many poor environments.

One night, we admitted a 20-year-old woman with shortness of breath. I taught the students on call that this was an urgent indication to obtain a chest X-ray because she might have a pneumothorax (a localized rupture of the lung resulting in air in the pleural space between the lung and the chest wall). Sometimes a valve mechanism results so that with each breath more air leaks into the chest cavity, compressing the lung, pushing the heart and other structures to one side, and, at worst, ending in respiratory and cardiovascular collapse. This emergency is called a tension pneumothorax and requires urgent placement of a chest drain to evacuate the air. Sometimes just inserting a small needle into the chest to let the air out can be life-saving.

The students were impressed when the difficult-to-obtain chest X-ray showed the patient did indeed have a pneumothorax. Her condition deteriorated, she was developing tension, and we scoured the hospital for a chest drain. Having found one after an hour of search and duly placed it, her condition immediately improved. When I passed by the next day to check on the young woman, no longer under my supervision, I could not find her. I was told that she had become distressed, likely indicating displacement of the tube and further tension, but nothing had been done. No consequences or discussion followed this unnecessary death.

Along the same lines, I recall a conversation with the eminent chest physician John Murray visiting from San Francisco when I was working in West Africa a decade later. He expressed shock to me that a young professor, in discussion with Murray, had shrugged his shoulders when interrupted by enquiries from a patient's relative, explaining that a patient in her 20s had died overnight. Murray was surprised; at his home institution, he said, the death of a young person would be the talk of the hospital and would stimulate extensive review.

I cannot explain these differences and certainly infer no superiority in values or capability in the North. Neither is it simply due to workload, which is excessive everywhere in medicine. Workers in resource-limited settings face stress from relentless, systemic inadequacies in the working environment, which, along with poor remuneration and shortages of staff, supplies, and drugs, conspire to erode quality and standards. Rewards and recognition for work well done are rare, doing things well may seem to make no difference, and corrupt systems undermine quality. There is neither stick nor carrot to drive improvement, and strong forces militate against change. Yet, low expectations and the occasional indifference to suffering and preventable death can be surprising. Fighting all this is essential for incremental progress, but unrealistic expectations are not helpful either. I used to say to critics of Kenyatta National Hospital that if what you seek are the standards of the Massachusetts General Hospital, go to Boston.

A specific, under-recognized category of problems complicates middle-income environments or privileged facilities in poor settings aspiring to complex work not done elsewhere in the country. Cardiothoracic surgery was introduced at Kenyatta National Hospital, renal dialysis was developed, and the hospital had a large intensive care unit. Outbreaks of HIV have been recognized in specialized facilities of some middle-income-country hospitals, reflecting their sophistication but inadequate performance in infection prevention and control.[28] The poorest of settings would not suffer such events because they do not have dialysis units, and richer countries have stronger systems in place to prevent them. Years later, cases of Ebola occurred in a dialysis unit in Conakry, Guinea. I never knew whether the story of patients dying on the intensive care unit at Kenyatta when domestic staff disconnected ventilators to plug in cleaning equipment was true or a local urban legend.

Tropical and Liver Diseases

I was anxious to see the classic tropical diseases that I had studied in Liverpool. Nairobi has a temperate climate because it is situated at an altitude of approximately 5,000 feet. The vector of malaria, principally *Anopheles gambiae,* does not breed there. For most other tropical infections, either the vectors or intermediate hosts were absent or ecologic conditions did not support transmission of these diseases. However, patients did attend the hospital from all over Kenya and brought their pathology with them, so one had to know the distribution of disease to make sensible diagnoses.

Depending on where patients lived, some diagnoses were either likely or impossible because of local ecology. The pathologist Michael Hutt, one of the world's experts who worked in Uganda in the 1960s, coined the term "geographical pathology" to refer to this interplay between disease and the broader environment. Makerere University in Uganda provided East Africa's first medical school and contributed enormously to the development of medicine in the region. Hutt worked with several colleagues in different disciplines in astonishingly productive collaborations that resulted in the first descriptions of several diseases, such as Burkitt's lymphoma and the heart condition endomyocardial fibrosis.

A few months after my arrival in Nairobi, I met a colleague critical to my subsequent work, the British pathologist Sebastian Lucas, who had worked closely with Michael Hutt in the United Kingdom. Hutt recommended that Lucas come to Nairobi, and he joined the hospital as a senior lecturer some months after I did. He was deeply committed to autopsy work and teaching, and we developed a close collaboration and friendship. He and his family also had to wait to be allocated university housing, just as I did, and in the meantime stayed in a hotel frequented by sex workers. Lucas was in the elevator with his 4-year-old daughter, Flora, when a young woman offered him "a good time." "Daddy, can I have a good time too?" piped up Flora.

Splenomegaly, enlargement of the spleen, can result from a wide variety of causes and is an unusual physical sign in patients in the industrialized world. It was long recognized that spleno-megaly was more frequent in tropical climates, and in some cases, the spleen becomes massive. It was often thought to be re-lated to malaria and, in the 1960s and 1970s this association was clarified by work at Mulago Hospital (now Mulago National Re-ferral Hospital) in Kampala, Uganda, again involving Michael Hutt, and in Papua New Guinea. The term "tropical splenomeg-aly syndrome" was coined to refer to this chronic enlargement of the spleen related to malaria, but diagnostic criteria were imper-fectly defined, and many other potential causes of splenic enlarge-ment remained. I was intrigued by this condition when I learned about it during my tropical medicine course.

Malaria received three full hours of lectures at Liverpool, all de-livered by the dean, Herbert Gilles. A dapper man originally from Malta, Gilles was an excellent lecturer who communicated clearly to us the overwhelming role malaria played in medicine in the tropics. There were four principal species of the malaria par-asite, but one, *Plasmodium falciparum*, accounted for the great majority of severe illness and deaths. Gilles' practical teaching provided a series of logical questions guiding the way forward. Is this malaria? Is the patient from an area of drug-resistant malaria,* at that time requiring quinine rather than the staple drug chloro-quine, to which resistance was spreading? Is the patient severely ill, requiring intravenous treatment? Partial resistance to chlo-roquine had just been reported for the first time in East Africa and, a few years later when back in London, I wrote up the first recognized case of complete resistance in a patient just returned from Kenya.[29]

---

* Chloroquine is no longer used for treatment of malaria in Africa because of extensive resistance. Standard treatment today is with artemisinin-based combination therapies.

Other parasitic diseases associated with chronically enlarged spleens included schistosomiasis (also referred to as bilharzia, after Theodor Bilharz who discovered the parasite) and leishmaniasis, the disease that Piet Kager and Philip Rees studied. A group of expatriate researchers worked on these tropical diseases, but few Kenyans did; most of the latter were more interested in subspecialties like cardiology. In 1979, the CDC sent Harrison Spencer from Atlanta, GA, to Kenya to initiate long-term malaria research. The US Army had a group already present there for 10 years working on leishmaniasis and malaria, the motivation being that American troops could face these infections in international deployments. Anthony ("Tony") Bryceson from the London School of Hygiene and Tropical Medicine conducted therapeutic trials on leishmaniasis.

A loose affiliation formed between these different researchers who felt sorry for me because of my poor remuneration and heavy clinical and teaching burden. I marveled at their sophistication and level of support, as well as the quality of their housing. Harrison Spencer* and I became friends, and he introduced me to his visiting supervisor from the CDC, Robert Kaiser. I had difficulty understanding at that time what this agency did, so committed was I to clinical medicine rather than public health. Yet again, serendipity played its role. Harrison would later become dean of the London School when I was on the faculty there, and I would eventually work for the CDC, including in Kenya. Harrison was sent to Kenya because Kaiser had worked there years before, met his British wife there, and had lasting affection for the country. Without that, the CDC's long and productive presence in Kenya might not have occurred.[30,31]

---

* Harrison Spencer died under tragic circumstances in 2016. (Obituary. Harrison Clark Spencer. Lancet. 2016;388:1154)

Schistosomiasis in Kenya results from infection with two different species of parasite, *Schistosoma haematobium* and *S. mansoni*. These flatworms have a complex life cycle that involves different species of snails as intermediate hosts; human infection results from exposure to water where the snails are living. Once the worms develop in the human body, their eggs are deposited in the genitourinary system, especially the bladder, in the case of *S. haematobium*, and the intestine and liver in the case of *S. mansoni*. The body's long-term reaction to these eggs can cause disease, including, for *S. mansoni*, portal hypertension (obstruction of blood flow through the liver) and enlargement of the spleen.[32]

Although schistosomiasis is one of the commonest causes of portal hypertension worldwide, it receives little interest from research donors. The variety that affected the bladder occurred at the Kenya coast and in the southern part of Kenya's Eastern Province,* whereas the intestinal variety was found in Eastern Province as well as around Lake Victoria.

Leishmaniasis is a more acute disease that causes massive enlargement of the spleen and is associated with fever, wasting, and anemia. Children were often affected and if untreated, could die. I taught the medical students about the importance of examining the retina with an ophthalmoscope in all patients, especially those with fever, because different diseases can have ophthalmic findings. Doing this on a febrile patient with an enlarged spleen, later diagnosed with leishmaniasis, in the crowded AOW, I nearly choked with surprise when I saw large hemorrhages at the back of his eye. We documented this in the *American Journal of Tropi-*

---

* Kenya's 2010 Constitution divided the country into forty-seven counties, replacing the former organization of eight provinces. The former Eastern Province was divided into eight counties, the southernmost being Kitui, Machakos, and Makueni.

cal Medicine and Hygiene,[33] but only after discovering that this finding had been described in China in the 1920s. It was a humbling reminder that there is enormous historical experience that physicians are often unaware of, and that most academic publications fade away into history.

The longstanding treatments used for leishmaniasis, antimony-based drugs, were toxic and difficult to administer safely. As for most parasitic diseases, drug development for leishmaniasis was lacking because the pharmaceutical industry had no financial incentives to undertake research on these diseases of the tropics. Money was to be made from drugs for diseases of the rich; as a pharmaceutical executive once said, there is no incentive to develop drugs for people who cannot afford to buy shoes. An instinctive reaction is to criticize Big Pharma, and sometimes criticism is justified for excessive profits made. Overall, however, the problem is that the global economic order is not suited for development of drugs for which there is no market. For diseases of the poor, or for rare diseases, special mechanisms for research and programs need to be developed.

Over the years, I saw successful advocacy for such diseases, including the establishment of WHO's program on neglected tropical diseases, a term that now encompasses some twenty-one diverse conditions, some infectious (e.g., yellow fever, rabies), and some not (e.g., snakebite).[34,35] This is a ragbag of different diseases not obviously associated other than that they afflict the poor, but the list is too long to be easily remembered. Mass treatment of certain helminthic infections without individual diagnosis has been an important programmatic advance.

The long-term utility of the term "neglected" is questionable because funding has increased for some of these conditions, and they are not all equally neglected. I recall sitting on a grant review panel in the United Kingdom years later when one wag suggested rejecting a proposal for study of rare fungal complications of AIDS on the grounds that the diseases in question were not rare enough. Nonetheless, that there are diseases affecting hundreds of millions of people and causing immense suffering and tens of thousands of deaths, and that little funding goes toward control of or research on these conditions are important and unacceptable.

Clinical experience in Nairobi exposed me to several of the major tropical diseases, including malaria, schistosomiasis, and leishmaniasis. Conditions we rarely saw were trypanosomiasis (sleeping sickness), filariasis (elephantiasis), and onchocerciasis (river blindness). Leprosy was not only rare but was looked after by the dermatologists and the tuberculosis program.

Human African trypanosomiasis is transmitted by the tsetse fly. An endemic focus in western Kenya had been largely extinguished, although the condition remained present in Uganda. The Democratic Republic of the Congo is heavily affected and by the 1990s, with the breakdown of systems there, levels of sleeping sickness were back to where they were before Belgian colonialists began campaigns against this disease in the early twentieth century.[36] A lesson applicable to virtually all infectious diseases is that control efforts must be continuous, along with ongoing surveillance.

Filariasis, the cause of extreme leg swelling referred to as elephantiasis, was largely restricted to the Kenya coast. When we did have patients with elephantiasis, the cause was noninfectious, though mostly obscure in origin (Figure 3.2).[37] A leading theory is that noninfectious elephantiasis results from obstruction of lymphatic channels by silica, the result of years of walking barefoot on soil rich in this compound. Onchocerciasis, another worm infection referred to as river blindness, also had largely been controlled in its Western focus.

A Dutch parasitologist who worked in Kenya for much of his career described the difficulties of field work on filariasis. The parasites circulate in the body and become detectable in the blood at night, requiring, at that time, nocturnal blood samples to be

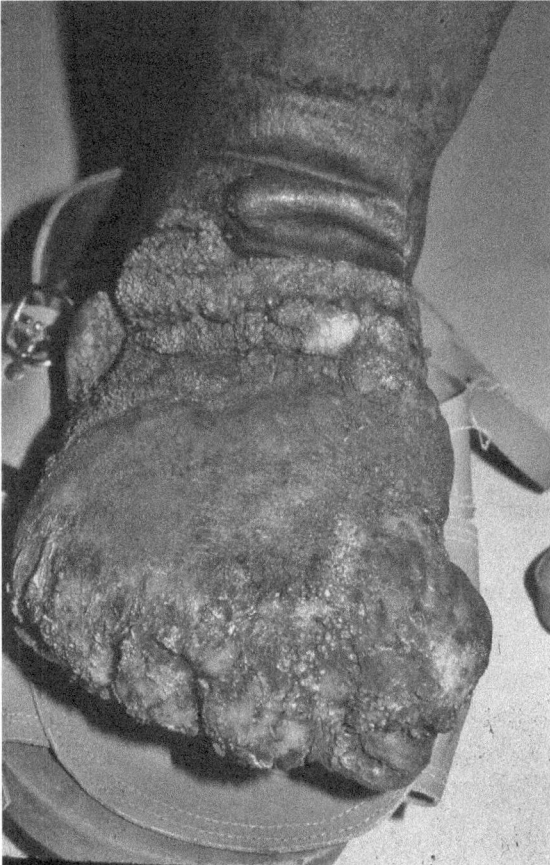

Figure 3.2   Nonfilarial elephantiasis.
(Kevin De Cock, personal collection)

examined for diagnosis. The people of the Coast, many believing in witchcraft, required much persuasion to allow blood to be taken by this white man visiting them at night. He reassured his study patients by taking their blood, examining the specimens under his microscope in the household, and leaving all blood and specimens behind as he bid adieu and continued on his way.

Other than some of these tropical conditions, splenomegaly resulted principally from liver disease, the commonest cause of which was cirrhosis. Working with Rees, Kager, Lucas, and, later,

Michael Hutt, I embarked on a study of patients with chronic splenomegaly at Kenyatta National Hospital, not only to determine the different causes of this condition but also to propose a diagnostic algorithm. Amidst a heavy clinical and teaching load, I sought out patients with splenomegaly, collected serum from every patient, and stored it for later testing for evidence of prior exposure to these different infectious agents, and to evaluate the utility of serologic testing for them.[38]

Leaving Nairobi

It was early 1982 and I was facing having to leave Kenya. Personal attachments and the intensity of clinical work stopped me leaving, while the desire to undertake further training, spend medical time in America (the "BA": "been to America"), and write my dissertation on chronic splenomegaly pushed me away. The Wellcome Trust graciously agreed to support me for 6 months to work with Michael Hutt in London while I conducted the laboratory work and writing. I had extended my 2-year contract with the University of Nairobi for an additional 6 months, then for a further 3 months, but I now sadly accepted it was time to go. Having decided to leave Kenya, I chose the first day of spring to depart.

The bureaucracy of leaving the university and the numerous forms to be signed before receiving the necessary plane ticket seemed endless. Some international colleagues had put together a whole file of steps required that was supremely helpful but indicative of administrative obstacles to work in a setting not one's own. An immigration officer at the airport spotted some notes of Kenyan currency in my shirt pocket and demanded they be surrendered to him before I could board the plane, adding to my gloom.

Sue Lucas, wife of my pathologist colleague who left Nairobi some months earlier, met me at Heathrow Airport and drove me to south London to the first of three residences over the next 14 months. We commiserated about the weather and difficulties of settling back into this drab environment. Return from extended field work is notably stressful. Few people understand the intensity or relevance of the overseas experience, colleagues' interest is limited, and it takes time to find one's equilibrium in the process of re-integration. Were it not for the intensity of effort that I committed to laboratory work and writing, I could have sunk into depression.

I had no background in laboratory work but was guided with kindness over the following months by staff at St. Thomas' Hospital and the London School of Hygiene and Tropical Medicine. My principal objectives were to assess the diagnostic utility of serologic assays for malaria, schistosomiasis, and leishmaniasis in patients with chronic splenomegaly, as well as to determine the proportion of chronic liver disease attributable to hepatitis B.

I was anxiously aware throughout my work in Nairobi and subsequently that safeguarding specimens and completing the laboratory work were critical to the whole enterprise: if I had no specimens, I had no study and no dissertation. Ever since, I have emphasized to younger colleagues conducting field work how critical it is to assure the integrity of specimens and quality of laboratory work, ideally by participating in work at the bench.

My supervisor, Michael Hutt, facilitated my introductions to other departments and seniors, such as Jangu Banatvala, head of Virology at St. Thomas', and Chris Draper, who oversaw seroepidemiology at the London School. Lucas instructed me in the reading of liver biopsy samples, which I did on specimens anonymized so as not to bias interpretation based on knowledge of other results. All this was done before the introduction of personal computers, and I managed the data by painfully entering results in pencil on large, lined paper charts that Lucas referred to as my railway timetables.

Michael Hutt gave me what may have been the single most important piece of advice I received: to start writing immediately. I have passed this on to others; if one waits to start writing a dissertation, or even a paper, until all results are in, the task may seem insurmountable. Large pieces—background and methods, but even some discussion and conclusions—can be written from the beginning or as one goes along.

We confirmed the association between malaria and tropical splenomegaly syndrome, and positive malarial serology is an essential element of the diagnosis.[38-41] With Tony Bryceson and Michael Hutt coordinating, we gathered an international group of researchers to recommend a change in terminology. Henceforth, a more specific name was adopted, hyper-reactive malarial splenomegaly,[42] which communicates its pathophysiology: an abnormally strong immunologic reaction to malaria. It was rewarding to see this proposed nomenclature adopted internationally.

During this ongoing work, the great tropical physician Philip Marsden spent time at the London School and gave the prestigious Heath Clark lectures. He spoke on three consecutive days, covering his own research in Brazil on malaria and Chagas's disease, the South American form of trypanosomiasis. He cited my own work in his lecture, mentioning these discussions on terminology, and, at my young age, this meant a great deal. Marsden led an unorthodox life that a career in global health can entail, and he became firmly entrenched in Brazil with a new family partnership, disregard for formality, reputed fondness for cognac, and impressive scientific productivity on parasitic diseases of the poor. He was a legendary figure and his lectures only enhanced his reputation.

Introducing his first talk, he broke down and wept as he thanked family and colleagues for support and collaboration. This left his audience moved by his sensitivity but, this being Britain after all, uncomfortable. When Marsden gave his second talk, he again thanked others and tears again flowed, though more controlled. This time people looked at each other in puzzlement. At the third lecture, listeners sat on the edge of their seats to see what would happen, but he mercifully got through his introduction without excessive emotion.

He reminded me of my own surgeon father's proclivity to weep at public events. Such cultural differences were highlighted to me by Marc-Alain Widdowson, a later colleague at the CDC. He and his wife, a Brazilian, studied at the London School in the early 1990s. Foreign students were given a talk on cultural adaptation to England and the English that included the advice, "Above all, don't touch them."

We showed in our studies that schistosomal serology was useful in the diagnosis of chronic splenomegaly in that negative results reliably excluded schistosomiasis as a cause (high sensitivity and negative predictive value).[43] For leishmaniasis, positive tests confirmed the diagnosis (high specificity and positive predictive value).[44] The work clarified the different causes of splenomegaly, and the proportion associated with portal hypertension.[45-47] As a cause of intestinal bleeding, portal hypertension was much more common in Kenya than in industrialized countries, accounting for about 20% of cases. Of those, one-fifth were due to schistosomiasis, a disease that today could be largely eliminated as a public health problem through mass drug administration to populations at risk.

We showed that a disproportionate number of patients with splenomegaly were from Kenya's Eastern Province, and the same was true for almost all causes of liver disease. Despite the intense investigations conducted, there remained cases of splenomegaly and portal hypertension whose causes and nature remained obscure.[48,49] There is need for further research into these subjects, especially in the region southeast of Nairobi, formerly the Eastern Province, but it is difficult to find funding for such research.

Over the years there have been repeated outbreaks in this geographic area of aflatoxin poisoning, with high death rates from acute liver failure. Aflatoxin is a toxin produced by a fungus, *Aspergillus flavus*, that grows on damp maize. Whether aflatoxin exposure is related to the high rates of chronic liver disease in the former Eastern Province is an important but neglected question.

The Wellcome Trust generously extended my grant, with carefully chosen words, "for a further and final three months." I learned from this experience that I could ask pertinent questions, synthesize information, draw generalizable conclusions, and write them up—in sum, conduct research. Within a year of returning to London from Kenya, my dissertation was bound and delivered to the University of Bristol, and later to the medical school library in Nairobi, and I felt ready to leave for America and further training.

The defense of my dissertation was held in December 1983 in the Department of Medicine in Bristol, with Professor Read overseeing the event. The chief and second examiners were, respectively, the eminent liver specialist Roger Williams and Tony Bryceson. Williams probed about the leishmaniasis work and its serology, but this was not his area of expertise. Professor Read expressed amusement and satisfaction at my successful defense.[49]

CHAPTER 4

Hepatitis and HIV in the City of Angels

First Awareness of AIDS

I remember where I was sitting in the University of Nairobi's medical school library in early 1982 when I first read of AIDS. My usual seat overlooked the car park, facing the meager bookshelves I had come to know, across from the white librarian's desk. Few white people worked in the hospital now, and each had a story of why they were there when most of the staff were African. The librarian was married to a Kenyan and now was settled in this country with children. Some medical staff in the hospital had been trained in Russia during the Cold War and came back with eastern European wives, though never husbands.

I read an article describing *Pneumocystis* pneumonia, Kaposi's sarcoma (a rare cancer), and other unusual infections generally restricted to people with impaired immune systems in gay men and people who inject drugs in California and New York City. The first reports of *Pneumocystis* pneumonia in homosexual men had been in the *Morbidity and Mortality Weekly Report* (*MMWR*),[1] the weekly public health bulletin published by the CDC, on June 5, 1981, but I had not heard of it.

I moved to London from Nairobi in late March 1982. The term AIDS had not been introduced when 37-year-old Terrence Higgins died at St Thomas' Hospital in London on July 4, 1982. Higgins had worked at the House of Commons across from the hospital. He was known to be gay but was otherwise not unusual except for the devastating nature of his illness and his young age. It was at St Thomas' that Professor Michael Hutt was based. Lucas was destined to follow Hutt as Britain's leading infectious disease pathologist. He watched a routine autopsy on Higgins and was surprised to find pneumonia and an obscure brain disorder as causes of death.* This was one of the first AIDS deaths in the United Kingdom. Friends of Higgins set up an organization in his name, the Terrence Higgins Trust, now the largest nongovernmental organization in the United Kingdom committed to HIV and sexual health.[2]

I occasionally heard this new syndrome discussed in infectious disease circles in London later in 1982 and early '83, but always as an obscurity. I pursued my interest in liver disease in which the dominant infection remained viral hepatitis, especially hepatitis B, which mainly affected gay men and people who inject drugs. Hepatitis B was to gay men what HIV would later become, a source of worry and stigma, illustrated by an article in the gay press describing a young man's shame and guilt about his infectiousness for this virus.

During 3 months as locum on the Infectious Diseases Unit at Northwick Park Hospital in north London in early 1983 I saw patients with a broad range of infectious diseases, some in passengers sent straight from Heathrow Airport, but no cases of AIDS. A television documentary on the new "gay disease" aroused interest but no sense of local relevance. I was due to leave London for a fellowship in liver disease at the University

---

* Lucas told me that the cause of the pneumonia was toxoplasmosis but that this was only recognized when the autopsy specimens were reviewed much later when AIDS pathology was better understood.

of Southern California (USC). My last residence in London was in a house south of the River Thames owned by a gay opera singer. A straight housemate, a trainee psychiatrist, and I would occasionally come home to find a dinner party for a dozen or so young men in full swing. At the last such gathering I recall, there was talk of the "gay cancer" that, according to one of the Australian guests, had "now arrived in Sydney." I departed for Los Angeles in May 1983, unaware of how AIDS was to dominate medicine in coming years.

Liver Disease in Los Angeles, 1983–1986

To a novice, Los Angeles is a frightening metropolis with confusing, intersecting freeways for its backbone. Its citizens have been described as "quadrirotor man"; it was impossible to survive there without a car. My sister Jacqui lived in La Jolla, some 110 miles south, providing useful support for adapting to this new world. I was now used to the routine of moving and its sequential priorities—find a short-term place to stay, buy a car, find a permanent residence, organize essential utensils and appliances, and start work. My reliance on mattresses on the floor and bricks and planks for bookshelves typical of student life lasted longer into adulthood than for most of my colleagues. I felt inwardly pleased when, at my next move, from Los Angeles to Atlanta in 1986, the moving agent looked around my apartment in Pasadena and commented "You travel light."

The USC Liver Unit was based in two hospitals: the vast County Hospital, the Los Angeles County–University of Southern California Medical Center downtown and a facility farther south, Rancho Los Amigos Medical Center, best known as a rehabilitation center for people with spinal injuries. An incidental claim to fame for Rancho was its hosting the wheelchair basketball scene in the

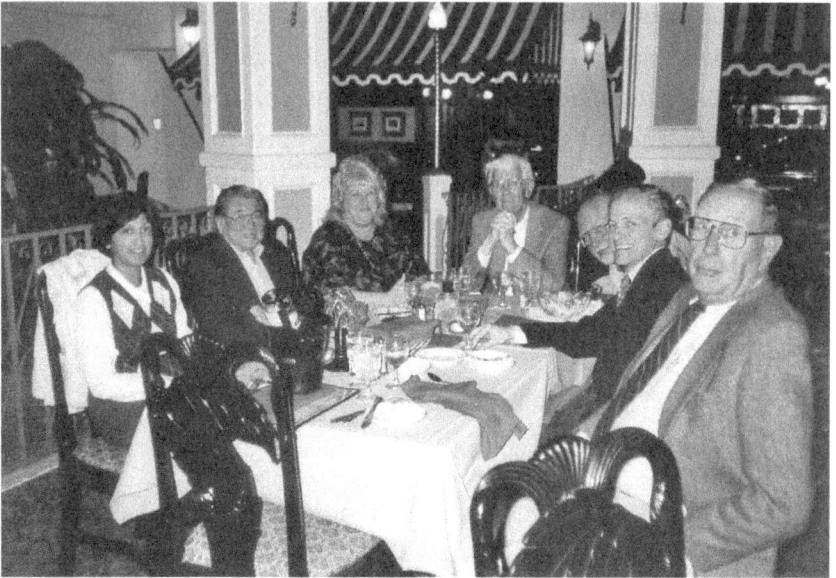

Figure 4.1   Staff of the Liver Unit, my leaving dinner, 1986 (*Left to Right*). Sugantha Govindarajan, Sy Yamada, Rita Musick, Telfer Reynolds, Oliver Kuzma, Kevin De Cock, Allan Redeker.
(Kevin De Cock, personal collection)

1978 anti-Vietnam war movie "Coming Home," starring Jane Fonda. Life on the Liver Unit entailed a lot of driving, with clinics and consultations at "Big County" but inpatients transferred to "the Ranch."

A triumvirate of seniors ruled this unit, possibly the largest clinical facility for liver disease in the world. It was somewhat incongruous that USC, a private and very expensive university, had the public county hospital as its medical teaching facility. Telfer ("Pete") Reynolds was the undisputed leader, a tall, lean man with a shock of silver hair that contrasted with his nickname from earlier years, "Black Pete" (Figure 4.1). He was absolutely committed to work, was intolerant of any pretention, treated the rich and famous who consulted him with the same directness as the poor, and was viewed with fear, admiration, and affection in equal measures. Reynolds had trained under the famous Sheila Sherlock in London in the 1950s and had met his English wife, an anesthetist, there.

Allan Redeker, tall, quieter, and more reserved, seemed over-shadowed by Reynolds but was his close friend and important advisor (Figure 4.1). Robert ("Bob") Peters directed the clinical and pathology laboratory that supported Rancho Los Amigos. Each of these three was recognized as a world expert, Reynolds in general liver disease such as cirrhosis and its complications, Redeker in viral hepatitis, and Peters in pathology. The latter had two stalwarts supporting his domain, senior laboratory technologist Mary Aschavai, and younger pathologist Sugantha Govindarajan ("Su Rajan") (Figure 4.1).

Helen Gronquist and Rita Musick (Figure 4.1) were the respective administrative assistants to Reynolds and Redeker, without whom neither could function. Deep friendships developed and the authority of both these women was immense. Both were tremendously capable and well organized, as captured in the comments of a senior colleague who said either could have run General Motors. Gronquist recounted that when she got married, at not that young an age, Reynolds sat poker faced at the back of the church, afraid his lifeline was to be severed (it was not). I learned how important it was to select the right people for management and administrative support.

The unit attracted residents and fellows from all over the United States and internationally, and dozens of trainees went on to occupy senior posts in hepatology around the world—a remarkable and enduring legacy. Longstanding relationships with other institutions meant a constant stream of young physicians coming for specialist training. I worked with outstanding colleagues such as Hugh Harley and Neville Sandford from Australia, and Paul Pockros from California, with whom I became firm friends. Harley's and my non-American medical backgrounds led to solidarity and mutual support, as well as deep discussions on cultural and medical differences. We found our American colleagues much quicker to order complex and expensive investigations and tests, and to rely less on clinical deduction and traditional bedside medicine.

Two other differences were striking. In the United Kingdom, clinicians involved families and loved ones in decisions but more readily withdrew medical support for terminally ill patients. In the United States, we were surprised at the aggressiveness of investigation and treatment in patients with hopeless outcomes. Secondly, specialist referrals seemed to be requested for the most ordinary of problems in the United States, fragmenting care and disempowering individual internists.

We were shocked by the lack of social support for the poor attending these US university hospitals. Some patients only had abandoned cars for a home. Expensive emergency care for destitute patients led to discharge back to the same streets whence they had come, in this, the richest country in the world. My foreign friends and I found this disturbing, but it seemed ordinary to our native-born colleagues. Yet, positive contrasts also existed with experience in the United Kingdom, where I had seen discrimination and bias against people of color in the medical profession. I found a greater disregard in Los Angeles for social background, color, or country of origin, refreshingly different from the hierarchy of Europe. My Australian friends and I passed the tests of diligence and knowledge and were readily integrated into this medical community that had people from all over the world except Africa.

Our 2-year fellowships were senior training positions that involved clinics, overseeing residents and students, taking care of inpatients, teaching, and research. The breadth of pathology was astonishing, the clinical responsibilities extensive. The ravages of alcohol and drug injection seen daily were extreme. I could recall virtually every patient with liver disease I had cared for in England; viral hepatitis was rare, and alcoholic liver disease at that time was an occasional diagnosis, often in a middle-aged man working in the hospitality industry.* By contrast, alcoholic liver disease was a daily presentation in Los Angeles, sometimes in people not long out of their teens. Our patients were seriously ill, yet some still had alcohol smuggled into the hospital.

The hours were long, exhausting, and full of novelty. LA County's Emergency Room had a unit called "the Red Blanket Room," because critical cases were covered in a red blanket as a sign of priority. I saw more gunshot and knife-wound victims there in one day than I had in my whole life. Most of our patients were poor and lacked medical insurance, more than half were Hispanic, and many were undocumented and spoke no English. Sometimes disparagingly referred to as "clinical material" or "County patients," our impoverished patient population provided the training ground for the vast medical workforce that Los Angeles attracted.

Big County in Los Angeles reminded me of Kenyatta National Hospital, except that it was possible to investigate patients with all the technologies of modern medicine. Yet, the social support for patients was equally lacking, the streets of Los Angeles no more protective than those of Nairobi. Medicine owes a great debt to the poor, who disproportionately educate the world's doctors.

Individual patients and their tragedies linger in the mind: end-stage liver disease in a teenager indicating years of drinking; ascites (fluid in the belly) so severe a patient could not move; young women who had moved to Los Angeles to find fame in the movie industry, only to end up at County in despair with life-threatening alcohol or drug-induced disease.

---

* The incidence of liver disease in the United Kingdom has increased greatly since my training (Williams R, Alexander G, Armstrong I, et al. Disease burden and costs from excess alcohol consumption, obesity, and viral hepatitis: fourth report of the Lancet Standing Commission on Liver Disease in the UK. Lancet 2018;391:1097–1107).

Lives saved and care given can be overshadowed by mistakes a clinician remembers for life, and as I age, I have found mistakes featuring more prominently in my mind than successes. I had carried out hundreds of liver biopsies, an important investigation that can be complicated by bleeding. A critical question is whether a patient has adequate reserve to undergo surgery to stem bleeding should it occur. One patient of mine suffered a postbiopsy hemorrhage and did not survive her operation; the surgeon's criticism remains with me to this day.

I referred a gay man with cirrhosis due to chronic hepatitis B infection for abdominal surgery to repair an aortic aneurysm, a weakening of the wall of the body's largest artery that posed a risk for a tear or rupture.* Perhaps I misjudged the competing risks between current liver disease and possible future aortic catastrophe, but my patient died of liver failure after surgery. The questioning of my judgment from Telfer Reynolds still stings, just as the patient's trust still haunts.

Some failures were technical, some human. Long ago, in Bristol, I correctly diagnosed a dissecting aortic aneurism on chest X-ray in a woman admitted as an emergency. I damaged an artery in her arm while attempting central venous access and then had to seek urgent help from a vascular surgeon who quickly repaired the lesion. The surgeons, however, deemed her aortic aneurism inoperable, and I failed this anxious woman in not providing comfort and information in her final hours as she correctly insisted her major problem was in her chest, not her arm. Perhaps the only consolation is that the only way to avoid mishaps is not to engage in the field at all, and the only recourse is to try to do better the next time.

---

* A torn aortic aneurysm caused the death in 2010 of the eminent American diplomat Richard Holbrooke, who was among early government officials warning about the severity of AIDS in Africa.

Sometimes my conscience was plagued not by mistakes but the unknown. An 11-year-old Hispanic boy presented to County Hospital with fever, wasting, and an enlarged liver. We failed to find the cause of his illness despite exhaustive investigation and opinions sought from the older colleagues I most respected. We settled, reluctantly and with little confidence in the equivocal diagnostic tests, on a possible diagnosis of Q fever, an infection acquired from ruminants. The great hepatologist Sheila Sherlock was visiting from London and we presented her this case. She doubted the diagnosis, had no definitive answer, and suggested the boy likely had a lymphoma or similar malignancy. I fear she was right and remember the accusing eyes of the boy's mother and her hurtful words, "You are a bad doctor," as she discharged her son against medical advice, never to be seen again.

I stayed 3 years on this Unit, my third year as an assistant professor in the USC Faculty of Medicine. The experience gave medical and scientific, and also human, insight. From early on I was struck by the close working relationship and evident mutual understanding between the pathologist Bob Peters and his senior technologist Mary Aschavai. My suspicion of a more significant relationship, which I had never articulated, was strengthened in the investigation of Peters' fatal and still unexplained stabbing outside his Pasadena house upon returning late from work in February 1984. The police never found the murderer.

Academic departments rise and fall, and so it was with the USC Liver Unit. Reynolds and Redeker, who were both in their 60s when I was there, intended to continue working until they dropped and had given inadequate thought to, or were unable to face, necessary transitions. Younger leadership was not groomed, and promising candidates went elsewhere for lack of space and opportunity. The most important developments in hepatology were in molecular biology and liver transplantation, but the unit was on the periphery of both. Su Rajan had done excellent work with

Peters and Ashcavai on developing molecular and serologic diagnostics for hepatitis viruses, but the Unit did not attract academic grants and was dependent on commercial payment for services. The County Hospital system could not support transplantation for indigent or undocumented patients, and this most important advance in liver disease flourished elsewhere.

The lack of involvement in liver transplantation was painful for Allan Redeker because of his engagement in the topic in earlier years. Redeker was friends from medical school with the pioneering transplant surgeon Thomas Starzl whose driven life is recounted in his autobiography *The Puzzle People*.[3] Starzl and his team, initially in Colorado and later in Pittsburgh, Pennsylvania, did more than any other group to make liver transplantation a reality. End-stage, previously fatal liver disease and acute, fulminant liver failure from causes such as viral hepatitis or drug toxicity became routinely curable by provision of a donor liver. Because of the liver's remarkable ability to regenerate, partial livers were also able to be transplanted, including in children and from living donors.

The determination and self-belief required to develop this field were remarkable, considering how initial results were appalling and essentially all patients died. Redeker had a framed letter of appreciation in his office bearing the seal of a deposed eastern European royal family. He had looked after the exiled former king who was dying of alcoholic liver disease. The end was near, but the family was desperate for something to be done. Redeker called Starzl to discuss the possibility of a transplant. After weighing the options, they agreed on surgery, Starzl closing the conversation with the memorable words: "I've never done a king before." A liver was transplanted, but the king died.

A decade later, in late 1997, I attended a dinner meeting in Los Angeles that brought together Sherlock, Reynolds, Redeker, and Starzl in honor of Reynolds' contributions to medicine. Starzl had been invited to give an after-dinner speech, but his technical talk on the use of cyclosporine, a novel drug preventing transplant rejection, and the ability of transplant organs sometimes to become recognized as "self" was drowned out by chatter. It was the wrong talk, for the wrong audience, on the wrong occasion. It was both inspiring and sad to see these medical and scientific pioneers in the evening of their lives, and it demonstrated the importance of planning closure of even the most productive careers.

Telfer Reynolds died of lymphoma in 2004, aged 82.[4] He worked to the end of his life. Redeker visited Reynolds in the hospital in his final days. Weaving in and out of consciousness, Reynolds suddenly looked up in panic to ask who was overseeing the liver clinic. Redeker died in early 2021, aged 96[5]; he also continued to work until he was very old. A few months before his death, he received a prestigious award in California for his contributions and gave a cogent speech summarizing his career that included our work on hepatitis. Sherlock had died in 2001, aged 83[6]—all these people founding members of the discipline of hepatology, remembered for their research and technical contributions and excellence in teaching.

A memory from my time in Los Angeles that meant much to me was generous comments from Reynolds speaking at my leaving lunch at Rancho Los Amigos in 1986, as I was heading for the CDC. He referred positively to my diverse experience and background, wondering where this move would take me. I recall thinking I was equally uncertain.

Viral Hepatitis, 1983–1986

We now recognize five distinct hepatitis viruses named hepatitis A through E, respectively. Hepatitis A is transmitted by contact with fecal material, as is hepatitis E. Hepatitis C had not yet been characterized but was identified a few years after I left Los Angeles; previously it was referred to by the cumbersome name "non-A, non-B hepatitis," meaning it was due to neither A nor B. Allan Redeker's extensive bank of serum specimens from patients with hepatitis contributed to the recognition of hepatitis C.[7] Most of my work concerned hepatitis B and D.

What is today recognized as hepatitis A was referred to in Redeker's early life as "infectious hepatitis." In low-income countries with poor hygiene, infection with hepatitis A is acquired early in life and results in lifelong protection, mostly without evident illness. Hepatitis A does not result in long-standing infection. Epidemic spread can occur and has resulted historically in large outbreaks, such as in institutions or military camps.

Illuminating but controversial studies conducted from 1955 to 1970 in the Willowbrook State School by Saul Krugman and colleagues provided basic information upon which much subsequent understanding depended.[8] This large facility on Staten Island, New York, was an institution for mentally and physically disabled children; hepatitis was frequent among both children and staff. Krugman reasoned that because one-third to one-half of the six thousand children in Willowbrook would acquire hepatitis within one year of their admission there, it was justified to conduct studies that involved intentionally infecting them and assessing methods of prevention. In an article published 30 years after the experiments, Krugman vigorously but controversially defended his work, arguing that research to understand and develop control measures was necessary.[8]

The research clearly identified that two distinct forms of hepatitis were circulating in the facility. "Serum hepatitis" (hepatitis B) was transmitted by intimate contact, oral exposure, and inoculation; and antibodies ("immune globulin") derived from patients who had recovered from hepatitis prevented infection. The research provided fundamental knowledge for later research and practice, including for hepatitis B vaccine development, but today would be considered unethical.

Hepatitis A was not a major focus of our work in Los Angeles, but it often provided insightful experiences. The illness was usually mild, even if we saw occasional cases of fulminant hepatitis, which tended to have better outcome than other causes of acute liver failure. In people with preexisting liver disease, hepatitis A could cause surprisingly severe illness because of lack of liver reserve.[9] Older people always seemed to do worse than younger ones—a truism in medicine overall.

Hepatitis A was also a risk, along with other intestinal infections, among gay men. The increasing incidence of diverse enteric infections more usually seen in the Global South but now common in gay men had led the New York physician Harry Most to publish an article in 1968 in the *American Journal of Tropical Medicine and Hygiene* entitled "Manhattan—a tropical isle?"[10] It was a prescient warning of increasing rates of sexually transmitted infections in this population and a harbinger of the subsequent AIDS epidemic.

Sometimes the source of hepatitis A infection was apparent, such as when a particular restaurant was quoted by individual patients, resulting in inevitable punishing follow-up from the Los Angeles County Health Department. In my last year in Los Angeles, we saw cases of hepatitis A in people who injected drugs, most of whom reported injecting a form of heroin referred to as "black tar."[11] Hepatitis A can be transmitted by needle sharing when the infectious source has virus in the blood, but this period of viremia is short. This evident outbreak of hepatitis A in drug users was never satisfactorily explained, though we wondered about fecal contamination of drugs circulating on the streets or person-to-person spread through sex or close contact. This experience was replicated over the years in different parts of the world, and black tar heroin has also caused clusters of botulism.[12]

The aphorism ascribed to Louis Pasteur that chance favors the prepared mind—in this case, Allan Redeker's—was illustrated by our experience with hepatitis E. Over a 10-month period in the mid-1980s, we saw three young Pakistani men who had recently travelled to the United States from their home country and who presented shortly afterward with acute hepatitis not associated with laboratory markers of hepatitis A or B.

Redeker ordered collection and freezing of the patients' stool, remembering that in the 1950s, a widespread outbreak of hepatitis had occurred in Delhi, India, after contamination of the city water supply with raw sewage. Initially thought to be due to hepatitis A, it was later concluded that this was not the case, after testing of stored serum with newly available diagnostics. The causative agent in the earlier Indian epidemic was unknown but given the daunting name "enterically transmitted non-A, non-B hepatitis." We wondered whether this was the agent responsible for the illness in our Pakistani patients.

We collaborated with Daniel ("Dan") Bradley in the CDC's Hepatitis Laboratory in Atlanta. He found virus particles in the stool specimens of the three Pakistani men, and all three patients had antibodies in their blood reacting to these particles. A marmoset was experimentally infected with this stool and subsequently also developed specific antibodies. These were the first recognized cases in the United States of what today is called hepatitis E. We published our results in the *Annals of Internal Medicine* in 1987 and suggested that recognition of this infection in three unrelated patients at our institution over such a short time suggested it was highly prevalent in Pakistan.[13]

Since then, large outbreaks of hepatitis E have been described in different parts of the world, including in refugee camps in East Africa. The infection is more widespread than previously thought and may be the most common cause of acute hepatitis in the world. Some patients appear to develop chronic infection and acute mortality as high as 20% has been documented in pregnant women. Development, evaluation, and ensuring availability of a vaccine are high priorities.

Hepatitis B and Hepatitis Delta Virus Infections, 1983–1986

Almost 300 million people worldwide live with chronic hepatitis B virus infection (HBV), almost 60 million with hepatitis C virus, and annually there are more than a million deaths from cirrhosis and primary liver cancer due to these virus infections.[14] Hepatitis B is transmitted predominantly through blood and other bodily fluids, so HBV disproportionately affects people who inject drugs, as well as blood transfusion recipients, people with hemophilia (before donor screening became universal), and persons at risk for sexually transmitted infections, especially gay men. Health care workers also are a vulnerable population. I stuck myself with a needle from a patient with hepatitis B for whom I was caring in England in 1978 and remember the painful injection of prophylactic globulin (immune antibodies) I received in my buttock.

Allan Redeker had started a hepatitis clinic years before. Individual patient details were recorded on duplicate, handwritten cards jealously guarded in the clinic and his office, and blood was collected for standard diagnostic tests and long-term storage. In today's digital age, Redeker's cards seem naively unsophisticated, but they served the unit well. I have often been struck how technological advances such as electronic data management do not always translate into deeper scientific understanding or even increased productivity.

About one-half of adults infected with hepatitis B suffer no specific illness and most never know they were infected. Perhaps one-fifth of this group, 10% of all infected, remain persistent carriers of the virus (the chances of chronic infection are greater in infants and children). Hepatitis B carriers are at risk of developing cirrhosis and liver cancer over the long term. Approximately 1% of adult HBV infections lead to acute liver failure from fulminant hepatitis, a condition associated with 90% mortality in the era before liver transplantation. The rest suffer the typical symptoms of acute hepatitis of fever, nausea, loss of appetite, tiredness, and jaundice. The weakness and tiredness I saw in some patients were memorable; even getting out of bed was an overwhelming challenge. The most useful clinical indicator of hepatitis severity, Redeker taught us, was nausea and vomiting; if patients with hepatitis were unable to keep down fluids, they were seriously ill and were at risk for fulminant liver failure and required hospitalization.

Through collaborations with Bob Peters' laboratory and the endeavors of Su Rajan and Mary Aschavai, tests had been developed to distinguish acute from longstanding hepatitis B, as well as to diagnose infection with the delta agent, hepatitis D. Hepatitis D virus (HDV) is an unusual microbe, discovered in 1977 by an Italian physician, Mario Rizzetto; that discovery propelled him to world fame.[15] An incomplete virus that requires HBV for its own replication and survival, HDV can coinfect with acute hepatitis B infection or superinfect individuals chronically infected with HBV. The delta agent is related to nonhuman infections. At a conference organized by Rizzetto in Italy in 1986, I recall a plenary speaker saying with a flourish "and here is the patient," as he showed a picture of a wilting potted plant.

Hepatitis D essentially makes everything worse, increasing the severity of acute hepatitis and progression of chronic liver disease. A memorable example was presented at a meeting organized by Sherlock at the Royal Free Hospital in London, where wealthy patients consulted from all over and were not exempt from being used for teaching purposes. A pair of Spanish identical twin brothers was presented, both drug injectors chronically infected with HBV. One was well, but the other suffered from progressive liver disease, an unexpected finding, because their identical genetic makeup predicted a similar clinical course. The explanation was that one was superinfected with HDV.

Redeker took me under his wing for what became a fruitful 3 years and a respectful friendship. Indicative of my background and the times, I called him Dr. Redeker to the end of his life, and never by his first name. We were systematic in our search for delta hepatitis in all patients with hepatitis B and quickly accumulated the most extensive clinical experience with hepatitis D in the United States, perhaps in the world. My push to retrospectively test all stored serum specimens was painful to Redeker, who saw his precious serum bank diminishing. Combined with prospective vigilance, this work gave extensive insight into the natural history and clinical manifestations of this unusual infection.[16-25]

Overall, 5% of all our patients with acute hepatitis B and 23% of our hepatitis B carriers were also infected with HDV[18]; in about two-thirds of all our patients with hepatitis D infection, that infection was associated with chronic hepatitis B. We came to know these patients well as individuals, and it was distressing to see their frequently adverse course.

Based on testing of stored specimens, we demonstrated that delta hepatitis had been present in Los Angeles as early as 1967,[16] so this was not a new agent, and other research had shown delta antibodies in immune serum globulin collected from US soldiers in 1944.[26] All this illustrated how a pathogen could circulate unrecognized for many years despite causing severe disease, and that "new" infectious diseases are often not new but newly recognized.

Describing hepatitis D in gay men was important because conventional wisdom had been that this infection was blood-borne and essentially restricted to people who inject drugs or received blood products.[27] Three-fourths of our drug-injecting patients with chronic hepatitis B were superinfected with HDV, but so were

14% of similar gay patients. This experience differed from else-where in the world, and we struggled to have this accepted by the scientific community. This exemplified the resistance to acceptance of new or alternative evidence-based findings that is remarkably common in academic circles. Our initial reports of likely sexual transmission were treated with skepticism by some, reminiscent of how heterosexual and mother-to-child transmission of the AIDS virus were also not accepted early on.

We documented a convincing case of heterosexual transmission in a young, recently married immigrant from Lebanon with severe acute hepatitis D.[28] His new bride was chronically infected with hepatitis B and D, as were another five of ten cousins tested. Another cousin had died 4 years earlier of liver failure. This family graphically illustrated how HBV and HDV could cluster in families and be sexually transmitted.

During these years, there was intense interest and competition to develop a vaccine against HBV. The global importance of hepatitis B was related not to its epidemic spread through Western communities of drug injectors and gay men but because of chronic infection that affected close to 10% of populations in Asia and Africa, and the risk this conferred for cirrhosis and liver cancer. The American epidemiologist Palmer Beasley had followed a cohort of civil servants in Taiwan and demonstrated that the risk of later development of liver cancer was 223 times greater in those with chronic hepatitis B compared with those without.[29] In many parts of the world, primary liver cancer, a uniformly fatal condition, was the most common form of cancer in men.

A vaccine for HBV given in infancy or early childhood would prevent the establishment of hepatitis B and therefore prevent chronic liver disease. In adulthood, vaccination would be useful for gay men and persons at risk of parenteral infection, including health care workers. The importance of hepatitis B vaccination in health care workers was demonstrated by a review of experience at LA County Hospital that I presented at Grand Rounds. Three medical residents were known to have become infected over the prior decade. One was a patient of mine, who had a self-limiting but unpleasant illness. Of the two earlier cases, one resident became a chronic carrier and the other died of fulminant hepatitis.

Gay men contributed enormously to vaccine development for hepatitis B, not only donating blood from which the virus could be recovered and modified for development of a prototype vaccine but also participating in trials to show the product was efficacious. When results from the first trial were ready to be presented by the Polish-born, immigrant epidemiologist Wolf Szmuness working at the New York Blood Center, Sheila Sherlock flew from London on the *Concorde* specifically to hear the results.

The successful outcome of the trials showing protection against hepatitis B were a triumph in public health research. Advances in molecular biology subsequently allowed manufacture of viral surface protein without requiring a human source, allaying fears about possible transmission of other infectious agents. Skepticism about public health impact because of cost was proven unjustified in the longer term, and the HBV vaccine is now part of routine immunization programs all around the world.[30]

HIV/AIDS, 1983–1986

Many of our patients with hepatitis were also at risk for the still-undiscovered AIDS agent, and they became increasingly concerned about it as the epidemic spread. Because most of our clinic patients with chronic hepatitis were well, their routine check-ups were generally friendly, stress-free encounters that offered opportunity for broader discussion. Much of the time was spent talking about AIDS.

With no diagnostic test for HIV at this time, the first indication of infection was usually the onset of illness. We watched helplessly as Joe, the gay man who helped administer our clinic's card and blood specimen system, developed mouth ulcers, lost weight, and faded away. Certain patients exhibited signs not understood at the time but that, in retrospect, most likely indicated HIV seroconversion illness and HIV-associated lymph node swelling ("persistent generalized lymphadenopathy"). This was the tableau in a young Kenyan woman studying in Los Angeles, referred to me by Philip Rees from Nairobi,* where AIDS had not yet been reported.[31] Another patient, a gay man, exhibited a mononucleosis-like illness with features of meningitis. This most probably was HIV seroconversion illness that was later described by David Cooper and colleagues in Australia.[32] Controversy about how to use the HIV test when it later became available was intense, but its earlier absence was stressful in a different way, for patients as well as clinicians.

I asked many of my gay patients about their "coming out," or lack of it, and when in their lives they had recognized their sexual orientation. Most replied they had always known that they were "different" from siblings or friends, and the vast majority were sure about their orientation before young adulthood. I am always reminded of these conversations when I hear homophobic suggestions, including in Africa, that same-sex attraction is a choice.

Stigma, denial, and lack of a diagnostic HIV test at this time caused suffering and delay. A middle-aged man presented with a respiratory infection, which, after some delay, was diagnosed as *Pneumocystis* pneumonia, indicative of AIDS. I had noted his

---

* I last saw Philip Rees when he visited me at the World Health Organization in 2007. His article on 25 years of HIV/AIDS in Nairobi[31] was characteristically original and with provocative insights. He was an excellent diagnostician and clinician whose practice was greatly influenced by his own experiences, such as use of antiretrovirals and corticosteroids in patients with advanced HIV disease. He died of heart failure in 2012, aged 76.

middle-aged, never-married status, but he initially denied same-sex relations, out of shame. Another patient, a flamboyant young Hispanic man, was seriously ill with fever and abdominal abscesses. He was surrounded at his hospital bedside by equally colorful male friends who all vigorously denied being gay, but the patient was found to have disseminated *Mycobacterium avium,* an AIDS-defining infection from the same family of organisms as tuberculosis. This powerful reluctance to disclose sexual orientation even in the context of critical illness was striking.

John Leedom was the senior infectious disease doctor at County Hospital, a cynical, world-weary, stocky physician who rapidly became the local expert on AIDS. He was an excellent physician and diagnostician, and I frequently sought his counsel. I learned of the role of the CDC and its responsibility for outbreak investigation and disease surveillance. By 1983, there had been thousands of cases of AIDS in the United States, but the cause remained unproven. With extraordinary largesse, the CDC sent anyone who asked sets of slides on current AIDS epidemiology and public health advice, all free of charge, and in these early days these resources were updated every 2 months. In this way, and by reading the CDC's *Morbidity and Mortality Weekly Report,* one had the very latest information at one's fingertips.

I also learned about the CDC through our hepatitis work. Allan Redeker invited me for a drink with Jim Maynard, head of the CDC's Hepatitis Branch in Atlanta. A large man with a determined, strongly opinionated manner, Maynard was interested in HDV. Tropical medicine textbooks described "Labrea fever," an old disease causing small but lethal outbreaks in the Amazon River basin, whose cause was unknown. It was thought to perhaps be yellow fever, but now was being discussed as possibly due to hepatitis D. A similar illness in northern Colombia was referred to as Santa Marta hepatitis, and HDV had been found in Yupca Indians in Venezuela.[33] Hepatitis D appeared to be a problem for indigenous, rural populations in different countries of South America.

Maynard, with his extensive contacts and characteristically ambitious thinking, wanted to organize an expedition with the Brazilian navy to sail up the Amazon, conduct epidemiologic and serologic investigations of hepatitis B and D in the riverside villages, look for cases of Labrea fever, and try to elucidate its cause. He needed someone with knowledge of liver disease and asked Redeker if I could be made available. My career plans were vague and entailed perhaps going to the National Institutes of Health in Bethesda, MD, for further laboratory and research training, but this sounded more intriguing. If this was what the CDC staff got involved in, I reasoned, then I wanted to learn more about this organization.

Maynard told me about the CDC's Epidemic Intelligence Service (EIS) program, the 2-year field epidemiology training program that is a major professional entry path to the CDC. As a footnote, I learned later that further data suggested Labrea fever was, indeed, a form of HDV infection,[34] but I do not know if Maynard's ambitious study was ever done. My evening gin and tonic with Jim Maynard was productive not only because it set me on the path to the CDC but also because of a side conversation. I asked him what the thinking was at the CDC about AIDS and its possible cause and origin. He said unhesitatingly that he thought it was due to an infection, probably a virus, that was spread like hepatitis B and had originated in Africa. Even before HIV was discovered and a blood test introduced, this suggestion provided a unifying hypothesis that phylogenetic and other work later proved correct.[35]

Tracking HIV

A blood test for HIV infection became available for research before its widespread introduction for blood screening and other public health use in 1985. Once again, Allan Redeker's hepatitis serum bank proved its value. We pulled the almost one thousand stored specimens from patients with acute and chronic hepatitis B in Los Angeles and tested them for HIV.[36] A gay man with chronic hepatitis B was positive for HIV in 1979, 2 years before the landmark description by the CDC of *Pneumocystis* pneumonia in Los Angeles in 1981.[1] By 1983, about one-third of gay men with acute hepatitis B in Los Angeles and almost one-half of those with chronic hepatitis B were infected with HIV. In 1983, 21% of gay men who were previously HIV-negative became positive, indicative of the HIV epidemic raging in this population.[36]

There was by this time strong evidence that gay men most at risk for HIV were those who had the greatest number of sex partners. Of our gay patients with hepatitis B who also had HDV, 70% were infected with HIV, compared with 23% of those without HDV.[36] This association suggested that acquiring hepatitis D also was more likely in the most sexually active men, reinforcing our earlier conclusions that HDV could be sexually transmitted. Years later there were other outbreaks in gay men with diverse agents, including syphilis, hepatitis C, and mpox,* all occurring more frequently in those with HIV.

We published our HIV study in the *American Journal of Epidemiology*,[36] a highly respected journal, and herein also lay a lesson. Our paper contained important and newsworthy information, including documentation of HIV on the American West Coast as early as 1979. Unfortunately, academically prestigious as it was, this journal was not widely read, and our paper was not as widely cited as I had hoped. I learned to choose carefully where to submit research.

I left Los Angeles in June 1986 to speak at a conference on HDV in Italy and attend the second International Conference on AIDS

---

* The name for monkeypox was changed to mpox in 2023.

in Paris. I was warmly welcomed by CDC staff at the Paris conference who knew that I would be joining them in Atlanta the following month. AIDS in Africa drew much more interest than before, and Jonathan Mann, director of the CDC-sponsored research site Projet SIDA (French for "Project AIDS"), in Kinshasa, Zaire (now the Democratic Republic of the Congo), was a media attraction. The awfulness of the epidemic and disease were now more evident, and I left for Atlanta convinced that there was no greater global health emergency than the spread of HIV in Africa.

When I saw Allan Redeker again over a decade later, I asked him about HDV and its trends in Los Angeles. He was rueful, describing how delta was now rare. Hepatitis B was now less frequent in people who inject drugs. Many patients had died of their liver disease, and if not of that, then of AIDS, which had decimated our gay patients.

These experiences with HDV illustrated that infectious diseases emerge but can also recede, including because of the death of their hosts. Were it not for this body of work, the passage of HDV through Los Angeles could have gone undetected despite its substantial impact.

PART II
EPIDEMIOLOGIST

I was always drawn to subjects that required or allowed an approach at individual clinical as well as the population level. Hepatitis B, for example, was interesting because of personal experience with patients as well as its global public health importance as a cause of chronic liver disease and hepatocellular carcinoma. Nonetheless, I did not expect to leave clinical medicine.

Epidemiology is extraordinarily elegant in its dissection of causes and effects, giving insight into avenues for prevention. Yet, it can appear dry and academic, far removed from the reality of ill patients or populations requiring health services. The CDC was intriguing to me in how it combined analytic approaches and academic communication with a real-world emphasis on practical problems, their measurement and evaluation, and their resolution.

Epidemiology is, by nature, a science of comparison, looking for differences between groups—persons exposed to a risk factor or agent, and those not exposed; or people who are ill versus those who are well. A joke is that if you ask an epidemiologist "How is your spouse?" you might get the answer "Compared to whom?"

Epidemiology seeks truth, which sometimes can be discomforting. Its essence is to highlight differences by undertaking comparisons, so it is discriminatory in its work. The word discriminatory refers to differentiation between groups, but it can also describe prejudicial speech or actions. And therein lies one of the potential unintended consequences of epidemiology: providing fodder for stigma and discrimination.

Highlighting differences can accentuate impressions that it is "those people" who are the cause of our problems. But hiding differences is not what science does, and softening truth does not serve public health. Scientific conclusions need to be interpreted in their broader context, including their social and political implications, and they need to be conveyed thoughtfully. The CDC and Epidemic Intelligence Service (EIS) highlighted for me the importance of clear communication of scientific and public health information and being mindful that our goal is to promote health and reduce disparities.

The EIS offered 2 years of practical training in field epidemiology. Henceforth, I called myself a physician as well as a medical epidemiologist. Although CDC work covers most of public health, its original emphasis was on control of communicable diseases, and infectious diseases continue to claim the limelight even though they are no longer the leading causes of death in the United States. Within its public health work, the CDC is best known for investigating and responding to outbreaks, especially infectious disease outbreaks, and implementing disease surveillance. Both were emphasized in EIS training. The etiology of outbreaks is not always immediately apparent, and the biology of pathogens affects the nature and impact of investigation and control activities. In this regard, I have found my experience in clinical medicine persistently useful in public health work.

Epidemic Intelligence Service officers are expected to be polyvalent, able to direct their skills and training at whatever problem the CDC is asked to assist with. Much of my work for the CDC has been international, mainly in sub-Saharan Africa. Section II of this book describes experiences with various investigations and disease outbreaks, the equivalent in public health to emergencies in clinical medicine. A sobering conclusion was that often, as in clinical medicine, the acute emergency was just the consequence of underlying factors that medicine or public health alone could not resolve. The final chapter of this section deals with the COVID-19 pandemic, including consideration of our work in Kenya as well as observations from afar of the CDC's domestic travails during this complex, politicized pandemic.

The experiences described illustrate the intensity and challenges of field work and outbreaks, and the importance of human relations in this work. Many think of global health in terms of where power is concentrated, such as in Geneva or Washington, DC. It is in the field, however, in remote places, that global health plays out and affects the lives of real people. Field work is the essential currency of global health.

CHAPTER 5

Chance and the Prepared Mind

To the CDC and the DRC

Early Days

I arrived in Atlanta on July 4, US Independence Day, in 1986 and began to address the essentials of finding a car and somewhere to live. Villa International is a tolerant, multidenominational guest house down the street from the CDC's campus and caters to predominantly foreign visitors. The director took pity on my homeless, penurious state. Although the house was full, he allowed me to sleep in his office while I searched for an apartment.

The EIS is a 2-year training program in field epidemiology that produces the CDC's "disease detectives."[1,2] It was established in 1951 at what was then called the Communicable Disease Center.* Its original focus was on investigation of and protection against biological warfare agents at the time of the Korean war. The program has always prioritized practical application of epidemiology linked to strong laboratory support, with an emphasis on investigation of outbreaks and disease surveillance. Today's CDC operates in all areas of public health, including noncommunicable

---

* The full name of the CDC, today the Centers for Disease Control and Prevention, has changed several times since its establishment in 1946, but the abbreviation CDC has always been maintained.

("chronic") diseases, injuries, and reproductive and environmental health.

The class of 1986 comprised fifty-one individuals, mostly physicians with a few other disciplines represented such as nursing, anthropology, and epidemiology. A handful of the new arrivals were foreigners. The class had met at the annual EIS conference in April earlier in the year, at which time "the match" was held, allocating the incoming officers to their 2-year professional assignments. For many of our group, this was the beginning of a long-term connection to the CDC or productive careers elsewhere in public health.

Two conclusions became evident to me. First, I realized at the match that it was more important to be rigid about what you did not want to do (in my case, any noncommunicable disease work) than what appealed the most; I have found this observation useful in other spheres of life. Second, it slowly dawned on me that if I pursued what from the outset was inspiring work at the CDC, I was going to be stepping out of clinical medicine to which I had been deeply committed.

Although I had expected to be working in viral hepatitis, that group had no free positions and I was attached to the unit specializing in viral hemorrhagic fevers, dangerous infections caused by agents such as Ebola, Lassa, Marburg, and other viruses mostly restricted to tropical environments. The head of the group, the Special Pathogens Branch, was Joseph ("Joe") McCormick, one of the three people who influenced me the most during my 2-year introductory period at the CDC (Figure 5.1a).

Joe was a short man whose tilted head and quizzical face gave the appearance of constant curiosity. He was remarkably capable across diverse subjects, having deep medical knowledge from his pediatric training, strong skills in field epidemiology, and expertise in the laboratory. He was fluent in French from time spent studying in Belgium and then teaching with a missionary

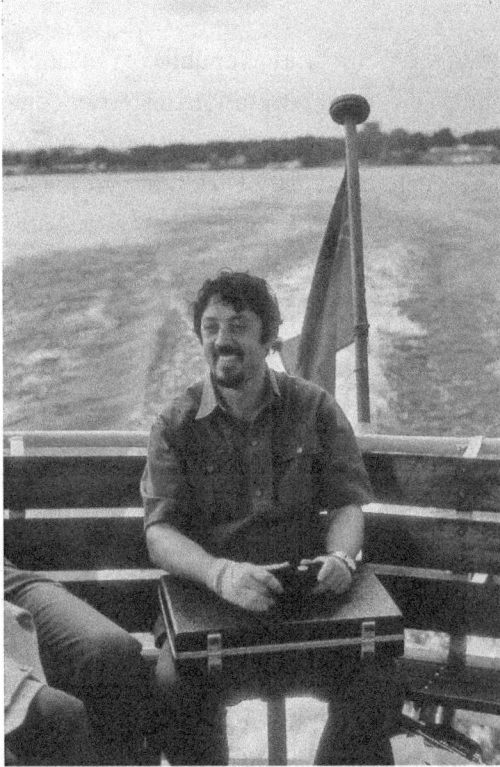

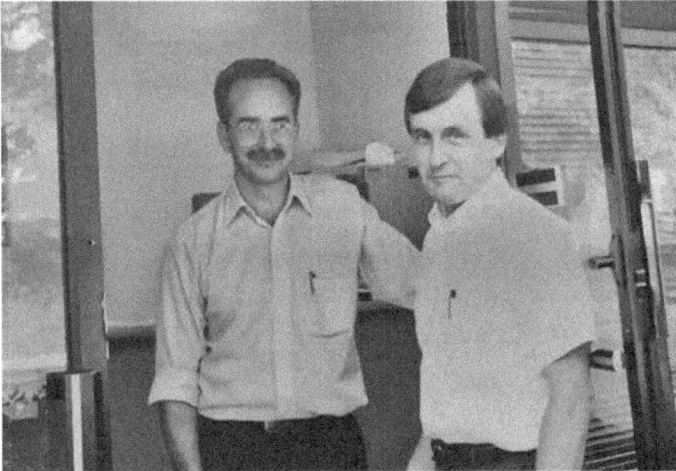

Figure 5.1 *Top*: Joe McCormick on speedboat from Kinshasa to Brazzaville, November 1986 and *bottom*: Jonathan Mann (*left*); Jim Curran (*right*), circa 1986.

(Kevin De Cock, personal collection)

organization in the Democratic Republic of the Congo (DRC). He had set up the CDC's research station in Sierra Leone in West Africa studying Lassa fever, where his practical bent extended to electrical and mechanical work to develop laboratory and other infrastructure. I felt rather inadequate being supervised by someone so broadly competent. Joe, however, was a supportive and kind supervisor, but he did not suffer fools gladly and expected his EIS officer to just fit in and get on with what had to be done.

A second person I met early on who had longstanding influence was James ("Jim") Curran, the head of the CDC's HIV/AIDS work (Figure 5.1b, *right*). What had started in 1981 as a small group with a cumbersome name—the Centers for Disease Control Task Force on Kaposi's Sarcoma and Opportunistic Infections—grew exponentially and was administratively renamed several times.[3] Curran led all the CDC's HIV/AIDS work until he moved to Emory University in 1995 to become dean of its public health school. He had an uncanny ability to rapidly get to the essence of any problem at hand, frequently offering a perspective or insight others had not seen. McCormick and Curran had a respectful relationship, Jim controlling the HIV/AIDS work and funding but recognizing that Joe and his group offered access and experience in Africa.

Epidemiology—the study of disease distribution and its determinants in human populations—is an extraordinarily elegant and powerful discipline. The EIS program taught it as a practical tool indicating avenues for prevention—that a restaurant should be closed because it caused a hepatitis outbreak, a drug to be withdrawn from the market due to toxicity, or a food supply chain blocked because it caused a multistate outbreak of intestinal infection. Some of the outbreaks investigated by the CDC over the years have legendary status in the annals of public health.[2] I have always regretted not obtaining a specialist degree in epidemiology and biostatistics, but I have been impressed by the impactful

Table 5.1

	Disease present	Disease absent	Total
Risk factor present	a	b	a+b
Risk factor absent	c	d	c+d
TOTAL	a+c	b+d	a+b+c+d

The 2 × 2 table is a fundamental concept in epidemiology. Read horizontally, (a+b) represents individuals exposed to a risk factor (e.g., drug exposure, dietary preference, sexual behavior), and (c+d) represents those unexposed.

In follow-up ("cohort") studies, disease incidence can be compared between the exposed (a/a+b) and the unexposed (c/c+d).

Read vertically, in a case-control study, the frequency of a risk factor can be compared between those with disease (a/a+c) and those without disease (b/b+d).

This way of presenting data is also useful for evaluating the performance of laboratory tests (sensitivity, specificity, positive and negative predictive value), beyond the scope of this discussion.

careers of diverse, respected CDC colleagues whose formal training also was restricted to the EIS program.

One of the first basic concepts taught was that of the two-by-two table, a way of presenting data on the presence or absence of disease in relation to the presence or absence of a risk factor (Table 5.1). If the joke from an EIS teacher that all epidemiology could be reduced to a single two-by-two table was not entirely accurate, it at least conveyed that relatively simple training and concepts can give insight and avenues for action for most public health needs.

Rigor is always required in medicine and public health, but purism can impede practicality. Years ago, the *British Medical Journal* published a satirical paper in its traditionally irreverent Christmas issue on the lack of controlled trials on the efficacy of parachutes.[4] Simple, limited observations can still be important, illustrated by publication in the CDC's *MMWR* of five cases of *Pneumocystis* pneumonia that heralded the AIDS epidemic.[5] The jibe that before epidemiology there was common sense conveyed need for rigorous analysis but also attention to practical implementation.

We had a month of teaching before being dispatched to our specialist groups within the CDC or to state health departments throughout the country. Michael Gregg, the patrician editor of the *MMWR*, emphasized the importance of precision with words. He told the story of a university president who attended a crowded concert on a rainy evening, gave his hat and umbrella to the attendant, received a ticket, and then went into the auditorium. When he emerged from the concert, the attendant returned the items even before the president showed his ticket. "Young man, how did you know those are mine amongst the hundreds of others?" the president asked. "Sir," replied the attendant, "I do not know these are your hat and umbrella, but I am certain that they are the ones you gave me."

We were sent on a field exercise to conduct a survey of seat belt use in Atlanta, feeling vulnerable and foolish as we stood on street corners peering into people's cars. This experience furthered my sense of inadequacy as I saw colleagues entering and manipulating data in real time using portable computers, at that time as big as suitcases, while I could not even type. Although I had published more papers than my classmates, everything published had been transcribed by a secretary from my handwritten submissions. I immediately went out to buy a teach-yourself-typing book and diligently applied myself. I spent a whole Sunday writing a first draft of a paper on HIV and hepatitis in Los Angeles[6] and switched off the computer, unaware of the concept of electronic saving of work. Even more drafts of the paper were required than usual. My knowledge of epidemiology increased similarly by self-teaching through the reading of basic textbooks from cover to cover.

The Viral Special Pathogens Branch was housed in the sub-sub-basement of a building destined for demolition. As the name of that floor suggests, our office space resembled a cave. What the working environment left to be desired was made up for by the competence and friendliness of staff, the camaraderie among EIS officers, and the intellectual stimulation of epidemiology at the CDC. I thought many people would be surprised that world experts such as my seniors worked under such adverse conditions, or that the CDC's high security laboratory was located there. (Two decades later, a large infrastructure project completely modernized the CDC campus, including its laboratories). McCormick and I had some preliminary discussions about my work after our introductory course finished. He proposed a study that was audacious in concept and initially seemed to me to be completely unrealistic.

Ebola's Insights into HIV

A legendary epidemic of Ebola hemorrhagic fever occurred in the fall of 1976 around the mission hospital of Yambuku in the former Zaire, today the DRC.[7] Of 318 people diagnosed with Ebola, 280 died, including 11 of the 17 hospital staff. By coincidence, a smaller outbreak had occurred in Nzara, South Sudan, a few months earlier, but these outbreaks, the first recognized occurrences of Ebola, were not related. Several of the protagonists in these dramatic events have written books detailing their experiences, including Peter Piot[8] and McCormick.[9]

In response to the 1976 epidemic in Yambuku, extensive field investigations were conducted by American, Belgian, and Congolese scientists, and hundreds of blood samples were collected from villagers in the surrounding areas to study Ebola and its spread. When the work wound down and the investigators returned to their countries of origin, the blood samples were shipped back to the CDC and frozen for long-term storage, their future use uncertain.

In the early 1980s, after recognition of AIDS in gay men and drug injectors in the United States and Europe, McCormick began to hear from colleagues working on tropical virology of unexplained cases of wasting and unusual infections such as fungal meningitis. Wealthy African patients were being seen in Europe, the origin of their AIDS-like illness unexplained because they were not homosexual and did not inject drugs. In the fall of 1983, McCormick led an investigative team that travelled to Kinshasa, the capital of the DRC, and clearly showed an ongoing epidemic of AIDS in heterosexual people.[10] McCormick reported back to Curran and CDC Director Foege in Atlanta, and a decision was made to set up a research project in Kinshasa to study this new disease. Jonathan Mann (Figure 5.1b, *left*), an ex-EIS officer and now the state epidemiologist in New Mexico, was recruited to head this venture.[3] Politics and institutional rivalries were intense, and the establishment of Projet SIDA became a complex undertaking involving the CDC, the US National Institutes of Health (NIH), the Belgian Institute of Tropical Medicine, and the government of what then was called Zaire. The CDC provided overall direction and oversaw epidemiology, the NIH ran the laboratory, and the Belgians provided a clinician. Projet SIDA became operational in 1984.

A commercial blood test became available for HIV in 1985, but the CDC had been working on in-house diagnostics developed from a virus isolate provided by the French scientists who first identified HIV in 1983. McCormick, impressed by the early investigations in Kinshasa showing a severe epidemic, reasoned that HIV was likely not a new agent but one that had been circulating for some time. He remembered the serum specimens collected a decade earlier in the rural and remote villages around Yambuku, pulled them from his freezers and tested them for HIV. To his surprise, but also gratification that his suspicions were correct, he found that 5 of 659 (0.8%) were positive.[11] He had shown that HIV was circulating in one of the most remote areas of Central Africa years before the AIDS crisis became apparent in the United States.

Many people might have left things there, content with this finding that likely would attract worldwide attention. However, McCormick sent Don Forthal, his then EIS officer, to Yambuku in 1985 to trace the people who were HIV positive. When I joined in 1986, McCormick told me to also travel to Yambuku, find people who had been HIV negative in 1976, collect blood samples from them, and determine if any had become infected in the interim. This was my introduction to the CDC and field work, an experience that, in many ways, more closely resembled a Graham Greene novel than the scientific investigation later reported in the August 1988 *New England Journal of Medicine*.[11] It was this experience that first led me to comment, as I have often done subsequently, that there is much that never gets into the Materials and Methods section of a scientific paper.

Kinshasa and Beyond

I was to travel to the DRC but first went to meet colleagues at the Institute of Tropical Medicine in Antwerp, Belgium. My task was to go to Yambuku, conduct a serosurvey in the villages, and see how many people I could find from whom we had serum from 10 years before so we could take a fresh specimen and assess HIV incidence, that is, the rate of new infections. I had no idea whether any of this was feasible, and my superficial written proposal was little more than one paragraph long.

My trip and this field work were being paid for by the CDC's AIDS Program and, before leaving, I was summoned by Wilmon Rushing, Jim Curran's quiet, no-nonsense administrator. Rushing asked me to explain what the study entailed. He listened patiently, but as the interview progressed, increasing concern crossed his face. I left his office feeling he was uncertain whether this plan was brilliant or plain crazy. My own worry increased when Joe McCormick mused one day that perhaps we should test monkeys for simian viruses. I asked how I was supposed to catch monkeys, and he replied, "Shoot them." Fortunately, this part of the plan was not taken up.

I stopped off in Belgium on the way to Africa and visited the virologist Guido van der Groen at the Institute of Tropical Medicine in Antwerp. Guido, a close friend and collaborator of Peter Piot, gave me a briefing about the Congo and Yambuku. They had arranged for me to meet a Belgian priest, Father Carlos, in Bumba, a town along the great River Congo, collect a vehicle, and proceed from there. Guido advised me to carry whiskey for Carlos and chocolates and salami for the nuns in Yambuku, which, based on the enthusiasm with which these were received, proved excellent advice.

I arrived in Kinshasa's disorganized, frightening airport late one September evening and was met by a dispatcher from the US embassy. In other countries this was a luxury not availed to junior staff such as I, but this was one airport where it was necessary to avoid being shaken down by opportunistic officials. I got out without difficulty, was driven into town, and fell into bed at the Hotel Memling, an old facility that had seen better days.

I woke up later than intended the following morning and hurried to dress and leave my room for a meeting with Robin Ryder, Projet SIDA's new director who replaced Jonathan Mann. I shut the door to lock it and found I held the door handle in my hand. After a nervous few minutes reassembling the door, fearful of theft if the room was not locked, I found an impatient Dr. Ryder pacing up and down. We had a conversation about my plans, and I returned to my room, exhausted and eager for a shower. I turned on the water and was now holding the tap in my hand. I realized nothing could be taken for granted.

Bob Colebunders, the Flemish clinician working with Projet SIDA, showed me around Mama Yemo Hospital (now Kinshasa General Hospital), a facility analogous to but poorer than Kenyatta National Hospital in Nairobi where I had worked some years earlier. The difference between the two hospitals was stark. Four years after my leaving Kenya, Mama Yemo offered an alien clinical experience. Rows of beds were filled with wasted, dying patients. This clinical picture was different from anything I had seen before and persuaded me that even if the causative virus was not new, the epidemic of AIDS certainly was. Ryder and Colebunders had quickly realized that a tour of the wards immediately and grippingly conveyed to foreign visitors the gravity of this emerging public health challenge. Henceforth, a visit to the wards was one of the first stops on the agenda for any visiting delegation.

Colebunders was energetic, driven, and full of novel ideas. He later helped me in my work in Abidjan and has been a friend since these early experiences in Kinshasa. He made important contributions describing clinical aspects of AIDS in Africa, showing their association with HIV and documenting their utility for diagnosing AIDS in these early years when serologic testing for HIV was not easily available.[3] I also met the internist Dr. Bila Kapita, a saintly man who labored under the most adverse conditions, fully committed to his patients. Kapita had watched the epidemic emerge in Kinshasa over the previous decade, noticing and documenting increasing numbers of cases of cryptococcal meningitis, an otherwise unusual fungal infection. He was not only a close collaborator with Projet SIDA but acted as senior advisor, mentor, and go-between with Congolese authorities.[3]

I spent about 2 weeks in Kinshasa before heading into the interior, taking a plane to Lisala, where I picked up a vehicle to travel on to Bumba. I was hospitably received in Lisala by the Congolese doctor working with WHO for the national immunization program. We went drinking on the Saturday evening at a large outdoor disco where literally hundreds of people were dancing and making merry, the men and women dressed in bright outfits whose elegance contrasted with the constrained facilities. Sanitation was lacking, and men and women relieved themselves quite openly in the rural setting as music blared. My host enquired whether he could arrange a woman for me for the night, an offer for which I thanked him but declined.

In the interior, money was scarce, and credit cards were nonexistent. I had been advised to get small denomination notes in Kinshasa that filled up a whole briefcase, the money dirty, malodorous, and so thin from use as to be almost transparent. I felt extremely vulnerable carrying this bulky, small fortune. The road to Bumba and beyond was unpaved and unmaintained, and I shot rolls of film capturing our four-wheel-drive vehicle negotiating difficult roads and fragile bridges (Figure 5.2). I frequently dis-

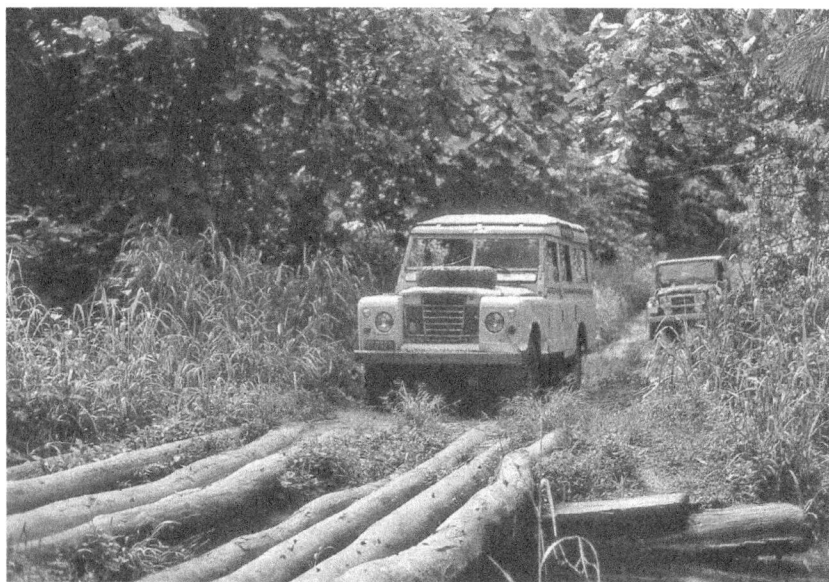

Figure 5.2   The Road from Bumba to Yambuku.
(Kevin De Cock, personal collection)

mounted and walked, my respect for the driver increasing by the hour as he negotiated this difficult terrain.

In Bumba, Father Carlos, the Flemish missionary my Antwerp colleagues had told me about, arranged for me to buy drums of fuel and provided a second car and driver. Carlos was a charismatic character, beloved by the people and a thorn in the flesh of the ecclesiastical authorities. He was the spiritual counselor to the town but also "Mr. Fix-it," to whom people turned for solutions to whatever their problem might be. In some ways he was more powerful than any politician, and certainly closer to the people. Missionaries like him, working in remote parts of the world that most would avoid at all costs, deserve their own place in heaven, whatever their human failings. Carlos gratefully accepted his whiskey, and I set off from Bumba to Yambuku with two vehicles laden with several drums of fuel.

Twenty years or so later I was reminded of this special bond that many Belgian missionaries had with the DRC. I visited my elderly cousin in Wetteren, the Flemish village where my surgeon father was born and where he operated once weekly in the 1950s. The nuns who ran the hospital had dwindled and aged, and a rest home had been built for them, overseen by the local priest. My cousin and I attended a service every year at the rest home to commemorate his late wife and daughter. The old priest raced through the Mass, explaining his speed by asserting that half the nuns were deaf and the other half asleep.

"Père Louis" had spent three decades in the DRC earlier in his priesthood, years that he looked back on as the highlight of his life. He now supported and stayed in contact with members of the Congolese diaspora in Belgium, spoke Lingala with them, and sometimes asked them to prepare Congolese cuisine for him. His eyes lit up when I explained my own work and showed my interest in his Congolese experiences. He talked of diverse health challenges he had faced working as a pharmacist, often pushed into responsibilities beyond his training. He described an outbreak of a respiratory disease that remained undiagnosed but killed dozens of people in a village he served. And reminiscing on how he was asked to treat all kinds of maladies for which he was not prepared, he said wistfully, "Imagine, doctor, I had never even seen a naked woman before."

Yambuku

Four Flemish nuns and two priests made up the mission of Yambuku in 1986, which now supported a school and small clinic but no hospital. Sister Marcella, the Mother Superior, and another sister were survivors of the 1976 Ebola epidemic (Figure 5.3). Being able to converse with them in Flemish, I was welcomed like a family member, and I spent evenings listening to their stories of their lives in Congo. Sister Marcella had served there for almost three decades and, with her colleagues, lived in an atmosphere reminiscent of my childhood in Flanders. They had adapted to their environment but never became completely part of it. They remained separate from the local population that they loved deeply and served faithfully, but probably never fully understood.

Mealtimes were an important occasion in the day, and the nuns had adopted Congolese cuisine served alongside Flemish food in imaginative combinations. "When you travel in Congo," they said in a statement that I took to heart, "you know when you will leave but you never know when or where you will arrive." I thought that, like many expatriates who had stayed in Africa a long time, they would find it difficult reintegrating into a Belgium that had changed so profoundly in their absence.

Ten years after the epidemic, Ebola remained a major topic of local discussion, reminding me of how World War II was a constant reference in adult conversations during my Belgian childhood. "The epidemic" was a frequently used phrase by villagers

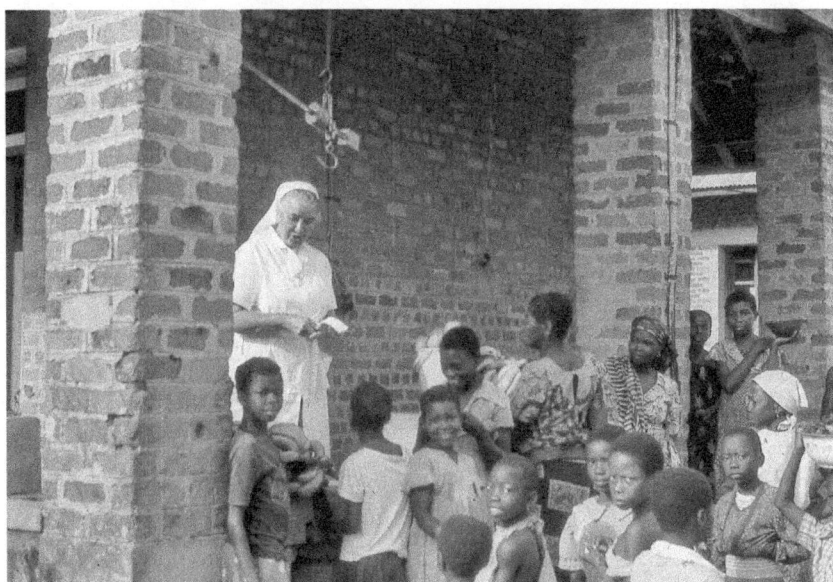

Figure 5.3   Sister Marcella with schoolchildren and mothers, Yambuku 1986.
(Kevin De Cock, personal collection)

that served as a marker in time: before the Ebola epidemic, or after the epidemic. The fear the nuns and priests felt as colleagues died from this unknown disease, the sense of duty to stay while patients fled the hospital, the sense of isolation and abandonment— all these were vividly recounted by Marcella.

When news of the outbreak reached Europe and the cause was clear—Ebola transmitted through reuse of unsterilized needles in the hospital—hostile commentaries appeared in the European and Belgian press. "Can you imagine," Sister Marcella said, "they called us murderers, but we did not do anything different from anybody else." I felt for her, and she undoubtedly was right that reuse of needles was rife throughout the country. It was, however, her facility that had the misfortune of admitting a source patient with Ebola, and reuse of unsterilized needles should not have been considered acceptable practice.

Two priests remained in Yambuku, Father F and Father G. Father F worked with the community in development ventures such as agriculture and derived his name from the local term for a bush taxi, "foula foula," that drove at high speed. His frenetic nature and peripatetic activities led to the community giving him this name, typical of Congolese humor. Father F was an enthusiast whose intentions did not always work out. He imported cattle for cross-breeding to improve local livestock, but the resulting calves were too large for the cows and regularly had to be delivered by cesarean section. He was generous to me and invited me every evening after work for a large bottle of cold Congolese beer.

The situation of Father G was more complex. A classic bush priest, he resembled any one of several characters in literature, tempted while extraordinarily committed. He spent his time travelling through the villages offering baptism and catechism, confession, care for the sick, and assistance to the dying. His fondness for local brews was famous, and when he arrived in a village, he would be offered a hut containing a large flask of alcoholic drink on the floor. Several mixed-heritage children were evident in local villages and questions were asked about Father G. I do not know whether any of these insinuations were correct, but I was inspired by his humanity and care for the community.

Father Carlos was deeply worried about Father G, who was ailing, and asked me to see him medically. I examined Father G and advised he return to Belgium, which he did within a relatively short time, dying not too long after. Knowing about his liberal alcohol intake, I interpreted the abdominal masses I found on examination to be an enlarged liver and spleen and described them as such in my referral letter. I later heard indirectly that he may have died of renal failure, and I wonder to this day whether I made the classic error of mistaking bilaterally enlarged kidneys for enlargement of the liver and spleen.

I had met earlier in Kinshasa with Dr. Melinda Moore, a CDC assignee to the US Agency for International Development for child survival work, and she had usefully advised me on sampling approaches for my study. In addition to trying to find people who had provided blood specimens 10 years previously, I was to undertake a random survey of the population to determine the current prevalence of HIV, the proportion of adults in the community who were infected. Moore shared with me a methodology called cluster sampling, which is often used to measure vaccination coverage.[12]

The good sisters introduced me to the community health worker *Citoyen* Agbote (in the days of Mobutu, all Zairois had to be addressed as *Citoyen* [Citizen] to emphasize dignity, independence, and support of the government), who was assigned to Yambuku. He and I worked together for the next few weeks, tracking people down and going to selected houses for our survey. I had brought with me, again at the advice of field-experienced colleagues, a small tape player with speakers and this was very popular wherever we went, despite my limited collection of music cassettes. Agbote was pleased when I left it with him when departing Yambuku. My shortwave transistor radio, essential for listening to international news, I did not part with.

To my surprise, my list of names and villages from 1976 was coherent and it was possible to find people. The community was isolated, migration was infrequent, and everyone knew everybody else. I marveled at this, thinking that it would be impossible to trace people in this fashion in Europe or America at that time. The epidemic of Ebola was so vivid in the memory of the community that many wanted to speak about it, and there was understanding of the value of medical research.

One of my photographs from this experience was of a schoolteacher tending his wife's grave a decade after she had died of Ebola virus infection. I located and drew blood from ninety people

on my list so we could perform a second HIV test and see the proportion newly infected over this 10-year period. I also did my random survey, collecting blood sampled from more than three
hundred people selected by chance to see if the overall prevalence
of HIV had changed. To avoid bias, I selected households for inclusion by the time-honored practice of spinning a bottle on the
ground and following the direction indicated.

Every night I would return to Yambuku, separate serum (the
yellow liquid left over when blood clots) into smaller tubes I had
carefully labelled for each person sampled, and place the precious
specimens in the freezer compartment of a domestic refrigerator.
This was not ideal esthetically, but appropriately wrapped, pack-
aged, and placed in a clean container, my specimens posed no
health challenge. I realized the nuns would have been horrified,
but field work offered little other choice.

Around the same time I was in the field, Peter Piot and Marie
Laga from the Institute of Tropical Medicine were exploring the
region to look for cases of AIDS in the hospitals and collect blood
from sentinel groups such as female sex workers and pregnant
women. Terminology can bedevil technical discussions. "Prostitute" became a term considered pejorative and was replaced by
"female sex worker," and later just "sex worker." "Prostitute" suggests a dichotomous view of sexual behavior, which ignores a
spectrum of transactional relations. In the DRC, *femmes libres*
(free women) were sexually active women who were unmarried
and who may have engaged in transactional sex, but who were not
sex workers as understood in the Global North. Pregnant women
were included in early studies on the assumption that they were
representative of the general population and who, by definition,
were sexually active. It was later recognized that extrapolating
from pregnant women to the general population tends to overes-
timate the prevalence of HIV, but pregnant women, nonetheless,
have remained an important sentinel group for surveillance.

I completed my field work, drove back along the same bad roads to Bumba, and took the flight back to Kinshasa. The flight was extraordinarily bumpy, and my Congolese colleague Dr. Malebe was even more frightened than I was, this expedition being his first experience of flying. The monkey and other bush meat he was carrying back from the famous meat market near Yambuku contributed to the nausea we both felt as the plane lurched over the dense jungle below.

Kinshasa and Brazzaville

I returned to Projet SIDA and was relieved to hand in my specimens. Losing or failing to assure the integrity of laboratory samples can sink a field investigation, and it is always a relief to know that specimens have reached the right hands. Skip Francis, the laboratory director, immediately took them and the HIV testing was completed within a few days. Projet SIDA's laboratory was a state-of-the-art facility in the compound of the run-down Mama Yemo Hospital, with superbly trained and capable Congolese technicians. It was ironic that in this neglected and mismanaged country existed the best AIDS laboratory at that time on the African continent. The scientific output from Projet SIDA was so prodigious that in those early years, the DRC was, for a time, the most cited country in the world for AIDS research.

Once back in Kinshasa, I was able to communicate with my American mother in Belgium who was deeply worried that she had not heard from me for some weeks. Imagining the worst, she had telephoned all over the world, even trying WHO in Geneva. When she spoke with Projet SIDA's director, Robin Ryder, he both alarmed and comforted her. "I suppose you are right," he said, "we haven't heard from him for a while," causing her to panic. But when he ended the conversation, he endeared himself by asking her to call at any time, saying "It's all right, Madame De Cock, I also have a mother."

Alan Greenberg was an EIS officer in the year above me studying malaria and its interactions with HIV in Kinshasa.[3,13,14] The malaria group at the CDC was tight-knit and depended on Jim Curran to fund these kinds of studies with AIDS money. Curran would play tricks on them with his characteristic humor. When they went to present their work and their funding requests to him, he would ask the most taciturn of the group, a laboratory scientist, to describe the political situation in the then-Zaire, leaving the poor fellow stuttering.

Greenberg did a series of studies to show that HIV in children was often acquired from blood transfusions given for malarial anemia. He recounted with excitement how during a study assessing whether malaria was more frequent in HIV-infected children, he saw a child who attended the emergency department on two separate occasions over a period of a few weeks. He remembered the child because the mother was so striking in appearance. The 6-year-old was negative for HIV on the first occasion but positive on the second visit.

Greenberg was concerned that laboratory or labeling errors had confounded his work but during the night suddenly woke up with a *eureka* moment, wondering whether transfusion of HIV-infected blood could be the explanation. He immediately ventured out to the hospital to check the case records and was overcome when he found that his hunch was correct. His senior colleague Phuk, a quiet malariologist of Vietnamese origin, did not appreciate being woken up with this news, despite its importance.

When I think of Alan, I am always reminded of hearing him on National Public Radio recounting this experience with emotion. This episode again illustrated how a single observation or case report can be critical to initiate a study or hypothesis in public health, but it takes the prepared mind to recognize it. Alan told another story showing the difficulties of work in the environment of Kinshasa. He was trawling through Mama Yemo Hospital charts for his malaria work, when he realized some were missing because, at that very instant, the nurses near him were burning them to cook their supper.

Projet SIDA had become the most famous research site on AIDS in Africa and had a constant stream of visitors. Robin Ryder was settling in as the new director, feeling the weight of responsibility of replacing Jonathan Mann, who had put Kinshasa on the world scientific map. In mid-1986, Mann joined WHO to establish the Special (later the Global) Programme on AIDS.[3] These were big shoes to fill, and Ryder was determined to show success. He organized a scientific review to discuss research priorities and planned studies to assess the prevalence of HIV infection in Mama Yemo's workforce and to determine the frequency of transmission of HIV from mother to child.

More extensive involvement of colleagues in Atlanta led to several young epidemiologists frequently travelling between Atlanta and Kinshasa, which was exciting but could be profoundly wearing. Several colleagues cried on my shoulder in later months, exhausted by grueling schedules, the rough and tumble of daily life at Projet SIDA, and the harsh city of Kinshasa. The scientific output was prodigious and showed the power of the EIS network, but it took a toll.

Writing It All Up

I returned to the United States on a Pan American flight that hopped from one capital to another across the African continent and on to New York. We pulled the disparate elements of the expedition together into one coherent story. In 1985, Don Forthal had tracked down what happened to the five individuals whose 1976 specimens had tested positive for HIV. Three had died from illnesses that could have suggested an AIDS diagnosis. Two were alive and were again found to be HIV positive, and a virus was isolated from one specimen that later contributed to the study of HIV evolution. There were no new infections in the ninety people on whom we had 10 years of follow-up data. The HIV prevalence of 0.8% in the general population of rural villages around Yambuku from our random survey in 1986 remained unchanged over this 10-year period. The epidemic, however, was slowly encroaching: 11% of *femmes libres* were infected, as were 2% of pregnant women, and there were a few patients with AIDS in local hospitals. HIV was not a new virus; it had existed in this remote region, and who knew where else in Central Africa, well before AIDS appeared in the United States.

These observations illustrated the classic concept that infectious disease epidemiology reflects interaction among the agent, the host, and the environment. An epidemic of HIV infection had emerged in the bustling city of Kinshasa, but not—or not yet—in this remote, rural area of Central Africa. Our paper was published in the *New England Journal of Medicine* in 1988[8] and was covered in the *New York Times* by medical reporter Larry Altman, himself a physician and former EIS officer. In research and reviews on the history and evolution of HIV or the history of AIDS in Africa, this paper is frequently cited. Joe McCormick's original idea is another example of Louis Pasteur's saying that chance favors the prepared mind.

I arrived back in Atlanta from the Democratic Republic of the Congo over a weekend in late November 1986. I passed by the Special Pathogens office and saw telegrams describing an epidemic of unknown cause in Nigeria. On the following Tuesday, I was told I was being sent to assist in the investigation and I departed on Thursday, heading back to Africa after just 4 days, this time to the western part of the continent.

CHAPTER 6

An Unknown Disease in Nigeria

Having just returned from AIDS work in the Democratic Republic of the Congo, I was instructed on Tuesday, December 2, 1986, to head for Nigeria, and I departed 2 days later. The World Health Organization had asked for CDC assistance in investigating an epidemic of unknown cause in eastern Nigeria, apparently with many deaths. The nature of the disease was uncertain, the extent of the epidemic unknown, and anxiety in Nigeria and internationally was rising. A possible diagnosis of yellow fever had been raised, and the CDC's Division of Vector-Borne Viral Diseases* in Fort Collins, CO, was contacted. This part of the United States is endemic for plague (a bacterial rather than viral disease), and this was one of the reasons for this Division being based in the Four Corners region of the country.

The Division did not have an EIS officer at this time and had contacted my supervisor, Joe McCormick, for assistance. I was to meet up with staff epidemiologist and ex-EIS officer Robert ("Bob") Craven, at New York's Kennedy Airport and continue to

---

* This division is still based in Fort Collins, but is now called the Division of Vector-Borne Diseases. It addresses arbovirus diseases, including dengue; bacterial diseases such as tularemia, Lyme disease and plague; and rickettsial diseases.

Nigeria. Craven was a seasoned field worker, having previously served at the CDC's Lassa fever field station in Sierra Leone and participated in many outbreak investigations. Typical of EIS responses, I read voraciously on the plane, trying to learn as much about yellow fever as I could so I would seem adequately knowledgeable on arrival.

We arrived in Lagos and were taken in hand by USAID's health officer, bought provisions at the US embassy commissary, and met with the WHO country representative over the weekend. Lagos was remarkably different from other parts of Africa I had seen. Busier, bustling, noisy, pushy—all these applied, but what was most striking was the infrastructure, so much more developed than in Kinshasa or even Nairobi. Highways and flyovers were not features of other African cities at that time.

The WHO representative was a retired military man from Ghana. He was generous, inviting us several times to his apartment for meals, where he was always accompanied by a young female colleague, with subtle evidence of a deeper relationship than was portrayed. Not everyone noticed, and I reflected inwardly on the importance of nonverbal clues, whatever the cultural context.

I observed over the years the occasional, somewhat inevitable, development of other relationships when international civil servants or humanitarian workers are posted far from home and family. It is an occupational hazard and human issue. Intense, stressful conditions throw people together over long working hours, sometimes leading to intimate relationships that would not have occurred under other circumstances.[1] Recourse to alcohol or other drugs is another hazard. And all this is very different from the exploitative sexual and other behaviors of some international civil servants or development workers that have come to light in recent years.[2]

The Ministry of Health, Lagos

It was astonishing how little was known at the central level in Lagos about the situation in the eastern part of the country, even though the outbreak had been going on for at least 2 months. According to the WHO official, a blood specimen tested in a reference laboratory by the respected virologist Oyewale Tomori in the first week of November, a month before our arrival, was positive for yellow fever, but we had scant other information, and the result could not be verified. WHO's Regional Headquarters for Africa, in Brazzaville, had been informed around November 10. At that time, four diseases were reportable on a mandatory basis to WHO: smallpox, cholera, plague, and yellow fever.

Benue State, in eastern Nigeria, was most affected, we were told. Media reports suggested an outbreak had started in early September and worsened in October. By the end of the third week of November, up to three thousand cases may have been identified, with 276 deaths. Cases were now being seen in the contiguous eastern states of Cross River, Imo, and Anambra. Little yellow fever vaccination had been conducted over the prior 10 years, so population immunity was likely to be low. If this was yellow fever, the population at risk in these states could be 20 million or more.

When Craven and I went to a scheduled meeting at the Ministry of Health on Monday, December 8, we were made to wait outside as a large group of Nigerian officials debated the way forward. The minister of health was the respected Olikoye Ransome-Kuti, brother of the legendary Afrobeats musician, Fela Kuti. There was evident sensitivity about the involvement of foreigners in the investigation and perhaps embarrassment that more was not known before a foreign team arrived. Such sensitivities are common in these outbreak situations, but eventually, especially if things are dire enough, CDC assistance is usually accepted.

After considerable waiting, we were invited into the meeting and formally asked to participate. I was surprised but pleased to meet Peter Tukei, a Ugandan WHO virologist sent from Nairobi. We knew each other from years before when I taught at the University of Nairobi and Kenyatta National Hospital and had been friends and tennis partners. This was an example to me of the importance of personal and professional networks formed early in life. High-level attention was now focused on the epidemic and difficult questions were being asked in the media. We met with the US ambassador, the seasoned diplomat Princeton Lyman, who was deeply interested and concerned.

Confusion and lack of clarity are common early on in such investigations. Rumors abound and it is difficult to dissect accurate facts from background noise. I thought back to my clinical days, reflecting that similar confusion and information of uncertain quality were frequent when I saw a seriously ill patient. It was time to get out into the field and see the situation on the ground—to extend the analogy, to examine the patient and review the diverse information available. The central task force at the Ministry of Health finally gave permission for travel to the affected area.

First Impressions: Oju, Benue State

Two teams were formed, Craven and I separating to ensure there was a CDC person on each team. Craven worked with a well-known Nigerian virologist, Professor Akinyele Fabiyi, and was to travel to Cross River State. I joined Tukei and the young Nigerian scientist who directed the Federal Vaccine Production Laboratories, Abdul Nasidi, and we were to assess the situation in Benue State. Both teams first travelled to Enugu, the capital of Anambra State, meeting with health officials there. As we left for our respective destinations for rapid initial assessments, we agreed to reconvene 4 days later at Enugu's Metropolitan Hotel.

Before parting, Craven and I discussed the priorities for field work. The first two questions when investigating an epidemic are: is there an epidemic, and if so, is it due to what you think it is or have been told?[3] A case definition is then formulated so that consistent decisions are made about what is a case and what is not, for accurate and unbiased reporting. We agreed that the priorities were to visit hospitals and clinics in our respective areas and review records to see if there had been a change in patterns of admissions and deaths over the previous year, particularly for fever with jaundice. We would examine current admissions for such illness and collect blood from active case patients and liver tissue from deceased individuals. If specific geographic locations appeared relevant, they would be targeted for later investigation. We also were to take note of yellow fever vaccine availability and use. All the while, the diagnosis of yellow fever remained a hypothesis rather than a fact.

Nigeria is a large and administratively complex country, and each level of the federal hierarchy needed to be consulted. In this way, my group found itself in Benue State's capital, Makurdi, talking to the health authorities. We felt we were closing in on the real problem, because these officials reported almost five thousand suspected cases in the state and one hundred and eighty deaths. It was still difficult, however, to know what really was occurring or what disease we were dealing with. To our knowledge, no specific laboratory confirmation of any pathogen had been made, and this remained an unknown epidemic, a classic challenge for field epidemiology. No case definition had been formulated and it was uncertain what was being reported. Another useful member joined our team, Paul Lichfield, a CDC Public Health Advisor seconded from CDC to UNICEF in Nigeria, specifically to work on immunization. Suddenly we had someone with us who had specialist knowledge of this critical area.

We reached Adum East, a village in the local government area (LGA) of Oju, Benue State, on December 12, 3 days after leaving Lagos, and realized we had stumbled into the heart of the epidemic, the epicenter. A so-called sick bay had been established in a dilapidated school room where we found twenty-two patients, men and women of all ages, some of them gravely ill, most of them jaundiced. New cases had presented that day, as they did the day after.

I cannot recall if it was on this first or a later day that I witnessed a nursing aide giving injections to neighboring patients without changing the needle or syringe. I spoke to the young man to explain that this was not acceptable practice and received a startling reply: "But Doctor, they are all jaundiced." Somehow, teaching about hepatitis virus and other pathogen transmission by injection had been unclear or only partially understood. I thought back to my discussions with the nuns in Yambuku and the Ebola epidemic that resulted from reuse of needles in the hospital.

Alex Ogba, a local teacher, told us that cases were first seen in July, 5 months previously, and that since then, several hundred people in the area had died. Other leaders were unable to recall a similar illness in living memory but graphically described the severity of the outbreak. "People were dying like animals," said one of our informants, and the dead were buried without ceremony or record. The local school had been closed in late October because seven children, 2% of the school population, had died over the previous 2 weeks. I wondered to myself how any school in Europe or the United States would react to seven student deaths from an infectious disease over a short period. The local authorities closed the market and restricted travel outside the area. We saw freshly dug graves, and new cases continued to present.

Oju LGA was a neglected and forgotten place, almost totally devoid of health care workers or facilities. Dr. J Enriquez, a Filipino doctor from Benue State's Epidemiology Unit, was the only physician on the ground. A total of four public sector sick bays had been established in different locations, and there was one fee-for-service mission hospital in the area. In our assessment, a priority was to assess essential needs for an effective response. Poor Enriquez, working alone, hoped for at least two other doctors, another sick bay, six vaccinators (he had assumed he was dealing with yellow fever), ten vehicles, night allowances for staff, and payment of delayed salaries. The local community representative expressed dismay about how Oju was overlooked—in his words: "Economic and social development inadequate, no roads, no health facilities, no decent water." We passed on these concerns and requests to national authorities but with limited expectations of a positive response.

Although none of our small team had ever seen a case of yellow fever, we concluded that this was the only unifying explanation for the outbreak.[4] From the data compiled with Enriquez's help, 286 cases of jaundice and 186 deaths had been recorded in Oju, and—this being the pre-PowerPoint era—we plotted these out in pencil on a graph showing cases and deaths over time, an epidemic curve (Figure 6.1a).* This convincingly showed that the epidemic was still ongoing. In addition, we reasoned that mass yellow fever vaccination was urgently required. Lichfield had the most logistics experience and argued that for an undertaking of this magnitude, and under such adverse conditions, only the armed forces had the capacity and resources to deliver what was needed.

We undertook the journey to Enugu for the prearranged meeting on Sunday, December 16, with Craven and other colleagues. They reported that in Cross River State there had been an outbreak, but new cases had reduced substantially. Collectively, we crafted a strongly worded message to be sent back to Lagos about the severity of the epidemic and the need for emergency assis-

---

* Our epidemic curve was unorthodox in that it portrayed a line drawing of cases rather than histograms.

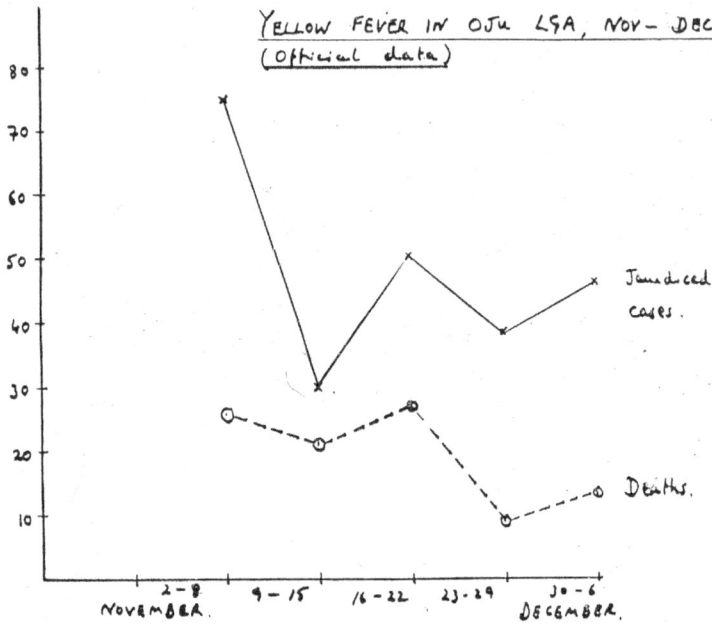

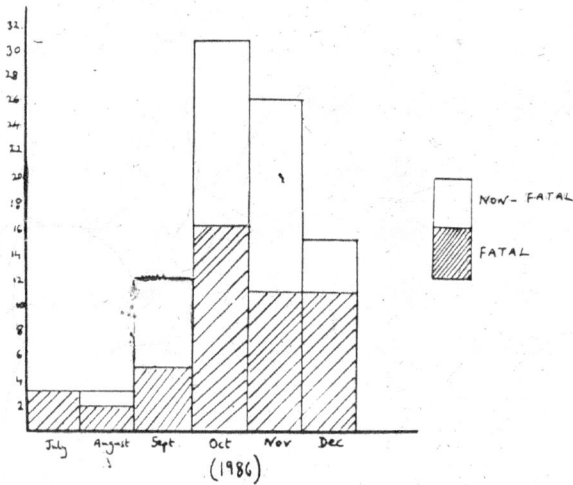

Figure 6.1 (a) Initial epidemic curve of yellow fever, Oju LGA, December 1986; (b) epidemic curve of yellow fever infections and deaths in nine villages, Oju LGA, July–December 1986, after serologic testing.

(Kevin De Cock, personal collection)

tance. "The epidemic of yellow fever in Oju Local Government Area, Benue State, including Adum East, is not under control," we wrote. "New cases and deaths continue to occur. . . . A critical shortage of supplies and facilities for acute medical care exists . . . Benue State and affected areas of Cross River State should be declared a Federal Disaster Area, requiring acute disaster relief. . . . [we advise] implementation of immediate mass vaccination in and around Oju."

We decided to visit the military governor of Benue State the following day to appeal for assistance from the army. Aware of the gravity of the situation in the state, the Governor agreed to see us without delay. I noted that security around him was tight, the doors to his office were always locked, and he had an escape exit behind his desk. We presented our case, explaining our crude, hand-drawn epidemic curve and what it meant. Our meeting lasted less than an hour and the governor agreed to mobilize the army to undertake mass vaccination. Elated, we returned to Oju. I felt intoxicated, reflecting that mobilizing the army in an epidemic response, all based on a few days of field work and limited but credible data, exemplified epidemiology for action.

Back in Oju, we were met by a middle-aged, wiry, fit-looking man walking around with an air of authority. This was Thomas ("Tom") Monath, director of the CDC Division of Vector-Borne Viral Diseases in Colorado. What he did not say, but I knew well, was that he was the world's leading authority on yellow fever. My stomach lurched, therefore, when he said to me, "It's bad, isn't it? But you know, I don't think this is yellow fever."

Field Investigations in Oju, Benue State

Monath was accompanied by a virologist from WHO headquarters in Geneva, the Venezuelan José Esparza, and we spent the next 45 minutes debating the diagnosis. As a first-year EIS officer who had never seen yellow fever, I knew to be careful about how I addressed the world expert. However, I did have an advantage: because of my background in hepatology, I quickly realized that I knew more than Monath about general liver disease and infectious causes of jaundice other than yellow fever. Whenever he raised another diagnostic suggestion, I would counter as to why that was unlikely or impossible. In fact, no other infectious disease or cause of hepatitis would have behaved in this fashion, and yellow fever was the diagnosis simply by exclusion, unless we were dealing with a newly recognized agent.

Fortunately, having looked around a bit more the following day, Monath agreed that we faced a severe yellow fever epidemic. He then confirmed the diagnosis by testing blood from affected patients using portable equipment he had set up in the kitchen of the house provided for us (Figure 6.2). Monath and his colleagues had developed enzyme immunoassays for yellow fever and other arboviruses in the laboratories at Fort Collins, and adapted them for field use. The assays showed acute immunoglobulin M antibodies to yellow fever virus, confirming the diagnosis.[5]

Monath was the third person at the CDC who made the greatest impression on me during my EIS training, along with Joe McCormick and Jim Curran. Deeply intellectual, Monath was widely read and broadly skilled in medicine, epidemiology, and laboratory science. Despite being so accomplished and recognized, he lacked pretension, was straightforward in his dealings, and appeared at ease in any environment. He exerted leadership through evident competence, quiet authority, gentle humor, and example. It was educational to work alongside him on this classic tropical disease.

Our living conditions in Oju were primitive. Our allocated house was minimally furnished and had no running water, and we depended on rainwater collected in a large drum outside. We used buckets to wash. One day, my Ugandan colleague Tukei asked me

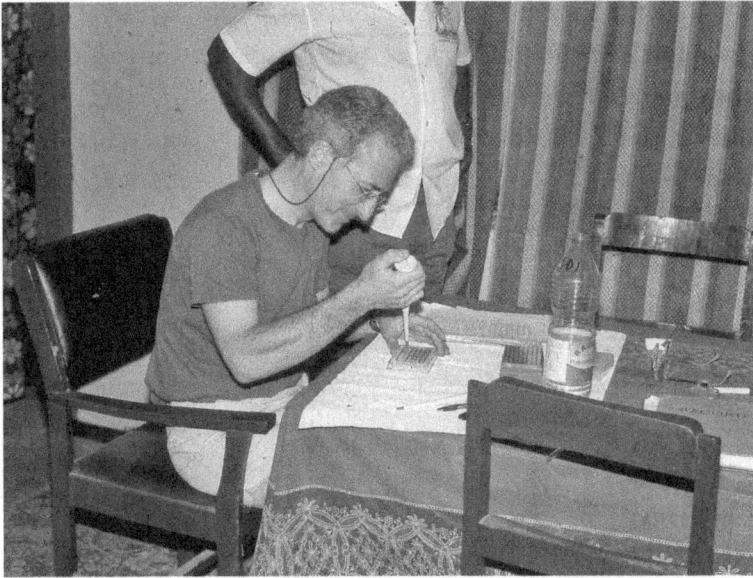

Figure 6.2   Tom Monath conducting yellow fever serologic testing in the kitchen of our housing, Oju LGA, December 1986.
(Kevin De Cock, personal collection)

a question he had been wanting to pose for some time. "Tell me, how do you wash using a bucket? What do you actually do?" I explained that I used soap and water to wash myself, dipping into the bucket, and at the end of the procedure poured the contents over my head. He roared with laughter, explaining that this was not the correct technique at all, and that only a white man would finish using dirty water to rinse himself.

We had no facilities or time for cooking, food was difficult to find, and we resorted daily to the grim local eatery that served watery soup that contained small, indeterminate pieces of meat. One night, Tukei prevented me from eating what I later understood were the genitals of an undefined animal. I cheered us up with the bottle of cognac I had bought in Lagos. Every night, Monath would ask the puzzled manager whether mango ice cream was on the menu.

Monath's brilliance was balanced by a maverick humor exemplified by a prank he told me he pulled while he was president of the American Society for Tropical Medicine and Hygiene. At the dinner for the annual conference in Denver, he had hired an actor to play the role of minister of Health from a South American dictatorship and invited as the guest of honor. The "minister" mingled with delegates and engaged several in conversations about collaboration, offering sponsored trips to his country, which a few accepted. The "minister's" after-dinner speech began in a monotone but became livelier with progressively more outrageous statements, such as that it was easier in his country to achieve results because the government could use guns. People slowly realized this was a spoof, the actor then chastising guests who had accepted promises of benefits from the "minister" and his despised regime. Some attendees thought the episode hilarious, some were offended; "archetypal Monath," I thought, though even he had to apologize later.

Investigation of the outbreak began in earnest. We visited villages throughout Oju to take a census of the population, ask about current and past illness and deaths using our case definition (Figure 6.1b), assess vaccination status, and collect blood specimens from each person for storage in liquid nitrogen, which would be shipped to Fort Collins for subsequent testing for yellow fever antibodies to assess the true extent of yellow fever infection.

Inevitably, we were consulted for other illnesses, and I was again humbled clinically when I failed to correctly diagnose a skin ulcer (the first time, but not again) due to guinea worm.[6] Dracunculiasis, as guinea worm disease is officially known, is a classic neglected tropical disease. It afflicts and debilitates poor people in remote areas who drink water contaminated by water fleas containing larvae of the parasite. A complex life cycle ensues in humans, which ends with female adult worms emerging from skin blisters upon contact with water, with release of larvae that are then ingested by the water fleas, and so the whole history is perpetuated. There is no drug therapy and no vaccine, and traditional management has involved careful winding of the worm, sometimes more than a meter long, around a stick and slow extraction over days or weeks, ensuring the worm does not break.

The CDC initiated elimination efforts in 1980 and the World Health Assembly, WHO's governing body, adopted a resolution in 1986 calling for eradication of guinea worm disease. Eradication means the causative pathogen has completely disappeared from the world—to date only achieved for smallpox. Two global eradication programs continue to this day, for polio and guinea worm.[6,7] They provide interesting contrasts, polio eradication depending on extensive vaccination and guinea worm on provision of clean drinking water. Both programs represent public–private partnerships, with Rotary International being a major supporter of the polio program and the Carter Center supporting guinea worm eradication. Both programs are frustratingly close but have not reached the end line, facing unexpected technical and other issues. For guinea worm, an unexpected obstacle to final success was recognition in 2012 of infections in nonhuman hosts, especially dogs. For both guinea worm and polio eradication, conflict has proven another challenge, limiting access to areas or populations in need.

Throughout our stay in Oju, we continued to see new cases of yellow fever; we were heavily affected by a man in his 20s who sought us because he was ill. Red-eyed and febrile, he was in the early phase of the illness, which shares many features with other acute fevers such as from malaria or dengue.[5] I was struck how rare it was for a physician of my generation to see a case of acute yellow fever. Sadly, the young man deteriorated and died before us over the course of a few days, another yellow fever death we were unable to prevent. Monath had participated in a symposium 2 years before in Brazil that focused on the clinical management of yellow fever,[8] but care of patients during epidemics in low-income settings of the

Global South generally received little attention. All of that was to change with AIDS and Ebola during the 2000s.

Another memorable experience was visiting a village where another young man had died a while before. For completeness, we wanted to collect liver tissue from fatal cases for later microscopic examination, a classic way of proving yellow fever. Having performed hundreds of liver biopsies in earlier clinical work, I was best placed to collect the relevant specimen. What I was not prepared for was to see a cadaver sitting upright in a chair, clothed in the expensive shirt of a famous British soccer club. I did not want to upset the decorum and, with the help of the understanding family, took the biopsy specimen with a needle, just as in a living person, but in this unorthodox position and under these unusual circumstances.

Christmas was approaching but our investigations were unfinished. Tukei had strong family commitments back in Kenya but was determined to stay until we all left. We ate in our hotel in Makurdi on Christmas Eve, memorable because the chicken stew gave me food poisoning and I was up all night vomiting; I was still queasy as we embarked on the long journey back to Lagos on Christmas Day. Monath and I had been asked by US Ambassador Lyman to report in with him as soon as we arrived. We gave him a full briefing, struck by the incongruity of sitting in the elegant diplomatic residence in our filthy field clothes, my uneasy stomach just able to accept the offered gin and tonic.

I again was educated by Monath, in this era that predated microcomputers and the internet. He rapidly synthesized all the information available and wrote a preliminary report, all by hand, with essential epidemiologic data and clear and specific recommendations for the Ministry of Health before we left the country. A final assessment of what occurred would only be possible once we had the laboratory results for the many specimens collected in the field. Monath encouraged me to spend time in his Division in Fort Collins to assist with the laboratory work, which I did in early 1987. The serum specimens collected also were tested for HIV, providing some of the first data on HIV from this large West African country.[9]

Our final assessment, written up in the journal the Lancet,[10] was that the epidemic in Oju had begun in July 1986, peaked in October when it came to the attention of the national authorities, and was still active when the combined field teams began investigations in December. We estimated from our laboratory and epidemiologic work that forty thousand people in Oju, 20% of the total population, became infected with yellow fever virus. Approximately 5% of residents of villages in Oju LGA developed clinical yellow fever, and half of those with disease died. This meant that a total of five thousand people in this locality died in this epidemic. Yellow fever also occurred in other nearby LGAs, and in at least one of them the intensity was probably the same as in Oju. This epidemic was one of the most severe in Nigeria's history, perhaps in the history of West Africa.

I was shocked that this severe epidemic took so long to be noticed and responded to, or that the deaths of thousands went largely unnoticed in the international press. The experience was a strong reminder of how lack of effective disease surveillance can allow dire consequences to unfold without reaction. This observation, unfortunately, also applied to my later experiences with HIV in Cote d'Ivoire[11] and Ebola in Guinea, Liberia, and Sierra Leone.

Another conclusion was that yellow fever vaccination should be incorporated into routine vaccination programs for children in endemic areas.[10] Monath and Nasidi later published a modeling paper showing that such a preventive approach in Nigeria would be cost-effective compared with traditional emergency control responses.[12]

Because yellow fever is a mosquito-transmitted infection, it is important to include entomologic expertise in the investigations to identify the mosquito vector. Working with the WHO-recruited entomologist Dr. Charles Ravaonjanahari from Sri Lanka, the vector in this outbreak was shown to be *Aedes africanus*, and the epidemic was transmitted between people, rather than involving monkeys as the host.

We worked hard to collate all the data for the *Lancet* paper but were frustrated by delays in receiving permission to publish from Nigeria.[10] Monath wrote a letter, on which I was a cosignatory, to the US ambassador asking for his assistance in resolving the logjam. I do not know who was offended in Lagos or who complained, but I was summoned by Stanley ("Stan") Foster, a kind and experienced international health epidemiologist at the CDC, and hauled over the coals for the audacity of writing to an ambassador. I pointed out my junior status in this saga, bemused by this upset over protocol but gratified that we achieved our intent.[10]

A prophetic concern was included in December's preliminary report to the Ministry of Health. The epidemic in Benue State and the lower-level transmission in Cross River all affected rural areas. Epidemics can occur in urban settings where a different mosquito vector, *A. aegypti*, is usually involved. The end of the year was a time of intense travel, and humans carrying yellow fever virus might introduce it into areas where the urban vector was present. Not only did this emphasize the importance of the mass vaccination campaigns recommended in eastern Nigeria, but it called for extreme vigilance. Unfortunately, we got the call from WHO in late April 1987 inviting us back for the very reason Monath had warned us about.

Urban Yellow Fever: Nigeria, 1987

The World Health Organization informed us in April 1987 of suspected yellow fever in five states in western Nigeria, the other side of the country from Benue. This time there was no reticence on the part of Nigeria inviting the CDC back in, and, in fact, the Nigerian Minister of Health reiterated the request for international assistance when he attended the annual World Health Assembly in Geneva, the annual meeting of senior international health leaders, in early May. Several members of the same team as before reassembled in mid-May, now much more conversant with what had to be done. Once again, containers of liquid nitrogen and laboratory supplies accompanied us as we flew to Lagos.

The epicenter of the outbreak was the town of Ogbomosho in Oyo State in the western part of the country. Nasidi had obviously learned from his experience in late 1986 and by the time he briefed Monath and me about the available data, he had a case definition, an epidemic curve, and cases broken down by age and sex, all essentials of descriptive epidemiology. By May 10, 1987, fifteen of Oyo State's twenty-four LGAs were affected. Monath concentrated on the investigation in Ogbomosho and asked me to rapidly survey hospitals in surrounding towns. I covered large distances, assessing eleven major hospitals in surrounding states and reviewing admissions and deaths over the previous year to detect any suggestion of epidemic activity. Fortunately, patterns of admission had remained stable, and numbers of cases of jaundice and death had not changed, leading us to conclude that the outbreak remained concentrated in and around Ogbomosho. The last official figures we saw indicated 361 cases were detected in Oyo State, of which 60% were fatal. Our own field investigations suggested the true incidence was at least ten times higher.[13]

Entomologic studies showed the vector to be *A. aegypti*, the classic vector for urban yellow fever. The density of infestation with larvae of this mosquito in water containers inside houses was 135 times greater than considered necessary to sustain an epidemic. Although there was no evidence of epidemic spread elsewhere, individual suspect cases were reported, nonetheless, from various locations, and we were anxious about the vulnerability of other major urban centers such as Ibadan. The most urgent of our recommendations concerned strengthening and better supervision of surveillance activities and mass vaccination. The occurrence of urban yellow fever for the first time anywhere in the world in 40 years was a significant event, and it was good fortune that other, larger urban centers were ultimately not affected.

Two other experiences stuck in my mind from this second sojourn in Nigeria. I had to return to the United States before Monath because I was presenting our work from the DRC on HIV at the upcoming International Conference on AIDS in Washington, DC. As I was returning from the field, dozing on and off in the front of the four-wheel-drive vehicle, I saw something lying on the highway as we sped by. I asked the driver what it was, and he replied, dispassionately, "A human body." It was not uncommon for individuals to be run down on the dangerous Nigerian highways and not have anyone stop, the bodies progressively pulverized. The health hazards from Africa's roads are vastly underestimated.

The second memory concerns a conversation I had on this trip with Dr. Edwin Beausoleil, a senior physician then heading communicable diseases for WHO's Regional Office for Africa. This WHO doctor from Ghana was short, round, and fat, and he chain-smoked. Despite his unhealthy appearance, he was extremely sharp, respected, and very witty. When Nasidi repeatedly mispronounced his name, making it sound like Beaujolais, he loudly corrected him, explaining his name meant beautiful sun and had nothing to do with wine.

Beausoleil and I were driving in the interior and stopped somewhere for coffee. He peered at me and suddenly asked, "Young man, what are you going to do with your career?" Unprovoked, he said, "You must not go to WHO as a young man. You will become a nincompoop." I do not know what stimulated him to say this but always remembered this exchange. When I worked at WHO many years later, and at a senior level, I thought of Beausoleil's comment, seeing for myself that people who went there too young could lose their way in the bureaucracy and protocol. By contrast, the leadership, simplicity, and technical expertise required for field work, demonstrated to me over the years by different mentors, can keep one grounded.

Conclusions

It is often difficult to explain the "why" of epidemics, and even more difficult the "why now?" Simplistically, epidemic yellow fever occurs when there is the coming together of the yellow fever virus (whose reservoir in nature is nonhuman primates), a susceptible human population, and an environment supporting virus replication in an abundant and effective mosquito vector. This mostly occurs in rural tropical settings, but urban spread can occur when the virus is introduced into susceptible populations in cities and towns with the required urban vector.

Mass vaccination combined with natural infection results in population-level immunity, which gradually declines over time as new and susceptible birth cohorts expand the population. Yellow fever in West Africa has tended to occur in 10- to 15-year cycles in large epidemics causing enormous suffering and death, and then recede and be forgotten until the next epidemic. Yellow fever was one of the infections that contributed to West Africa being labeled "the white man's grave" during early colonial times. Today, more than one hundred thousand cases with more than fifty thousand deaths are estimated to occur worldwide annually,[14] with 90% of the burden in Africa. That yellow fever has not been established in Asia, where the vector is present, is fortunate and unexplained, but should not be taken for granted.

An effective vaccine has been available since 1937 and gives lifelong immunity. Incorporating this vaccine into routine immunization practice could eliminate these kinds of dramatic outbreaks. However, as is so often the case, the mere existence of an effective public health intervention is no guarantee of its implementation. The epidemics of yellow fever in Angola and DRC in 2015–2016, which included urban transmission, were the world's largest over the past 30 years. More than thirty million people were vaccinated but vaccine supplies were still inadequate. Different international partners established the Eliminate Yellow Fever Epidemics Strategy in 2017 to enhance capacity for detecting, preventing, and responding to outbreaks, including through scale-up of diverse vaccination strategies.

In addition, there must be concern that maintenance of medical and entomologic expertise in yellow fever and other arbovirus infections (infections transmitted by arthropods like mosquitoes) like dengue or Chikungunya virus is inadequately prioritized. Just over the past decade, the world has seen major outbreaks of dengue, Chikungunya, and Zika, all transmitted by *Aedes* mosquitoes. The world cannot afford to allow erosion of technical and intellectual capacity in this niche area of infectious diseases that was so emblematic of earlier tropical medicine but became overshadowed by HIV/AIDS and other concerns.[15]

CHAPTER 7

Outbreaks in Kenya

An Outbreak that Wasn't

As taught in the EIS, the first questions when confronted with an epidemic are whether the apparent increase in cases is real and whether the supposed cause of the outbreak is correct.[1] The number of people reported with a disease may suddenly increase because of changes in reporting practices, laboratory errors, or altered working habits of personnel involved. A change in case definition is another potential artefact, as the CDC witnessed when the case definition for AIDS was changed in 1993 to include persons with a CD4 cell count below 200/mm³.[2] Suddenly, with no change in HIV or disease incidence, the number of people reported to have AIDS almost doubled, making analysis of trends very difficult.[2]

Michael Gregg was editor of the CDC's flagship publication, the *Morbidity and Mortality Weekly Report* (*MMWR*). I remembered his brilliant teaching in the EIS program, his eloquent use of spoken and written language, and attention to individual words in his role as *MMWR* editor. He and I once argued over my use of the term "gut." He thought it an inappropriate synonym for intestine in CDC guidelines on hemorrhagic fevers. "Skepticism is the chastity of the intellect," I recalled him saying at another time, "not to be surrendered lightly to the first comer"; a reminder not to take anything for granted in medicine and public health.

Anthrax

For some diseases, including anthrax, botulism, or hemorrhagic fevers, a single case is reason enough for an epidemiologic investigation. I was in Atlanta on Tuesday, September 11, 2001, in the offices of what was then called the Global AIDS Program, when the planes hit the Twin Towers in New York and the Pentagon in Washington, DC, and also crashed in Pennsylvania. Horrified CDC staff, some in tears, watched television monitors in the corridors. I drove around Atlanta fruitlessly the following day, trying to find a copy of the *New York Times* describing the tragic events.

I was supposed to return to Nairobi on the Wednesday, the day after the attacks, but all flights were cancelled. I succeeded in obtaining a seat on a flight out of Atlanta on Thursday, September 13. Although flights were overbooked, the airport was eerily empty, many people having annulled their travel. Passengers looked at each other warily.

A week after 9/11, the first letters containing anthrax spores were mailed to several news organizations in the United States, followed 3 weeks later by more such letters to two Democratic senators.[3-5] During October and November 2001, five people died and another seventeen became ill in these acts of bioterrorism. Eleven of the twenty-two patients had inhalational anthrax and the other eleven had the cutaneous form of the disease. The fatalities were all in those with inhalational anthrax. Twenty of the twenty-two case patients were mail handlers or otherwise involved in mail processing or distribution. A total of forty-three people had tests showing definitive exposure to anthrax, and about ten thousand were considered to have possibly been exposed.

The October 2002 issue of the journal *Emerging Infectious Diseases* was devoted entirely to anthrax as a tool of bioterrorism, and it captures the enormity of the anthrax investigations.[6] The biologic attack on the United States that followed the terrorist attacks of 9/11 profoundly altered public health, with long-lasting implications. Preparedness and stockpiles were subsequently oriented toward terrorism as much if not more than to other epidemic threats—a relevant consideration as we analyze the quality of preparedness and response to the COVID-19 pandemic.

Law enforcement was central to the anthrax investigations, and cultural differences between the diverse government agencies involved, including the Federal Bureau of Investigation (FBI), the US Postal Service, as well as health agencies and the CDC, were often apparent. The FBI eventually concluded that Bruce Ivins, a government microbiologist and anthrax expert at Fort Detrick, a biodefense facility run by the Department of Defense, was the sole culprit. Ivins committed suicide in late July 2008 before he could be charged.

Nairobi, Kenya

It was with an open mind and some curiosity that I went to the Ministry of Health in Nairobi on the morning of October 17, 2001, summoned urgently for a meeting described only as important, the agenda unknown. A large group of senior health officials had convened in the boardroom and was kept waiting for the Minister, Professor Samson ("Sam") Ongeri, a pediatrician with whom I had worked years before at Kenyatta National Hospital. Ongeri was late because he had been talking to the international press, including major outlets such as the BBC and the *New York Times*.

The Minister came in and announced to us, just as he had to the media, that Kenya was the victim of a bioterrorist attack with anthrax. A letter mailed from Atlanta to an unidentified recipient had been found to contain white powder positive for anthrax. At around the same time that this information was being shared, the fifth case of anthrax was identified in the United States in an employee of CBS television, so the topic was hot in the media. Posted on September 8, the letter to Kenya had been routed via Miami, was received in Kenya on October 9, and opened in Nairobi on October 11. The Minister's statements went around the world: Kenya also had been attacked.

Several other letters were suspected of being infected, including one received at the Nairobi headquarters of the United Nations (UN) Environment Program. The US Ambassador Johnnie Carson pledged support to the Ministry of Health. Assistance from the CDC to the Ministry was accepted, including for defining protocols on how to handle suspicious letters and packages. In the wake of the attacks in the United States, hoaxes and false scares were paralyzing mailrooms and post offices in America and elsewhere as suspicious powders in envelopes were investigated.

The causative bacterium, *Bacillus anthracis*, occurs in the wild, typically in herbivores that become infected after ingesting material containing anthrax spores. Anthrax can cause skin infections when skin is exposed to infected material such as animal hides, or more serious generalized infections when spores are inhaled or ingested. It is the long survival of anthrax spores in nature and the high lethality of inhalational disease that make anthrax such a powerful candidate as a biological weapon of terror.

Anthrax is endemic in parts of Kenya, and repeated outbreaks have occurred involving livestock, wildlife, and humans, the latter most commonly suffering cutaneous exposures and disease.[7] Nonetheless, bioterrorism-related anthrax in Kenya would seem, at the very least, surprising. Remembering Michael Gregg's dictum about skepticism, I leaned over to a colleague at the Ministry of Health meeting and said we should make sure this really was anthrax.

Nairobi is fortunate in having specialized staff and several laboratories capable of sophisticated microbiology. Julie Kiehlbauch was an academic American microbiologist who had previously worked at the CDC and with whom I had collaborated in Cote d'Ivoire.[8] She was in Nairobi conducting research with the Kenya Medical Research Institute (KEMRI), where our CDC group (CDC Kenya) had its offices and laboratories. Kiehlbauch's senior Kenyan counterpart was Sam Kariuki, a very respected microbiologist specializing in intestinal infections.

After careful consideration of basic microbiologic characteristics of the materials from various letters, it seemed unlikely to us that this was anthrax; other bacteria from the same family of organisms seemed more probable. As always, personal connections and networks were important, and we were able to reach out to CDC headquarters. Over the last 3 months of 2001, one hundred thirty requests for anthrax assistance or advice were received by CDC headquarters from more than seventy countries or territories outside the United States[9]; ours must have been one of the first. Despite the turmoil at the CDC that was in overdrive, trying to cope with the very real bioterrorism situation in the United States, laboratory colleagues in Atlanta graciously sent us specialized diagnostic reagents not previously shared outside of the homeland.

Within a week of Professor Ongeri's press conference, we were sure the letters sent to Kenya did not contain anthrax. Ordinarily, this should have been good news. Unfortunately, pride intervened, and the opportunity to convert a misjudgment into a "feel-good" story enhancing everyone's reputation was missed. Honor became the prime objective, and it was judged that rejection of an anthrax diagnosis was disrespectful.

Ambassador Carson and I were summoned to meet the Minister, to hear him complain that we were undermining him, and that I was disloyal to long-standing friendship. Kenyan journalists ran after us as we left the building, enquiring about what had transpired. Carson answered repeatedly that medical and technical collaboration between the United States and Kenya was outstanding.

Little more was said, and the story of bioterrorism-related anthrax in Kenya faded away. Tacit understanding evolved that it had all been a mistake or miscommunication, best forgotten. Nevertheless, two final events were noteworthy. The Minister left no stone unturned and ordered further testing. An old-fashioned diagnostic test was to inject material into experimental animals such as guinea pigs to see if they developed disease. The results were negative.

For myself, I was due to travel to the United States at the end of October 2001, and I looked forward to getting away, relieved that this distraction from our regular work was over. I glanced at the Sunday newspaper and a cartoon on the editorial pages caught my eye. Two men in white coats, one depicting the minister and the other a CDC scientist, were peering through magnifying glasses at open envelopes lying on a laboratory table. The minister was berating the scientist for not seeing the obvious while the expert professed nothing was there (Figure 7.1).

Ongeri later moved on to another ministry and afterward lost his parliamentary seat. We greeted each other in friendly fashion on the subsequent occasions that we met. Sam Kariuki, the quiet microbiologist whom Ongeri had looked to for vindication, much later became the KEMRI director. He expressed words concerning this episode that have stayed with me. "There are two types of science," he said, "medical science and political science." We were dealing with the latter.

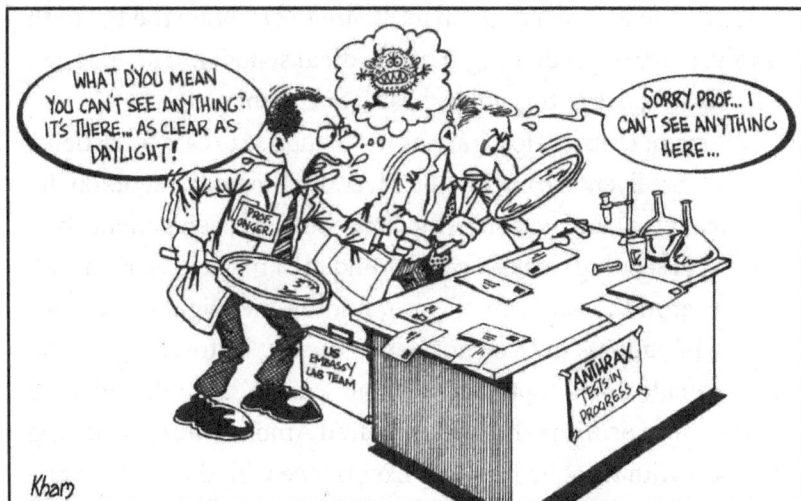

Figure 7.1   Cartoon depicting the Minister of Health arguing with a CDC scientist over anthrax diagnosis.

(Courtesy James Kamawira "Kham"; appeared in Standard, October 28, 2001)

Epidemic Aflatoxin Poisoning, 2004

Aflatoxin and the Field Epidemiology Training Program

We launched the Field Epidemiology Training Program (FETP), an international version of the EIS, in Kenya in the spring of 2004. In early May, just 2 weeks into the month-long introductory course for our first FETP cohort, we heard of an outbreak of jaundice with deaths in Makueni District, an hour and a half southeast of Nairobi on the way to Mombasa, in what was then Kenya's Eastern Province.

The Ministry of Health asked us to investigate, and a rapid assessment over the next few days made it evident that this was no small outbreak. Because of the urgency and magnitude of the event, the lack of experience of our FETP program, and feeling our group's credibility was on the line, senior CDC Kenya colleagues and I became more deeply involved than I had expected.

I was due to attend a reunion in Bristol to celebrate the thirtieth anniversary of graduating from medical school but abandoned the trip because of this public health emergency.

Makueni District Hospital was not equipped to care for patients with severe liver disease. I found several jaundiced patients on the medical ward and was informed that several such patients had died in preceding weeks. I was reminded of my field work on yellow fever in the 1980s in Nigeria, finding the plight of such severely ill patients in this poor health facility distressing. On the positive side, I was impressed with the "can do" attitude and drive of the supervising medical officer, Jared Amolo, who was making the best with what he had. The experience with this outbreak so affected him that he later applied for a position in the FETP, subsequently became an instructor, and later still was hired as resident advisor for the FETP in Nigeria, an example of capacity building as well as South–South collaboration.

We asked the usual questions—is there an epidemic and is it due to what we think it is—before formulating a case definition and describing cases in time, place, and person. Laboratory tests for yellow fever were negative, as were assays for hepatitis viruses and hemorrhagic fevers. Preliminary laboratory testing of maize from the affected area showed high levels of aflatoxin, and I felt confident we were facing an outbreak of aflatoxin poisoning.

Aflatoxin is a toxin produced by a fungus, *Aspergillus flavus*, that grows on maize and other produce such as peanuts, especially when damp. Consumed in large doses, it is toxic to the liver and can cause death from acute liver failure. Chronic, low-dose exposure can cause chronic liver disease and liver cancer and has been suggested to cause stunting in children and immune dysfunction. Studies decades earlier had incriminated aflatoxin as a causative factor for the high incidence of primary liver cancer in Kenya.[10] My thesis on enlarged spleens in Kenya showed a disproportionately high rate of diagnosed and undiagnosed liver disease in the former Eastern Province, a poor area that is the home of the Kamba tribe.[11] An earlier study had shown a higher incidence of primary liver cancer in this group compared with other tribes.[12]

I recalled going on a field visit in 1981, late in my tenure at Kenyatta National Hospital, to visit a rural homestead in this same geographic area where several members of one family had died of acute liver failure. Aflatoxin poisoning was incriminated and the twenty cases with twelve deaths were described by local investigators in an article in the *Lancet*.[13] I reflected on how, at that earlier visit, I had no practical epidemiology experience and could only ask clinical, not relevant epidemiologic, questions. What we were seeing now was similar but greatly magnified in scale and scope.

Aflatoxin Field Investigations

To determine the extent of the aflatoxicosis outbreak, we scoured the area, visiting hospitals and households with cases across seven districts.* Time was short and geographic distances were large, requiring us to mobilize resources from across all our programs. Multiple vehicles and staff left in different directions to conduct assessments. Cases graphed out over time suggested the epidemic had started in Makueni, the district most heavily affected.

It helped to be relatively senior and to know people, simply by virtue of length of service. We made an official request to CDC headquarters, through the Ministry of Health, for assistance. The CDC director at the time was Julie Gerberding, whom I knew from AIDS work; she had been a leading researcher in San Francisco and policy advisor on HIV infection in health care workers and its

---

* Before Kenya's new constitution defining forty-seven counties was introduced in 2010, the country was divided into eight provinces and forty-six districts.

prevention, and we always enjoyed a mutually respectful relationship. She took a personal interest in our work on this outbreak and her office provided $160,000 as emergency support.

I contacted colleagues in Atlanta who I knew worked on food- and waterborne infectious diseases, including the veteran expert, Rob Tauxe. He has always remained in mind because when I joined EIS years before he greeted me in perfect Dutch, knowing of my Belgian background. On our first call about this outbreak, he wisely involved colleagues from the CDC's National Center for Environmental Health. Epidemiologic and laboratory assistance was subsequently provided by specialists from this group, including Lauren Lewis and Helen Schurz Rogers, all under the leadership of Carol Rubin. Some of the colleagues sent out from Atlanta had little or no international experience and were shocked by the rural poverty and desperate circumstances faced by affected communities. The laboratory and toxicology support they provided, however, was critical to subsequent investigations.

The severity of the situation and the complexity of the problem meant that an extraordinarily diverse group of organizations became involved, including the Kenya Ministry of Health, the CDC's National Center for Environmental Health, the US Food and Drug Administration, Kenya's Office of the President, the Kenya Ministry of Agriculture, the US Foreign Agricultural Service, the United Nations' Food and Agriculture Organization, and, of course, the US embassy. This experience illustrated the importance of diplomacy in global health, including in emergency situations like an epidemic.

As we conducted active surveillance for cases, we also attempted to understand the reasons for the outbreak and how to contain it. In addition to finding contaminated maize in individual households, we detected aflatoxin contamination of maize that was being sold in local markets. This immediately raised a critically important question: Was the outbreak due to contamination of maize grown and stored in people's homesteads, which was then traded locally; or was there contamination of maize at a central level nationally, with subsequent distribution to markets from there? If the latter were the case, then dangerous aflatoxin exposure could be occurring all over the country, rather than restricted to these few districts. We learned a great deal about the market dynamics of maize, which were more complicated than I ever imagined.

The official upper limit of aflatoxin in food was 20 parts per billion (ppb), consistent with other international standards. This limit is probably well below any level of danger, and where monitoring of levels and application of regulations are weak, as in Kenya, it is quite often breached without evident harm. And here my environmental health colleagues gave me insight with the quote "It's the dose that makes the poison." That observation, attributed to Paracelsus (1493–1541), is one of the basic tenets of toxicology. Two other fundamental principles are that different chemicals exert specific, not generalizable, effects; and that because humans share biological features with other animals, studies in animals can contribute to understanding of toxicology in humans. Reports of unexpected domestic animal deaths in the affected region proved the latter point.

The acute outbreak uncovered extraordinarily high exposures to the A. flavus fungal toxin. Absence of disease, however, offered no reassurance that the level of aflatoxin exposure was safe, and chronic exposure could be inflicting major public health damage. This was an illustration of the concept developed and promoted by the English epidemiologist Geoffrey Rose: a weak risk factor affecting many people can result in more disease than a strong risk factor applied to fewer individuals.[14]

In a study of dozens of markets involving hundreds of vendors and maize products, we found that more than 50% of maize samples tested had aflatoxin levels above the acceptable limit.[15] More than one-third had levels above 100 ppb, and 7% had levels greater than 1,000 ppb, guaranteed to cause acute poisoning. Markets in Makueni, the district with the most pronounced epidemic, had the most contamination. Maize sold at the local level entered the complex market system and was further distributed, making it a risk factor for a widespread and continued outbreak. The only way to interrupt the cycle was to stop people from eating contaminated maize and have poisonous maize replaced with clean food.

If this was all a local problem, essentially restricted to southeastern Kenya and involving only locally grown maize, then this required food replacement for these rural areas. If it was a centrally driven, point-source epidemic, derived from central contamination of maize and national distribution, the problem was of a wholly different order of magnitude, possibly requiring a nationwide response.

Despite Ministry of Health involvement and multiple discussions, we felt the gravity of the situation was not well understood. I determined that I should brief the US ambassador and ask him to accompany me to alert the minister of health about the seriousness of the situation, which surely would have to be conveyed to the Kenyan president.

Ambassador Mark Bellamy, successor to Johnnie Carson, was a respected career diplomat who, like all ambassadors I dealt with over the years, was extremely supportive of the CDC's work. When he took up his post, I think he was determined to focus on traditional areas of diplomacy and development, and not lean so much toward AIDS and health as Carson had done. Inevitably, he was drawn into global health issues. We went together to see the minister of health, the veteran Kenyan politician Charity Ngilu, former opposition politician and the country's first female presidential candidate.

Once again, as years before in Nigeria dealing with yellow fever, I pulled out a piece of paper showing the epidemic curve

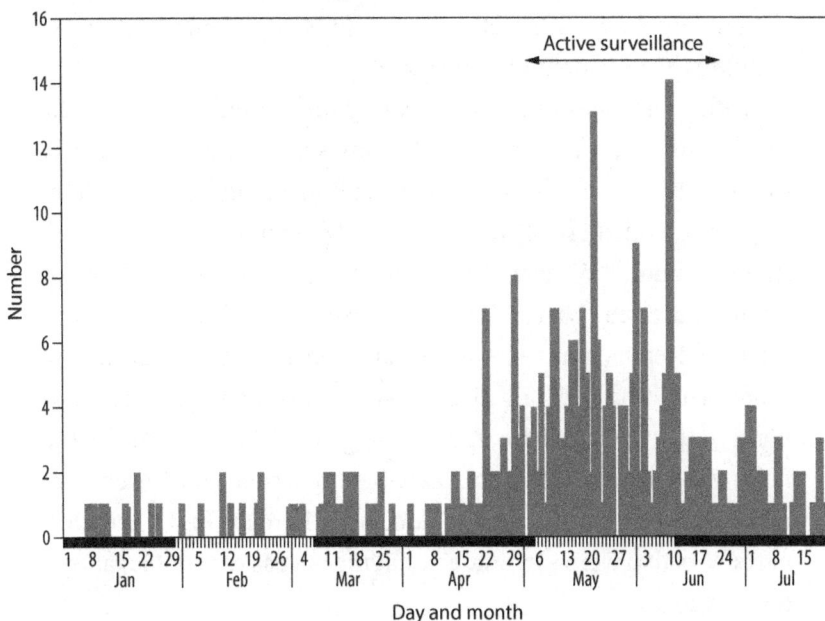

Figure 7.2 Epidemic curve of aflatoxicosis cases by date of reporting, Kenya Eastern and Central Provinces, January–July, 2004. (MMWR 2004;53:790–793)

(Figure 7.2) and described the situation and the relief needed. I explained the critically important question that still had to be addressed: whether the source of the epidemic was local contamination of homegrown maize or contamination from a national source. The implications were different, though neither situation was good. Makueni and other affected districts clearly faced a severe epidemic, but if the source was central, the whole country was at risk.

A look of panic crossed Ngilu's face as she realized two sets of political risk, which she did not vocalize but the ambassador and I well understood. First, she was the member of Parliament for Kitui, the second most heavily affected district, and the population might hold her personally accountable. Second, she might have a national public health crisis on her hands and would have to account to the president and the country.

Asking the right question, I was again reminded, is critically important. We mobilized staff from across our programs to rapidly investigate risk factors at the household level, conducting a case-control study that compared persons with disease and those without.[16] We were fortunate in the technical depth of our team; Laurence (Larry) Slutsker, director of CDC field work in western Kenya, had extensive experience in investigation of foodborne outbreaks of disease and led the study. Kim Lindblade, a skilled malaria epidemiologist, directed work in the field. EIS Officers Eduardo Azziz-Baumgartner and Karen Gieseker worked shoulder to shoulder with Kenyan FETP counterparts. We also were fortunate in having access to reliable laboratory testing.

The results clearly showed that consumption of homegrown rather than externally purchased maize was the most important risk factor for disease.[16] alleviating the concern of national-level contamination of food. Laboratory work determined that the levels of aflatoxin in some of the food specimens from affected households were hundreds of times greater than the internationally accepted safe upper limit, and an important early clue had been the deaths of domestic animals in some affected households.

The End of the Outbreak

Having until now concentrated on infectious diseases, I found this an illuminating but also jarring introduction to environmental epidemiology and the concept of environmental justice. Villagers often knew they were eating poisoned maize but had no alternative; they would have starved otherwise. By the time we ceased field work some 2 months after initial recognition of the outbreak, three hundred seventeen case patients had been detected, of whom one hundred twenty-five (39%) had died.[17] I was sure the true extent of the outbreak was much greater.

New, but fewer, cases were still occurring. The people affected by this outbreak, possibly the largest epidemic of aflatoxin poisoning ever described, lived a marginal existence in a neglected part of the country. Unseasonal rains had occurred early in February 2004, and villagers were forced to harvest maize prematurely. To prevent theft, maize was stored damp in dark households, and the combination of humidity and temperature promoted growth of *Aspergillus*, the production of aflatoxin, and a subsequent severe epidemic. Later laboratory studies showed the strain of *Aspergillus* was the S strain, which is associated with higher aflatoxin production.[18]

Necessary solutions were, in the short term, confiscation of contaminated maize and its replacement with clean food. In the longer term, public health requirements included surveillance for human aflatoxin poisoning, enhanced food inspection measuring aflatoxin levels, and implementation of appropriate agricultural practices for safe harvesting and storage of maize. All of this was out of reach for these rural populations that were bypassed by their political leaders.

Efforts to replace all maize in the two most heavily affected districts were handicapped by logistic weaknesses. The lack of a clear definition of who oversaw food replacement and of monitoring and evaluation of its implementation were the weakest part of the response. The decline of the epidemic likely resulted from the most heavily contaminated maize having already been consumed, rather than from widespread food seizure and replacement.

Institutional rivalries surfaced amidst these intense activities, distracting from the public health challenges at hand. WHO's Regional Office for Africa had sent a specialist in environmental health and toxicology to assist the Ministry of Health. She appropriately argued for local capacity strengthening but was wary about the CDC's deep involvement. Supervisors of the global FETP program in Atlanta, already stung by feelings of loss of control, were critical from thousands of miles away that we were not implementing agricultural interventions to enhance maize safety, something completely beyond our role or capacity. Some collaborations were excellent, such as with US government toxicology experts at the CDC, the FDA, and the Department of Agriculture.

To try to assist the affected population of Kenya's Eastern Province, Ambassador Bellamy and I persuaded the UN leadership in Nairobi to convene a meeting of different donors and agencies. I presented details of the epidemic and the need for acute food replacement but gained little traction. In a context of restricted international resources, the situation in southeastern Kenya was considered a Kenyan government responsibility and not severe enough to warrant multilateral intervention.

The need for replacement food for aflatoxicosis in southeastern Kenya in 2004 was subsequently overtaken by a larger, more widespread crisis of acute food shortage. In early July 2004, the president of Kenya formally requested international food aid in response to prolonged drought and food shortages affecting much of the country; shortly thereafter, he declared a national disaster. The plight of aflatoxin-affected villagers in eastern Kenya was easily forgotten.

Parting Thoughts

I realized that what we had been dealing with was not primarily a medical issue and that public health had little to offer as a solution. Perhaps our most important contribution, integral to the CDC's role and identity, was surveillance and outbreak investigation, simply bearing witness. We as medical epidemiologists could advocate for but not deliver the necessary food assistance or agricultural and regulatory interventions.

The outbreak of aflatoxin poisoning was a sentinel event indicative of structural and agricultural deficiencies and lack of social justice. Just as with HIV/AIDS, factors beyond individual choices, factors over which individuals had little control, left people vulnerable and put them at risk. The affected communities often knew they were eating contaminated food but had no alternative; some households were so poor they were even reluctant to give up small samples of maize for our laboratory testing.

Closing this experience, we persuaded WHO to convene a meeting in Geneva to discuss aflatoxin poisoning and review research and intervention priorities. A useful paper resulted,[19] but on the ground little has changed. Smaller outbreaks occurred in 2005 and 2006, and studies of aflatoxin levels in household maize, the staple food, in the same areas of eastern Kenya in 2005–2007 showed that up to 50% of samples tested had levels greater than the official limit of 20 ppb.[20]

Innovative use was made of blood specimens collected in 2007 for the Kenya-wide survey of HIV infection (the Kenya AIDS Indicator Survey) conducted every 5 years to study national aflatoxin exposure.[21] Evidence of recent aflatoxin ingestion was found in 78% of specimens tested, affecting all parts of the country. Median concentrations of aflatoxin products in sera from the former Eastern Province were more than twice those in specimens from the province with the next-highest levels. A comparable population-based study in the United States found aflatoxin exposure in only 1% of participants, and the highest level detected was more than twenty times lower.[22]

The threshold of 20 ppb for "safe" aflatoxin exposure may be more stringent than necessary, but it is widely ignored. Higher levels of exposure are widespread, unmeasured, and unaddressed. Aflatoxin levels in maize are highest in eastern Kenya, and that region remains at risk of acute outbreaks when aflatoxin levels rise rapidly under conditions of environmental stress. Concerning chronic, lower dose contamination of food, the risk of disease must reflect cumulative exposure, but the long-term impact remains unmeasured and understudied. It must be considerable.

The oral presentation on this outbreak by Azziz-Baumgartner at the 2005 EIS conference won the Donald C. Mackel Memorial Award, a prize given for the most effective combination of epidemiology and laboratory science in a field investigation. The published case control study was awarded CDC's Alexander D. Langmuir Prize recognizing excellence in a scientific manuscript.[16] I was gratified but also reminded of how our experience, careers, and reputations are built on the suffering and misfortune of others, often the poor who educate us in medicine and public health.[23] And compared to the magnitude of the public health challenges facing the communities we serve, the inevitable interpersonal and broader rivalries that arise seem trivial indeed. An adage that has helped me keep organizational competitiveness in perspective is that the feuds are often so bitter because the stakes are so low.

CHAPTER 8

From Exotic Infection to Global Health Priority

Ebola in West Africa

The political scientist Francis Fukuyama famously posited that after the end of the Cold War, Western democracy would spread and result in stable governance over a previously unruly planet.[1] History apparently had different designs, and today's world seems more fractious and divided than ever. I saw analogies in 2014 when optimism concerning global health and the Millennium Development Goals gave way to alarm about Ebola in West Africa and overall global health security.

First recognized in 1976 in the former Zaire[2] and South Sudan,[3] Ebola had caused some twenty-four recognized outbreaks by 2014, resulting in about twenty-five hundred cases across Africa, predominantly in the central part of the continent.[4] Ebola's fearsome reputation resulted from the nature of the associated illness and its high lethality: 41% to 90% of affected persons died. Because hemorrhage does not occur in all cases, "Ebola virus disease," or simply "Ebola," have replaced "Ebola hemorrhagic fever" as a name. After an incubation period of 2–21 days, disease manifestations include fever, nausea, headache, body aches, abdominal pain, vomiting, and diarrhea. Death results from multisystem failure and sometimes hemorrhage.

Treatment until 2014 was simply supportive—fluids, nutrition, bed rest, and treatment of complications—but the remote and underprivileged settings in which outbreaks occurred meant care was rudimentary. Recovery is thought to result in lifelong immunity. The management of outbreaks was simple, at least in theory: find and isolate the cases; safely bury the dead; follow contacts of infected or dead persons and isolate any showing symptoms; apply strict infection prevention and control (IPC) measures, especially in health care settings and for burial teams; and declare contacts clear if free of disease after 21 days*. In this way, chains of transmission are disrupted, and outbreaks contained. Outbreaks have also been extinguished simply by the high death rates of affected persons curtailing further transmission. If no cases had occurred within two incubation periods (42 days) of the last case patient's onset of illness, the outbreak was considered over.

Ebola's putative reservoir is a type of fruit bat common across Africa, but extensive field research has not yet proved this definitively. Ecologic searches for a source have been challenged by the enormity of the task, with uncertainty about Ebola's distribution, frequency, or seasonality precluding specific focus. In a humorous presentation (he described a snake escaping in his laboratory) at a 1996 colloquium on Ebola at the Institute of Tropical Medicine in Antwerp, Belgium, the South African virologist Robert Swanepoel presented a different approach, inoculating Ebola into different plants and experimental animals. Bats supported Ebola replication without themselves becoming ill.[5] The evidence for a bat reservoir is more definitive for Marburg virus.[6]

Spillover into humans is thought to result from contact with bats carrying the virus or with other infected animals, includ-

---

* "Isolation" refers to removing infected or ill persons from circulation. "Quarantine" refers to separating individuals potentially exposed to an infection, but who are well, from others.

ing mammals and primates hunted for bush meat. Person-to-person spread occurs through direct contact with ill persons, exposure to infected bodily fluids, or handling of an infected corpse. Ebola is essentially a disease of touch, highly contagious from contact with ill persons or their fluids, but not airborne and, therefore, much less infectious than measles or influenza viruses. Leaving aside occasional transmission from survivors, human-to-human transmission is largely or exclusively from ill individuals.[7]

Until the events of 2014, Ebola virus disease was largely a phenomenon of isolated, rural areas in Central Africa. Cases had never occurred outside of Africa, and the farthest west human infection had ever been observed was in Cote d'Ivoire, where a Swiss veterinarian became infected in 1997 after performing an autopsy on a chimpanzee that had died in the forest.

The Beginning

I was head of the CDC's office in Kenya where, in March 2014, colleagues and I began to follow reports of Ebola in Guinea with interest. It later transpired that the epidemic in Guinea had started in the Forest Region of the country in late December 2013.[8] Cases of Ebola were reported in the bordering area of Liberia and an epidemiologist in our group, Joel Montgomery, [9] was sent by headquarters to West Africa to investigate in early April. Case finding and contact tracing were initiated, and the Liberian outbreak seemed to be rapidly curtailed.

In late May 2014, Ebola was again reported from Liberia, and not only was the outbreak continuing in Guinea but cases were now also occurring in Sierra Leone (Figure 10.1). I read the reports with unease, struck by the differences of opinion aired. The medical charity Médecins Sans Frontières (MSF) raised alarm while WHO said all would soon come under control.

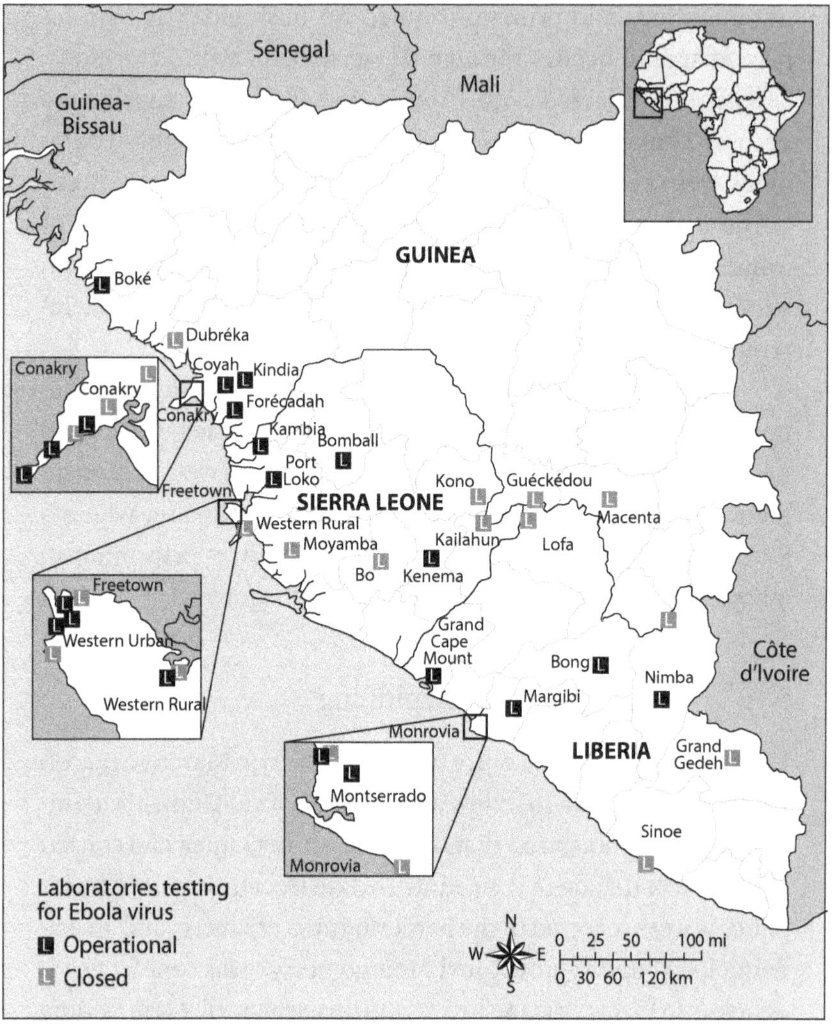

Figure 8.1 Map of Ebola-affected countries in West Africa, including Ebola laboratories, 2014–2015.

(Spengler JR, et al. Emerg Infect Dis 2016;22:956-963)

Atlanta, June/July 2014

The Emergency Operations Center (EOC) at CDC headquarters in Atlanta[10] could feature in a Hollywood movie. Row upon row of computer workstations fill a cavernous room dominated by large screens on the walls that show maps of ongoing crises, television news channels, or health-related data. Smaller rooms off the main floor house specialized staff, executive meeting space, mapping facilities, logistics staff, and a legion of other entities supporting 24-hour communications and response capacity for emergencies anywhere in the world.

Activating the EOC is a decision in the purview of the CDC director.[10] Reasons for EOC activation in recent years have included major events such as COVID-19 and the mpox outbreak (interestingly, the EOC has not been activated for the opioid epidemic, although more than one million Americans have died of drug overdoses since 1999, with almost three-fourths of such deaths being opioid-related). With EOC activation, an Incident Management System is implemented, with the incident manager in hierarchical control over the whole event, drawing in staff as needed from across the agency, and reporting directly to the CDC director. Sometimes more than one public health event is at play at the same time, and the EOC can be a complex place teeming with people and humming with activity relating to diverse emergencies.

I travelled to Washington, DC, from Nairobi in late June 2014 for a committee meeting to plan the following year's Conference on Retroviruses and Opportunistic Infections. It was always useful to stop by CDC headquarters in Atlanta to consult and remind headquarters of our work in Kenya. Montgomery and I had become concerned from our field perspective that a crisis was developing in West Africa. Already this was the largest Ebola outbreak ever, and three countries—Guinea, Liberia, and Sierra

Leone—were now affected. The CDC, however, including the Center for Global Health that I led from 2010 to late 2012, was silent, the EOC had not been activated, and no EIS officers had been deployed.

I was aware I was now a field person and no longer a senior official at headquarters, but I sent an email to agency leaders, including Director Thomas (Tom) Frieden.[11] Just at that time, on July 1, the Ministry of Health and Social Welfare of Liberia sent a message to the US ambassador in Monrovia asking for assistance from the CDC in epidemiology and surveillance, laboratory work, logistics, and coordination, and requesting deployment of a small team. Inger Damon,[12] the CDC's expert on smallpox and related infections and the overall lead in the Ebola response, was on leave but called me to ask if I would lead a team to Liberia.

Specialists in Ebola were housed in the Viral Special Pathogens Branch (VSPB), in which I had done my 2-year EIS training almost three decades before. VSPB comprised a hardy group of about forty experts, some of the best in the world, used to doing their specialized work independently and comfortable with responding to outbreaks in difficult places. I was briefed by Ute Ströher, a senior laboratory scientist, and talked with health security expert Ray Arthur, a seasoned epidemiologist with extensive connections at WHO and other agencies. Pierre Rollin,[13] a senior VSPB staffer and world expert, was on the ground in Guinea.

I drew several conclusions from the incomplete, uncoordinated information available. First, laboratory support in the field was limited, and assuring Ebola diagnoses would be challenging. Second, we had no idea about the magnitude of the outbreak, although cases had been reported in Liberia's capital city, Monrovia, and in the north of the country, in Lofa County. Third, our team would be stretched to the limit and individual resilience would be required. And I felt a gnawing concern that VSPB staff were more than hesitant about the larger scale involvement of other CDC staff that would become inevitable, especially with imminent activation of the EOC. The deep technical capacity of VSPB was desperately required, but the magnitude and implications of the epidemic, its international visibility, and the politics ensuing would inevitably mean VSPB losing its usual control over this response.

Monrovia, Liberia, July 2014

I arrived in Monrovia on July 16 to be met at the small but crowded airport by Christie Reed, a CDC epidemiologist assigned to the US Agency for International Development (USAID) to work on malaria. The support from in-country CDC colleagues is invaluable for making immediate connections when arriving for an emergency such as this, and Reed gave outstanding assistance. I had written to her before my arrival to ask for an early briefing on all available information and to secure urgent appointments, including with the US ambassador to Liberia, Deborah Malac*.[14] Essential logistics had to be assured, such as transport, internet access, and communications. We went immediately from the airport to the Liberia Institute for Biomedical Research (LIBR), the only facility performing Ebola testing, to meet its director, Philip Sahr.

The state of the institute reflected the turbulent and difficult history of the country itself.[15] Liberia, along with Sierra Leone and Guinea, were among the poorest countries in the world, and ranked toward the bottom of all assessments of human and economic development. Literacy in Liberia was barely 60%, and the country was still suffering the consequences of its brutal civil wars

---

* Once again, earlier connections were shown important. Ambassador Malac had worked for Ambassador Johnnie Carson when the latter was Assistant Secretary for African Affairs in the State Department. I interacted with them both while I was director of the Center for Global Health from 2010 to 2012.

that had destroyed national infrastructure, including the electricity grid. Walking around the grounds of LIBR, I saw chimpanzee statues and derelict animal cages. I recalled from my hepatitis days that the New York Blood Center previously had a collaboration with Liberia for studies involving experimental hepatitis infections in chimpanzees, and LIBR was where the research was done.[16]

LIBR and Liberia were fortunate to have scientists from the National Institutes of Health (NIH) and US Army Medical Research Institute of Infectious Diseases in-country for preexisting research. Lisa Hensley and Randal (Randy) Schoepp led and trained a cadre of Liberian technicians to perform Ebola polymerase chain reaction (PCR)* testing under rudimentary conditions. LIBR's Director Sahr warned me that the institute could not afford the 2000 gallons of fuel required to run the generators more than a month, and that even if funds were available to pay salaries for extending working days, only about thirty specimens could be tested daily for Ebola.

Initially, security to limit access to the compound and laboratory was lacking, specimens were left outside the laboratory's working area, and only a plastic curtain separated the "hot" area where potentially infectious specimens were inactivated from the rest of the laboratory.

A further challenge to rapid and extensive testing was LIBR's distance from the city, more than 50 km away. Liberia was colorful in its use of names. The area near the airport and LIBR was referred to as "Smell no Taste"; during World War II, American soldiers had been stationed here, and their food preparation was odorous and evident, but not shared. Another part of Monrovia

---

* PCR is a technique detecting genetic material of an infecting agent in the specimen being tested. It is highly sensitive and yields positive results before other assays such as serologic tests (i.e., it has a shorter window period, or time between infection and when testing can return reliable results).

was called Red Light, not because of any association with sex work but because it harbored the city's single traffic light.

Different CDC colleagues began to arrive in subsequent days, our core team expanding from an initial three (two EIS officers and me) to an eventual twelve: five EIS officers (Mary Arwady; Patrick Ayscue; Joseph ["Joe"] Forrester; Jennifer Hunter; Almea Matanock); a recent EIS graduate from VSPB (Ilana Schafer); another recent EIS graduate (Satish Pillai[17]); two specialist colleagues focusing on border security (Tai-Ho Chen[18]; Thomas George), emergency management (Edward Rouse[19]), and communications (Ben Monroe); and me.

For maximum efficiency of the team, it was important to impose some organizational structure, and I asked Pillai to assure the necessary coordination and delegation. The initial priority was to extract meaning from the chaotic and limited information available about the outbreak, rapidly see the situation firsthand, define what was known and unknown, and determine the most urgent interventions.

It was immediately apparent that a disaster was unfolding. Ebola was spreading in the community, ill people lay in hospital grounds or died at home, and bodies were occasionally seen in the streets. Monrovia was gripped by fear, and all of us were surprised by the intensity of the environment and the rapidity of events. Two clear priorities were trying to get deeper understanding of the full situation and strengthening case isolation, however the latter could be achieved. The ideal was to access Ebola Treatment Unit (ETU) beds, but these were scarce.

I fielded questions from headquarters in Atlanta about contact tracing that were appropriate for small outbreaks but were unrealistic in view of the large number of active cases not isolated. It made little sense to focus on people who were well when overwhelming numbers of people who were sick and potentially transmitting infection were not isolated. This was the first, but not only, time that expert but dogmatic advice from far away was incompatible with the reality on the ground. We immediately understood that conveying the gravity of the local situation to our distant headquarters was going to be difficult—it had to be seen to be believed.

The Ministry of Health and Social Welfare, Monrovia, Liberia

Our CDC team was in Liberia upon request from the chief medical officer, Berenice Dahn, through the minister of health, Walter Gwenigale. Meeting the seniors at the ministry was not only necessary protocol but essential for garnering support for subsequent work. Daily meetings of the "Ebola Task Force" were held in the ministry's auditorium, a large room with rows of plastic chairs. We attended the morning meeting the day after arrival, which was important because it yielded introductions to the diverse actors involved, including Ministry of Health officials, the WHO country representative, and partners from civil society organizations.

Key contacts now included Luke Bawo, responsible for surveillance and reporting at the ministry, Lindis Hurum, the emergency coordinator for MSF in Liberia, and the WHO country representative (the "WR"). We also met Ambassador Malac and senior officials at the US embassy. Not only would we rely on the embassy for logistical support but the State Department had to be kept informed of this evolving international crisis. The ambassador is responsible for all US government employees in-country, so maintaining good relationships is always critically important.

The task force meeting revealed new cases in nearby Bong County, as well as several deaths in Lofa County and Monrovia. Numerous logistic uncertainties were raised, and the meeting

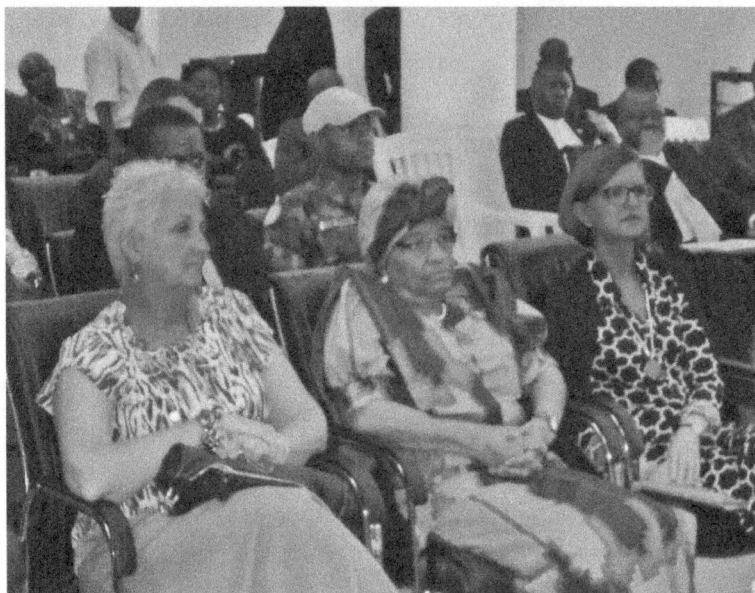

Figure 8.2   *Left to right*: Ambassador Deborah Malac; President Johnson Sirleaf; Karin Landgren, special representative of the secretary-general and head of UNMIL.
(Kevin De Cock, personal collection)

finished with a dozen or so items requiring follow-up. It was also announced that the director of WHO's Regional Office for Africa, Luis Sambo, would be visiting Monrovia at the end of the week. Attendance at the task force meetings on subsequent days gave disturbing insight. It seemed anyone could attend, and even the president sometimes came (Figure 8.2). Although an agenda was adhered to, action items were not followed up, and lines of authority and responsibility were unclear.

I met Minister Gwenigale on my second working day. He was a short and wiry surgeon who must have been almost 80 years old and who had been in the post since 2006. He had stayed in Liberia throughout its recent civil war, despite opportunity to leave for the United States. He later told me he did not know how old he was; to go to college overseas he had to give his birthday, which his mother did not know, so he arbitrarily chose the first day of an arbitrary year.

Having looked around a little and mindful of the priorities Atlanta had emphasized, I began to explain my thinking to the minister when he politely cut me off, suggesting firmly I let him define the country's needs. It was a gentle but humbling, useful rebuke that I will always remember. Two priorities the minister emphasized were defining epidemiology and assuring capacity for laboratory testing for Ebola.

Close collaboration ensued with Luke Bawo, the highly capable head of surveillance, instantly recognizable for his booming voice and severe limp from a motor vehicle crash in earlier life. By the time we commenced collaboration, some 173 cases of Ebola had been reported, but over the ensuing month, that total grew almost five-fold, with a mean of twenty-three new cases and twelve deaths reported daily, the maximum daily toll in this first month of field work being sixty cases and thirty-three deaths. The WR, who had experienced smaller outbreaks of Ebola earlier in his career, said in disbelief that we were heading for one thousand cases. The ultimate number was to be far higher.

Ebola in Liberia: From Exotic Infection to Global Health Security Concern

A series of events over the second half of July 2014 propelled Ebola to global media attention. On July 20, Patrick Sawyer, a politically connected Liberian American, flew from Monrovia to Lagos in Nigeria, via Lomé in Togo, despite being visibly ill. Although supposedly traveling on official government business, rumors were that he intended to seek help for his illness from an evangelical church. He collapsed on arrival in Nigeria and died of confirmed Ebola on July 25. Some 20 subsequent cases of Ebola ensued in

Nigeria over three generations of transmission, eight of them fatal, and there were 894 contacts needing investigation.[20] Ameyo Adadevoh, the physician who cared for Sawyer and made the correct diagnosis, herself died. This experience illustrated the danger of Ebola being exported to other countries in Africa with secondary spread, especially in health facilities.

The two organizations providing Ebola care in Liberia were MSF and Samaritan's Purse, the Christian relief organization directed by Franklin Graham, son of the evangelist Billy Graham. In an unlikely collaboration in view of their differing political philosophies, MSF worked with Samaritan's Purse to train the latter's workers in Ebola care. MSF's resources were stretched because they had been providing services in Foya, Lofa County, on the border with Guinea and Sierra Leone, as well as in Monrovia. One of my first visits in Monrovia had been to Eternal Love Winning Africa (ELWA) mission hospital, where Samaritan's Purse was expanding its Ebola treatment facility. I met the medical lead, Kent Brantly, the country director, Kendell Kauffeldt, and some other Samaritan's Purse staff, and was impressed with their commitment.

On Wednesday, July 23, Brantly woke up with fever and isolated himself in his house. He arranged for a blood specimen to be sent to LIBR but submitted it using a pseudonym. I was informed of these events on Saturday, July 26, at a meeting with WHO, after I had been asked by Samaritan's Purse to chase down Brantly's test result. His Ebola test was positive.

Shock pervaded the conference room as we learned of the first-ever Ebola infection in an international responder, with no clear protocols in place of how to deal with such an event. Almost unbelievably, a second Samaritan's Purse employee, nurse aide Nancy Writebol, was also confirmed to have Ebola after having been diagnosed with malaria a few days earlier and ill since July 22. We subsequently learned that a third Samaritan's Purse

staff member, Bobby Weh, who worked with Writebol, had become unwell on or before July 20 and died of Ebola on July 27.
This Liberian hygienist was little mentioned in the extensive
international communications and publicity around Ebola in
the missionaries.

An unexplained, perhaps coincidental, event had been a call
from Samaritan's Purse to Ute Ströher in VSPB, Atlanta, on Tuesday, July 22, to ask a hypothetical question about procedures in
case of contact with bodily fluids from an Ebola patient without
wearing gloves. I was never able to elucidate the relevance of this
call to subsequent events.

Joe Forrester, Jennifer Hunter, and Satish Pillai spent many
hours talking to Samaritan's Purse staff, including, when possible,
the infected individuals. Three points seemed important. First,
that Brantly, Writebol, and Weh all became ill around the same
time raised the possibility of a common source exposure—perhaps
all three were infected at the same time from some shared incident. I wondered whether some fault relating to spraying personal
protective equipment with decontaminant could have been responsible, because they all applied or received spraying for personnel entering the high-risk ward.

Second, Brantly had worked in the main ELWA Hospital at the
same time he was staffing the ETU, and we knew that other health
care workers at ELWA were infected in the main hospital around
the same time. Missionary colleagues of the two Americans later
reported various breaches of infection prevention protocols, but
no known exposure to infection.* In a statement released during
his later recovery, Brantly said, "When Ebola spread into Liberia,

---

* In his book describing his Ebola experience, Brantly described unpro-
tected contact with possible Ebola patients in the main ELWA hospital on
the night of July 14, nine days before his illness onset. (Brantly K, Brantly A.
*Called for Life: How Loving Our Neighbor Led Us Into the Heart of the Ebola
Epidemic.* Waterbrook; 2015)

my usual hospital work turned more and more toward treating the increasing number of Ebola patients. I held the hands of countless individuals as this terrible disease took their lives away from them." It was possible that the Samaritan's Purse physician was infected in the main hospital.

Finally, Samaritan's Purse staff believed that Weh, the Liberian hygienist, came to work while ill and that infections may have been acquired through direct contact with him at work (De Cock KM, unpublished).[21] We were unable to dissect out and incriminate any individual event but concluded that abundant potential exposures occurred outside of the ETU. Paradoxically, working in the ETU with its associated preventive measures was probably safer at this time than working in the poorly resourced general hospital. We documented these first-ever Ebola infections in international Ebola responders, who happened to be American citizens, in an article in the *MMWR*.[22]

A conundrum was how to treat the ill expatriates. Traditionally, in much smaller and localized outbreaks, the attitude was that any internationals who acquired Ebola would have to take their chances locally. Predictably, with this much larger epidemic, greater numbers of international responders, Samaritan Purse's political connections, and increased global attention, attitudes changed.

Arrangements were subsequently made with an American commercial company as well as different national militaries, and more than a dozen international health care workers were later evacuated from West Africa to Europe and the United States. The two Samaritan's Purse workers were the first to benefit, being admitted to Emory University Hospital, next to the CDC in Atlanta, in early August 2014. Both survived, to widespread publicity.[23]

Another early, less fortunate situation in August 2014 concerned a Spanish Catholic priest. His first Ebola test was negative and he was released from isolation. However, as for other infectious disease diagnostic tests (the most discussed probably being for HIV), there is a window period between establishment of infection and the test becoming positive. The priest did, in fact, have Ebola, and before a second test was positive, he infected others in Monrovia prior to his own medical evacuation.

A nurse in Spain who cared for him and for another evacuated cleric became infected with Ebola. Both priests died. The nurse had a dog, a mongrel called Excalibur, who had been exposed to her while she was symptomatic. Authorities decided to euthanize the dog, amidst widespread protest. Excalibur became one of the most famous early victims of the Ebola crisis, arousing comments about the contrasting silence on thousands of nameless deaths in West Africa.[24]

The CDC had no direct involvement in evaluation of experimental medicines for Ebola, but I knew that Lisa Hensley, running Ebola testing at LIBR, specialized in this area of work. I linked her to Samaritan's Purse, and we discussed potential options, later being questioned as to whether we were exceeding our mandate, a position I strongly rejected. Samaritan's Purse followed up with different private companies, and their infected colleagues were the first recipients of the experimental medicine ZMapp, a preparation of humanized monoclonal antibodies.[25]

Lance Plyler, another Samaritan's Purse physician who was caring for the very ill Brantley, felt that ZMapp was responsible for his clinical improvement, having tearfully told me in late July that he thought his patient would die. When Brantly reached Atlanta, he was able to walk unaided into the hospital, suggesting he was largely better when he arrived—the drug, the patient's relative youth, and time all potential contributors to his survival.

The attention accorded to these infected Americans was helpful in raising awareness of the gravity of the situation in West Africa and the need for a more robust international response. At the same time, we felt troubled by the privileged access to care the expatriate missionaries received compared with national staff. Some of us with more secular, strictly medical bents had unease about the religious tone of some of the discussions. Samaritan's Purse drew ranks after these events, their communications became less open, they shut down their longstanding Liberia operations for an unspecified period, and all their staff left the country.

Almea Mattanock had spent time in Liberia earlier in her training and knew several local doctors. She spearheaded the first systematic investigation of Ebola in health care workers, identifying ninety-seven infections in such personnel, or 12% of the 810 Ebola infections reported by the time of her analysis.[26] We identified ten clusters of cases and showed that most infections were acquired outside of specialized ETUs, in general health care or informal settings. Just as for the Samaritan's Purse staff, the general medical environment was more dangerous early in this large outbreak than the ETUs, with their protective measures and heightened awareness.

Liberia had only about fifty doctors in the whole country at this time, and the impact of each Ebola health care worker infection was devastating. Several prominent physicians lost their lives. In early August 2014, Liberia's President Johnson Sirleaf wrote a letter to President Obama asking for access on a compassionate basis to experimental medicines for several Liberian doctors infected. I was drawn into this chain of communication and ZMapp was provided by the manufacturer for Dr. Abraham Borbor, head of internal medicine at Monrovia's John F. Kennedy Medical Center, who nonetheless died. While still able but confined in the ETU, Borbor courageously offered to provide care for other patients in the unit. Another physician was luckier. He was admitted to an ETU, but it was later realized that his positive Ebola result was a miscommunication and he was, in fact, uninfected.

He survived his forced detainment and was subsequently honored internationally as a survivor.

Our team was humbled by the courage of the Liberian health care workers but also dismayed by the extreme vulnerability of the whole health care system to Ebola. EIS Officer Jennifer Hunter ordinarily worked for the group in Atlanta dealing with hospital infections. Her supervisor had told her that the CDC would not be getting deeply involved in the issue of Ebola in health care workers, but we quickly discerned that this was unrealistic. Indeed, one of my early, chilling realizations was that the whole African health sector was vulnerable if Ebola were widely exported, because of weakness of IPC in health care facilities across the continent.

Ebola that Wasn't

In early August 2014, midway through this first deployment, Almea Mattanock told me she felt unwell and intended to stay in the hotel. I sensed the worry in her voice and manner, and her unspoken fear she might have Ebola. She complained of diarrhea, did not have fever, but felt listless. She admitted that during a hospital visit she had shaken hands with a staff physician but had not had contact with anyone obviously ill. Rationally, Ebola was most unlikely to be the cause of her illness. VSPB staff were well aware of the risk of mild intercurrent illness, especially foodborne infections, during deployments to difficult environments.

Jennifer Hunter shared rooms with Mattanock, and they frequently ate together. When Hunter complained of similar symptoms, I further reasoned this could not be a secondary case transmitted from Almea, because the incubation period was not compatible. Although they most likely had a foodborne intestinal infection, I nevertheless remained uneasy, even waking up in the night with subliminal worry, until their symptoms resolved. I later told this story to Sheila Paskman, the seasoned deputy chief of mission at the US embassy, to convey the generally stressful atmosphere. My estimation of her went up when she snorted that if she suspected Ebola every time she had diarrhea in Liberia, she would never get any work done. This episode was a useful reminder that a priority for epidemic investigators is to protect personal health. Our team was scrupulous, for example, in adhering to malaria prophylaxis to avoid the distraction of febrile illness among responders.

Resistance, Security, and the Incident Management System

The attitude of the Liberian population in July 2014 was ambiguous and fluid. There was widespread skepticism about Ebola, some people suggesting it was dreamed up by the government to bring in foreign money. Hostility, and even violence, was shown by some communities toward health care workers bringing Ebola information or initiating investigations. Extreme sensitivity surrounded traditional funerals, where touching corpses was a major source of infection but also a cultural norm. As the situation worsened, denial was often replaced by impatience that the government was not doing enough. Conflicting behaviors included aggression toward health care workers collecting dead bodies and protest against delayed government assistance, expressed by dumping bodies in the streets or in wealthier neighborhoods.

Satish Pilai and I were dismayed by the daily task force meetings, ostensibly the pinnacle of decision-making, which we deemed inefficient. We proposed an Incident Management System that would streamline the response, institute clear lines of authority under the direction of an incident manager, and define specific responsibilities to different groups. We recommended that the daily meetings be limited in size, only attended by essential staff and key partners. A summary of the resulting outcome was later published in the *MMWR*.[27] Another important success was persuading CDC headquarters, in collaboration with the NIH, to support the rapid establishment of an Ebola laboratory in Monrovia to increase testing capacity. Pleasing to me was deployment of colleagues Barry Fields and Clayton Onyango from our CDC office in Kenya to help set up this emergency laboratory.

I arranged to discuss the Incident Management System with Minister of Health Gwenigale on Wednesday, July 23. No sooner had Pillai and I sat down when the minister's secretary interrupted to say the building was on fire and we had to evacuate. Thick black smoke engulfed Pillai and me as we descended the stairs from the fourth floor. I began to cough, and I realized this was a true emergency. We reached outside to find an atmosphere of confusion and the car park full of people. We rounded up CDC staff, ensured all were accounted for, identified our vehicles, and left for the safety of our hotel.

It later transpired that the fire resulted from arson in the task force conference room. A disgruntled family member of a boy who died of Ebola poured kerosene over plastic chairs piled together and set them alight. According to newspaper reports, this individual had attended the open task force meeting, had been prevented from speaking, and returned in frustration the following day to burn the building down. An unconfirmed story was that the arsonist was apprehended but escaped from his detainers by shouting that he had Ebola.

Concerned about Minister Gwenigale's safety because I had not seen him exit the building, I called him later that afternoon. He briskly told me he was fine, that he was seeing his daughter-in-law off at the airport, and that the conference room was no big loss because meetings would now be smaller. "Some sangfroid," I thought, wondering how ministers elsewhere would respond to such an event.

The physical security of our staff was a constant concern. Patrick Ayscue was working in Foya in Lofa County in late July, where one of the country's few ETUs had more than twice the number of Ebola patients than intended. Communicating with Ayscue from Monrovia was difficult because of inadequate cell phone coverage and limited email access. We were alarmed when he sent a brief message to say that Samaritan's Purse vehicles had been attacked, one car was destroyed by fire, and four health care workers were missing. Along with MSF staff, Ayscue had to cross the border into Guinea for the night, waiting for matters to calm down on the Liberian side.

To assess the geographic extent of the outbreak, I felt it important to conduct rapid assessments of all of Liberia's counties. The southeastern part of the country, difficult to access, had reported few or no cases. I asked Joe Forrester, a self-sufficient individual who had interrupted his surgical residency for EIS training, to investigate the situation in this region bordering Cote d'Ivoire. He recounted grueling travel and found no Ebola cases but conveyed that the area was woefully unprepared should infection be introduced.[28] The isolation of this part of Liberia simply from lack of transport infrastructure likely served to protect it from Ebola.

The UN Mission in Liberia (UNMIL) was established in 2003 to enhance security after the civil war. UNMIL assisted with transport to remote areas by helicopter—Russian machines dependent on line-of-sight for navigation, and flown on contract by Ukrainian pilots. I tried twice to visit Lofa County in the north of the country, the area where the epidemic had started, but each time, our lumbering helicopter had to turn back because of poor visibility. I was constantly aware of the need to pay attention to the safety of our staff and was relieved we had no adverse events other than occasional fright.

Liberia, August 2014: Piecing It Together

In the first half of August, international attention to Liberia increased and resources began to flow. Joanne Liu, MSF's international director, visited, and what she saw on the ground helped in powerful advocacy to world leaders and at the United Nations in New York.[29] Lindis Hurum and other MSF staff led ETU expansion in Monrovia, with the previously unimaginable reality of a tented facility with more than 100 Ebola beds at "ELWA 3" and with room for further growth (Figure 8.3).

CDC deployments were time limited as people had to return to their regular duties, and our first team disbanded in mid-August 2014, 31 days after I arrived in Liberia. The international airlines had mostly stopped flying into the affected countries of West Africa, and I left on the last Kenya Airways flight out of the country.

Ordinarily, one would expect an epidemic curve to convey the element of time in describing the outbreak. Despite my regular requests to our staff, this proved frustratingly elusive to produce because of inconsistent reporting and incomplete laboratory testing. Months later, for the annual EIS Conference skit in April 2015, I was asked to make a recording of increasingly impatient and expletive-ridden demands for an epidemic curve.

Nevertheless, we were able to piece together events characterizing Liberia's early struggle with Ebola.[30] I felt satisfied that we had made important public health contributions, the Incident Management System was operating, airport screening of travelers had been initiated by the CDC's Tai-Ho Chen, laboratory capacity had been increased, and good collaboration was underway for epidemiology.

Resurgence of Ebola had started in late May 2014 in Lofa County, a predominantly rural county bordering Guinea and Sierra Leone, and cases quickly began to be seen in Montserrado

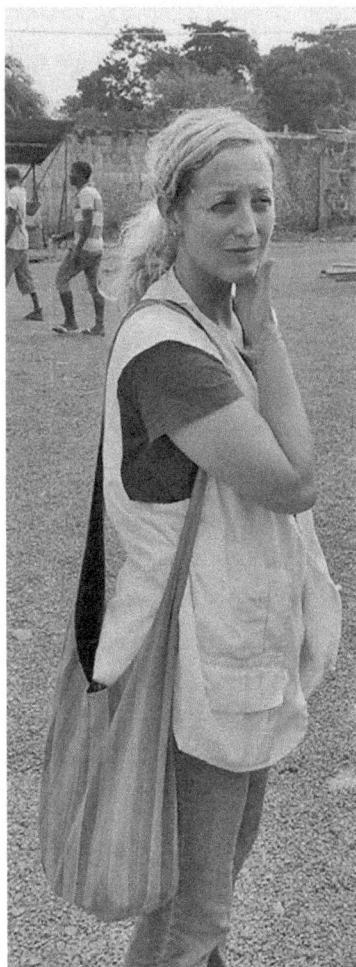

Figure 8.3   MSF Emergency
Coordinator Lindis Hurum.
(Kevin De Cock, personal collection)

County, which includes Monrovia. By August 15, 826 cases and 455
deaths (a 55% case fatality rate) had been reported. Just over half
of national cases were from Lofa, and just over a quarter were
from Montserrado. These two counties were reservoirs of infection for the rest of the country, where smaller Ebola clusters were
likely initiated by travelers and sometimes amplified in health
care settings. Only five of fifteen counties, predominantly those
in the hard-to-reach southeast, had reported no cases.

We summarized essentials for the CDC Atlanta headquarters, and here I later regretted adhering to protocol. I should have sent my summary to Director Frieden but instead went through channels, missing an opportunity to persuade him of the extent of the crisis earlier. Our recommendations covered data management (much more support was required, and the CDC's homegrown Epi Info program was cumbersome and not suitable for an epidemic of this magnitude); Ebola testing capacity (more was needed); coordination of field teams for specific technical areas such as case investigation, contact tracing, and burials (Atlanta's provision of staff needed to be better organized); patient care (more ETUs were needed, but investment in lower-level, but still safe, facilities would have to be considered in the face of unmanageable case numbers); and various other issues. Most importantly, we advocated for longer senior deployments, a county-based strategy with CDC teams allocated to each county, much greater investment in data management, and consideration of a CDC EOC in the field.

The events in the summer of 2014 in Liberia changed global perception of Ebola from a remote, tropical infection to a threat to global health security.[30] I warned colleagues that the epidemic might occupy the CDC for at least a year. As we left Monrovia in mid-August, we had no idea how this would all play out. The phrase that remained with me most strongly was uttered by Lindis Hurum, MSF's emergency coordinator. "There are three things you can never have too much of," she said, "chlorine, gloves, and body bags."

August–October 2014

A Worsening Crisis

Once I returned to Kenya, I received a supportive email from Tom Frieden whose tone suggested to me that Atlanta-based CDC staff were concerned about my judgment and thought I was exaggerating the situation. In a later CDC interview, to my irritation, Frieden said I was "imbalanced" from the experience.[11] I was not imbalanced; I was frustrated that I was unable to adequately convey the gravity of the situation, and I recommended that Frieden himself visit West Africa. His tour of the region in late August galvanized increased response, his communications when he returned to Atlanta very different: "I had never seen anything like I saw in West Africa. . . . It's like scenes from Dante."[11] When I spoke to him weeks later, he was gracious enough to say that he realized after his visit that everything we had said about the situation in Liberia in August was correct.

As the situation in Monrovia worsened, an ill-judged move by the government illustrated how Ebola could threaten the security of the state. West Point, a slum housing about seventy thousand people on the east side of the city, was placed under quarantine on August 22, 2014, with barbed wire and police and military forces preventing movement.[31] Residents protested, burning Ebola isolation facilities and associated supplies in their neighborhood. Further violence was triggered by inadequate access to food, water, and medicines resulting from the lockdown. The forces of order used tear gas and live ammunition to quell the rioting. It was quickly realized that communities had to be part of the Ebola response, and President Johnson Sirleaf backed down and lifted the blockade at the end of the month.

After his return from West Africa, Frieden immediately briefed the White House and on September 16, President Obama visited CDC headquarters in Atlanta, announcing increased assistance that included the deployment of some three thousand American troops to Liberia.[32] Cases in Liberia continued to increase and, in late September, Ebola reached America.

Thomas Duncan had had contact with an Ebola patient in Monrovia prior to traveling to the United States. He presented to

Dallas Presbyterian Hospital in Texas with fever, headache, and abdominal pain on September 25, 10 days after his exposure. He was sent away with antibiotics, only to present again, now more ill, days later, going on to die of Ebola on October 8. Two nurses became infected, both diagnosed the week after Duncan's demise. One had flown on a commercial airplane during her incubation period. Both nurses survived.

A firestorm erupted after these events, engulfing the CDC and its director.[33] Frieden had made two comments that were later perceived as injudicious. "Just to reiterate . . . essentially any hospital in the country can safely take care of Ebola," he said in a CDC briefing on October 2, 2014. He also suggested, perhaps impulsively, that that the nurses' infections must have resulted from a breach of protocol. The first comment seemed overpromising, and the second as blaming the nurses. The *New York Times* published a biting cartoon showing the CDC's director saying Ebola was transmitted by body fluids, blood, gaffes, and blunders. Until then, very visible in the media and usually a good communicator, Frieden disappeared from the airwaves for some time, with NIH's Anthony ("Tony") Fauci becoming ever more visible ([34]).

Frieden later told me that Fauci had been very supportive during this difficult period, and the latter recounts in his autobiography how he smoothed relations in Washington, DC, for the CDC. "I looked on Tom as sort of a very talented younger brother whom I had to defend every once in a while," wrote Fauci in a somewhat backhanded compliment that illustrated perceptions of agency hierarchies.[34]

Return to Liberia, November–December 2014

I arrived back in Liberia on November 9, 2014, after a circuitous flight on Royal Air Maroc, the only carrier apart from Belgium's Brussels Airlines still serving Monrovia. This interruption of air traffic to the affected countries of West Africa, imposed as a measure to restrict exportation of Ebola, hampered access for medical personnel and supplies.

I had just attended an HIV conference in Glasgow, where I was asked to step in for Columbia's Wafaa El-Sadr, who was to give the named Lock Lecture, supported by the Royal College of Physicians and Surgeons of Glasgow. El-Sadr was quarantined by her own university; she had just returned to New York after a brief visit to Sierra Leone and was instructed not to travel. That same week, the American Society of Tropical Medicine and Hygiene held its annual meeting in New Orleans, Louisiana, where the governor instructed that anyone from an Ebola-affected country was to stay away. These travel restrictions illustrated the irrational political responses taken, inconsistent with WHO and CDC guidance.

Liberia was a different place from the one I had left almost 3 months earlier. Despite epidemiologic uncertainty, different trends pointed to a declining epidemic. The fear and oppressive atmosphere I had sensed in August had gone, the state of emergency had been lifted, and the city felt more normal. Pressure was on to reopen the schools and plans for Senate elections in December were maintained. Joe Forrester and Satish Pillai, who had accepted my request that they redeploy, later commented on how it all seemed less stressful, despite individual concerns about security in the field.

The US Military

Blackhawk helicopters and Ospreys, the awkward craft that combined the attributes of a helicopter and turboprop, flew over Monrovia. The forces were from the Army's famed 101st Airborne Division under the command of Major General Gary Volesky, an officer with prior service in Iraq and Afghanistan. Lean and muscular, Volesky and his executive officer epitomized hardened soldiers, tough and of few words. US Ambassador Deborah Malac was visibly in the lead of American assistance, constantly interacting with the highest levels of the Liberian government. Mobilization of USAID's Disaster Assistance Response Team and the associated commitment of several hundred million dollars, the military deployment, the large CDC team, and establishment by the US uniformed Public Health Service of a sophisticated ETU for Ebola-infected health care workers from the region sent a clear message that the United States was there for Liberia.

The power of the military for construction of ETUs, training, and laboratory expansion was impressive. Disappointing, however, were the restrictions on troops' direct involvement in field work. When the possibility of military deployment was first discussed in August, including by MSF, I envisaged troops combing through communities looking for cases or assisting with contact tracing. In fact, they were under strict orders to avoid any situation where virus exposure was even remotely possible.

Our military colleagues were allowed to fly CDC staff into distant villages but not evacuate them after they had conducted their investigations, in case anyone had become infected. This was unnecessarily cautious because, even in the unlikely event of a CDC person acquiring infection, they would not yet be infectious. Sometimes this meant CDC workers had to hike for miles before being able to access transport back from remote field work. The military were also forbidden from transporting specimens, despite lengthy earlier discussions.[9,13]

I criticized this situation at a meeting of the Incident Management System, surprised later that the wide-ranging discussions had been recorded and leaked to the *New York Times*.[35] "Kevin, I'm very disappointed," Volesky said to me sternly. Despite these challenges, relations were generally excellent. One of my strongest memories is of flying in a Blackhawk helicopter over the Liberian rainforest with the doors open, reminiscent of war movies.

The Evolving Response

By now, the CDC was involved in the largest international response it had ever mounted, to Director Frieden's great credit; it would eventually draw in a cumulative total of more than three thousand staff, with more than twelve hundred deployed over time to the West African field.[36] The domestic and global political attention, EOC activation, and associated noise at CDC headquarters resulted in much of the energy and communication efforts flowing upward. In the field, with incessant demands for information and tighter control of deployed staff, we sometimes felt sight was being lost of what was happening on the ground.

The Incident Management System was functioning, even if not as streamlined as we originally intended. Tolbert Nyenswah was the incident manager and used his close connection to the presidency effectively, later writing a book about his experiences.[37,38] President Johnson Sirleaf remained closely involved, often calling Nyenswah for information and hosting a presidential advisory council in which the CDC participated. High-level international visitors trooped through town on a regular basis, including former British prime minister Tony Blair, WHO Director Margaret Chan, and UN Secretary General Ban Ki-moon (Figure 8.4). I sat next to Blair at an expanded partner meeting, impressed by the grip he held over the room with just brief remarks, his political charisma suggesting a British version of Bill Clinton.

Coordination of international assistance and of the almost one hundred different organizations operating in the Ebola response was challenging. WHO had replaced its country representatives in the three heavily affected countries, with Alex

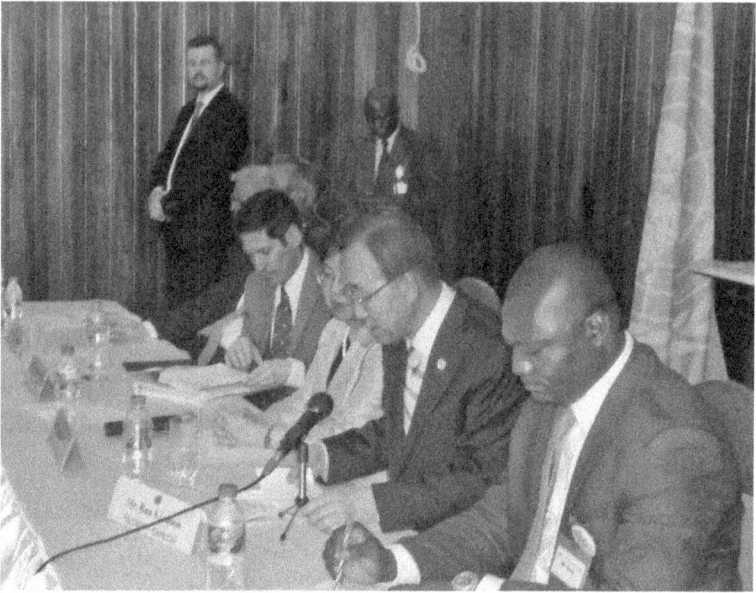

Figure 8.4   *Right to left:* Tolbert Nyenswah, Ban Ki-moon, Margaret Chan, Tom Frieden; Monrovia, December 2014.
(Kevin De Cock, personal collection)

Gasasira appointed the new WR in Monrovia.[39] His extensive previous experience and personal simplicity greatly facilitated collaboration between the CDC and WHO. Overall, however, WHO had been deemed slow to respond, and the UN secretary general had created the UN Mission for Emergency Ebola Response (UNMEER), the first ever UN emergency health mission.[40] UNMEER's role was to coordinate the overall Ebola response, but its organization and impact were unclear, and it was handicapped by having its headquarters in Accra, Ghana, far from the action. Adding in an extra layer of bureaucracy or a new coordination mechanism during an emergency is a desperate measure, and the move suggested lack of confidence in the existing structures such as WHO and the UN's Office for the Coordination of Humanitarian Affairs.

Frank Mahoney, a seasoned CDC epidemiologist highly effective in difficult situations, succeeded in streamlining daily decision-making. He persuaded the incident manager to convene a smaller group, consisting of staff from the Ministry of Health, UNMEER, WHO, the CDC, and USAID, henceforth referred to colloquially as "the Gang of Six." The group met early in the morning each day, ensuring coordinated activities, swift decision-making, and effective follow-up.

Epidemiology and Data Management

I took over as CDC lead from Frank Mahoney in November 2014. Earlier, he had been working in Nigeria on polio eradication and had been drafted into the Ebola response after Patrick Sawyer's journey to Lagos in July and the subsequent events. The CDC team in Liberia now consisted of some fifty-five people requiring a different management approach from our exploratory deployment in July. We now had specialists in diverse subjects and had to ensure appropriate liaison with multiple collaborators. Our earlier recommendation on the need for county-specific responses was acted upon, and staff were deployed to more than half the counties to work with local authorities and other partners.

Principal technical areas of focus included epidemiology and data management, border screening, IPC, laboratory coordination, dead-body management, and contact tracing. The work was more supervisory, the atmosphere more "normal." If the question in July had been "how big is this?" it now seemed "how small is this?" because cases had declined so precipitously.

The CDC was looked to for assuring data quality, but in each of the three heavily affected West African countries, data challenges persisted. The CDC's homegrown viral hemorrhagic fever data management application, the Epi Info VHF, was impossibly labor intensive for such a large outbreak, but its VSPB proponents remained reluctant to accept this.[41]. Peter Graaff, UN-MEER's director in Liberia, invited the famous Hans Rosling to come and advise, a veiled criticism of the CDC's data efforts.

Rosling was professor of Global Health at Sweden's Karolinska Institute, a member of the Swedish Academy of Sciences, an internet sensation with his TED Talks and YouTube videos, and a sword-swallower.[42,43] He proudly told me he was the eighth most followed scientist on the internet and had more than two hundred thousand Twitter (now called X) followers (almost four times more than Tom Frieden, he gleefully informed me). Rosling later exchanged heated words with Frieden concerning the CDC's Ebola modeling, which predicted (without interventions) 1.4 million cases in Liberia and Sierra Leone by late January 2015. He implied, to Frieden's irritation, that political and budgetary considerations had influenced the exercise.[44,45]

The CDC modeling had led me to being interviewed for *PBS Newshour* on the likelihood of Ebola spreading further afield.[46] The most important aspect of the model, however, concerned containment: if 70% of infectious cases were rapidly isolated, thus preventing further spread, the model predicted the epidemic would be controlled. This usefully focused attention on rapidity of case isolation as a key indicator of Ebola response performance.

Rosling inserted himself into a central role in the Ebola Surveillance Unit, dominating discussions and presentations in a professorial fashion. Despite imperfect health, his commitment and impact were unquestionable. He was harsh but humorous in his criticism of the CDC's short deployments and restrictions, likening the agency to Cuba ("nice people, terrible system"). Concerning the VHF Epi Info application, Rosling described it as "an antiquity—to be preserved but not used." He stayed in Liberia until January 2015, garnering widespread affection and respect locally for his commitment and simplicity. I was touched but saddened when he wrote to inform me in 2016 that he had been diagnosed with pancreatic cancer, from which he died a year later.

With fewer daily cases and more staff, linking disparate data became feasible. Bawo and Rosling drove an important innovation, starting all data reporting and analysis from individual positive laboratory tests and then linking those results to diffuse information available from ETUs and other sources, such as dead-body registers. Finally, we had a more accurate view of Ebola incidence and trends, and meaningful epidemic curves. All indicators showed reductions in new cases. In addition, there was a declining prevalence of Ebola infection in tested cadavers, a surveillance approach we proposed.

Ray Ransom and Terrence ("Terry") Lo worked feverishly with Rosling and Luke Bawo to improve data systems. Basic footwork— "shoe leather epidemiology"—by Paul Weidle, Michael Beach, and others convincingly showed, with Rosling orchestrating the presentations, that by mid-December 2014, about ten laboratory-confirmed cases were being recognized daily across the country, two-thirds of them from Montserrado County. The epidemic was drastically reduced but not finished, and it was now concentrated in the capital city.

The single explanation for reduced Ebola incidence from October 2014 onward was more effective and rapid isolation of cases, thanks to massive expansion of ETU beds, which, by early November, numbered almost seven hundred.[47] International commitments subsequently suffered from lack of flexibility in the face of changing epidemiology, which Rosling loudly criticized. Continued ETU construction began to yield empty beds while the epidemic became one of more widespread but isolated, smaller eruptions of infection (Figure 8.5).

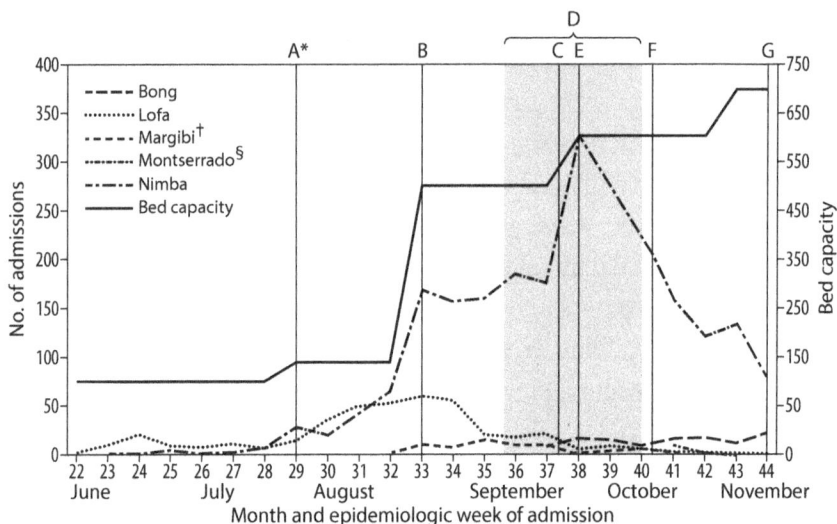

Figure 8.5 ETU bed capacity and numbers of patients admitted by county and week, June 5–November 1, 2014.

(MMWR Morb Mortal Wkly Rep. 2014;63:1082–1086. Erratum in: MMWR Morb Mortal Wkly Rep. 2014;63:1094)

Monrovia and Hot Spots

A new epidemiologic pattern was of sudden clusters of Ebola, sometimes in extremely remote villages, often initiated by a traveler from Monrovia. Kim Lindblade[48] commented: "As Montserrado goes, so goes Liberia," to which another colleague added, "And as Guinea goes, so goes the region." Both comments were fundamentally correct. Addressing these hot spots was demanding because villages were sometimes accessible only on foot or by helicopter.

I flew to Rivercess County to drop off two colleagues and pick two others up, humbled by how they had lived in tents in this forest area for almost 2 weeks. The villagers had initially been resistant but accepted Ebola assistance after thirteen people had died. EIS Officer Jose Laguana's investigation showed that thirty-three cases arose from one woman who had travelled from Monrovia and initiated infections in Grand Bassa and Rivercess Counties. He developed an illustration on his computer in the bush, combining information on transmission links, the locations where they occurred, dates of events, whether cases were confirmed, whether patients survived, and more. It would have served as an extraordinary teaching tool.

A strategy entitled RITE, Rapid Isolation and Treatment of Ebola, was developed to address hot spots.[49,50] After experience with a dozen such events, time to case isolation and safe burials decreased, numbers of transmission chains decreased, and time to extinction of outbreaks shortened. Kim Lindblade presented a slide of preliminary analyses that so impressed Tom Frieden that he used it in a briefing for President Obama. Despite the progress made, results were not equally good everywhere. In Grand Bassa County, Satish Pilai and Kristin Yeoman were pursued by machete-wielding men and had to run for half an hour to get away.

Although the basic strategy for Monrovia was the same as elsewhere, tactics had to be different. An Incident Management System for Montserrado County was established, the aim being to greatly strengthen local case detection and contact tracing. A persistent concern was the occurrence of unsafe burials that posed a risk to all who touched highly infectious cadavers. On August 6, 2014, the government had controversially decreed that all dead bodies in Monrovia should be cremated, not buried.[51] The original reason was twofold: to reduce risk of Ebola transmission and because of lack of safe burial capacity in Monrovia.

The high water table combined with heavy seasonal rains in August had resulted in macabre scenes of buried bodies floating upward above the earth's surface. We now heard rumors of bodies being exported from the city, such as from the waterfront slum of West Point, by canoe at night. Teams found that when they arrived to conduct a so-called safe and dignified burial, the body often had already been dressed or buried. From estimating the number of deaths expected in Monrovia, we surmised that not more than one-third of dead bodies were being collected by trained teams.

An innovative investigation was testing cadavers for Ebola through the use of oral swabs. Intense work was conducted to track Ebola infection rates in cadavers, assess burial trends, investigate attitudes, and sensitize communities to the dangers involved. This was an unusual opportunity for field work and research to translate quickly into public health policy and operational guidance. Manisha ("Mo") Patel was so captivated by the work, which was on the cusp of leading to major policy changes, that she extended her deployment, as several other team members had done in other areas of work.

I had a memorable conversation with Mosoka Fallah, a charismatic Liberian professional who had voluntarily returned from the United States to work on the epidemic.[52] In a group discussion he said that many people preferred to risk Ebola over seeing loved ones cremated. He animatedly explained the deep-seated attitudes concerning links to the dead, beliefs of continuity with ancestors, and the duty to honor and visit human remains. Cremation brutally ruptured these traditions and was culturally offensive; people were more affected by a body being burned, Fallah recounted, than by the death of the relative concerned. Weeks before I had bumped into Michael ("Mike") Ryan, a veteran of many Ebola outbreaks with WHO. He told me that he always included an anthropologist in his initial investigational teams to gain an early understanding of local cultures.

Leaving Liberia, December 2014

I left Liberia on December 19 after a 6-week deployment. Perhaps my most important feeling was one of admiration for the CDC deployers, their *esprit de corps*, and their technical excellence. Several were close friends and colleagues, like Larry Slutsker, who had acted as my deputy, and a disproportionate number of them over recent months had previously served in Kenya, which sometimes aroused unjustified comments that Kenya veterans were being favored for Liberian service. Another CDC Kenya veteran, Barbara Marston, was serving in the EOC at CDC headquarters coordinating international deployments to West Africa.[53] I appreciated Mike Ryan, the former WHO staff member, commenting when I met him in Sierra Leone, that it was MSF and the CDC "that had carried the water" in the response in West Africa.

If we had witnessed exponential growth of the epidemic in Liberia in the summer, Ebola's decline was equally precipitous. In late November 2014, the US embassy in Freetown invited me to brief Sierra Leone's President Koroma on lessons learned in Liberia*.[54] The president and many others were asking what explained Liberia's apparent success while the situation in Sierra Leone, and especially in the capital, was deteriorating. USAID's Justin Pendarvis and I travelled to Freetown and met with US embassy leadership, President Koroma and his senior advisors, and senior UK officials.

My suspicion that Freetown had delayed isolating the sick while waiting for ideal ETUs to be constructed was validated by a question from the head of their case management group. He asked what the ideal ratio was of ETU to case holding beds. I commented diplomatically that I did not see the issue in those terms; the pri-

---

* The US ambassador in Freetown was John Hoover, with whom I had worked some years before at the US embassy in Nairobi.

ority was to isolate patients immediately and offer whatever care one could under the local circumstances, and the key was early isolation.[55]

End of the Ebola Epidemic in Liberia

I arrived in Liberia for my third deployment on March 6, 2015. Ebola still had lessons to teach, this final visit giving insight into sexual transmission and the importance of survivors. Once again, I took over from Frank Mahoney, who, in the early new year, led innovative interventions for the last large, and difficult, cluster of Ebola.

The husband of a fatal Ebola case patient had collapsed in the street in the deprived Monrovia area of Red Light in mid-January 2015. Two youths, dubbed the "Good Samaritans," assisted him. Despite their biblical name, the Good Samaritans were drug-using gang members, one of whom shortly thereafter was stabbed by another member of the group. Roaming around the area over the next 2 days, the stabbing victim visited several health facilities, infected at least one health worker, exposed others, and died alone in a warehouse where he had sought refuge. The other Good Samaritan became symptomatic, was admitted to an ETU, and survived. The St. Paul Bridge cluster, as this came to be called, involved 22 Ebola cases over three generations of transmission, 15 deaths, and follow-up of 745 contacts.[56]

Exceptional field work by Fallah, Mahoney, and other staff resulted in vigorous support from the local community (Figure 8.6). Trusted interactions with group members who sported gang names like Spoiler and Time Bomb facilitated their successful quarantine (their detention was diplomatically referred to as "voluntary precautionary observation") without further Ebola transmission. In a National Public Radio interview, Mahoney described

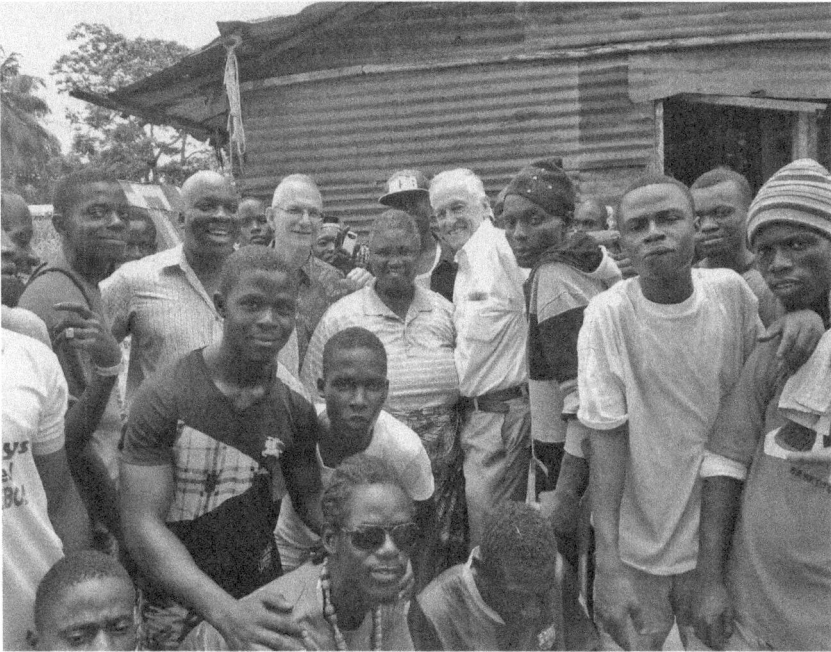

Figure 8.6   Field visit, Monrovia, March 2015.
(Kevin De Cock, personal collection)

the unorthodox approaches he and his colleagues used, including addressing the gang's drug-using requirements[57] in a way not covered in their dry epidemiologic report of the cluster.[56]

The CDC began to invest in longer-term staff in Liberia, analogous to my position in Kenya, assigning Desmond Williams[58] as lead. He and I attended Decoration Day celebrations in 2015 at the Presbyterian Cathedral in Monrovia, held annually on the second Wednesday of March to honor dead ancestors. Ebola was largely considered over, and the occasion was a memorable demonstration of Liberian resilience and spirited singing. "Because they died, because they died," thundered the officiating pastor, as he paid tribute to those who had perished from Ebola, urging congregants to meet their responsibilities and "talk to the man in the mirror."

"May we pause to remember all of those who lost their lives during this Ebola crisis; I say they were heroes and not victims," he boomed. "Had they not died, the international community would not have come. Had they not died the US government would not have sent all the US Marines they sent. . . . They did not die in vain." His words conveyed what is often overlooked, that many of those who became infected with Ebola likely did so through acts of love or assistance to family, friends, and even strangers who were sick. Williams and I were deeply moved by the event.

Ebola Survivors

Countries are declared Ebola-free when no further cases have occurred over 42 days, twice the maximum incubation period, and Liberia seemed on the road to success. Athalia Christie and I, while visiting Freetown, Sierra Leone, for discussions in late March 2015, were dismayed to receive a phone call reporting a new case. A 44-year-old woman was diagnosed with Ebola on March 20, 2015, and died 1 week later. Intense investigations of her circumstances failed to identify a source of infection or possible exposure. One intriguing finding was that she had had vaginal intercourse with an Ebola survivor 1 week before her symptom onset. In the absence of any other explanation, we wondered whether this was a case of sexual transmission.

Ebola was known to be able to survive in sanctuary sites and to be present in semen for as long as 82 days.[59] Sexual transmission, however, had not been reported, and precautionary health guidance after recovery from Ebola was to avoid sex or use a condom for 3 months. The survivor in question in Monrovia had been ill more than 6 months before. By coincidence, a filovirus meeting was going on in Washington, DC, around this time, attended by leading subject matter experts, some of whom had heard rumors about this case and were dismissive of our thinking.

As it turned out, a semen specimen from the survivor was positive for Ebola on PCR testing 199 days after his likely disease onset. Genomic sequencing of Ebola in the woman patient's blood specimen showed unique mutations that matched those in the genomic fragments derived from her partner, essentially proving sexual transmission (Frieden still insisted we temper the discussion by referring to "*possible* sexual transmission").

International conference calls were rapidly organized involving the CDC, WHO, and the Liberian health ministry. An article for the *MMWR* was urgently prepared, with Christie as the first author, to report this case and advise prolonged condom use or abstinence after recovery from Ebola.[60] More detailed analysis was published in the *New England Journal of Medicine*.[61] The implications of this case, borne out by later events, were that a declaration of freedom from Ebola after 42 days could not guarantee that there would not be local instances of resurgent transmission from survivors.

WHO declared Liberia Ebola-free in May and September 2015, but each time, local resurgences occurred, with similar experiences described in Sierra Leone and Guinea. We defined three priorities in the final stages of the Liberian epidemic: ensuring rapid detection of reintroduced or resurgent Ebola, strengthening IPC in health care settings, and re-establishing regular health services. Ensuring no missed diagnoses required sensitizing health care staff and communities to report suspected cases, continuing oral swabbing of dead bodies, monitoring health care workers for disease, and ensuring screening at the borders—all very challenging. Although unmeasured, more people may have died from suspension of care for maternal and child health and other health services than from Ebola itself, so return to normality in the health sector was urgent.

Ebola transmission in the region finally ceased in 2016. A new phenomenon was that of Ebola survivors, of whom there may have been close to twenty thousand across the region. A later regional analysis identified thirteen possible instances of Ebola transmission events from survivors, one resulting in four generations of cases.[62] Almost two-thirds of male survivors still had Ebola in semen at 4–6 months after illness, and one-quarter at 7–9 months, with declining proportions out to 18 months.[63] A case was reported of an HIV-positive Ebola survivor whose semen remained positive 565 days after recovery.[64] Later experience in Guinea showed that much later outbreaks might result from reactivated transmission.[65]

Almost half of survivors complained of one or more lingering symptoms affecting joints, vision, and mental health, all significantly more frequent than in control individuals.[66] Most striking were ocular abnormalities that included uveitis and cataracts, requiring specialist ophthalmological care. Several cases were reported of Ebola persistence in sanctuary sites such as the eye or brain in repatriated Northern Hemisphere health care workers,[67,68] making me wonder how often this might have gone undetected in West Africa. Equally or more detrimental to survivors were persistent stigma and discrimination that extended to families, the workplace, and housing. Clustering of Ebola in households resulted in a high incidence of orphanhood. Unexpected to me, some of these social effects were reminiscent of those associated with HIV, despite the extreme differences in the epidemiology and natural history of these two pathogens.

2015 and Onward

The urgency of addressing the epidemic overshadowed the question of research and its requirements. I facilitated discussions between the Liberian Ministry of Health and Social Welfare and the NIH concerning opportunities for research on Ebola as early as August 2014, linking Chief Medical Officer Berenice Dahn with my friend from HIV work, Cliff Lane, a senior scientist at NIH.[69,70] By end of 2014, many discussions had been held and protocols prepared, but specific research had not started despite discussions with President Johnson Sirleaf about the urgency of such investigations. Ebola incidence in Liberia had declined to such an extent by then that meaningful evaluation of interventions was no longer possible, though valuable research was conducted among survivors. Important results on vaccine and therapeutic interventions came from Guinea[71,72,73] and, years later, from the DRC.

WHO lifted its declaration of a Public Health Emergency of International Concern (PHEIC) on March 29, 2016. The CDC officially stood down its West African Ebola response on March 31, 2016 while continuing to provide field support. Ebola continued to grumble; the last known cluster of thirteen cases extended from late February to April 2016. It likely resulted from transmission from a survivor in Guinea with nine more cases locally and three related cases in travelers to Monrovia.[74] The West African epidemic of Ebola was considered over on June 9, 2016, after the occurrence of an estimated 28,646 cases and 11,323 deaths.[8] These estimates are probably lower than the true incidence and mortality, and accuracy of the available epidemic curves is uncertain.

How Did This Happen?

Inevitable questions arose after this unprecedented public health disaster. How did this happen, who was to blame, and how do we prevent this from happening again? Numerous after-action analyses and reports were published by multilateral, bilateral, civil society, and other groups, with one unifying conclusion: "never again." If there were heroes in this saga, it was the frontline responders, recognized as "Person of the Year" in an extraordinary gesture by *Time* magazine in its 2014 annual issue depicting the person who most influenced global events over the prior year.[75]

MSF received credit as the single organization that beat the drum to attract global attention from March 2014.

Reasons that the rest of the world delayed acting are various. The three affected countries of West Africa were isolated and neglected, events there seemed of little relevance to the rest of the world, and the sheer power and implications of unchecked spread of Ebola were underestimated. WHO was deemed in charge; because it did not ask for assistance, no measures seemed necessary. And Ebola outbreaks over the past 40 years had always been remote and quickly contained.

The West African epidemic showed the limitations of WHO's constitution and functioning, which promote independence of regional offices from headquarters. WHO in Geneva delayed declaring a PHEIC until August 2014, a declaration that demands a coordinated international response. Frieden had described tension and competitiveness from WHO concerning deployment of CDC staff to the West African field earlier in the year.[75] WHO's Regional Office for Africa overestimated and overemphasized its capacity and autonomy—basically, turf issues were responsible for earlier rejection of assistance from WHO headquarters as well as the CDC. Peter Piot, then director of the London School of Hygiene and Tropical Medicine, and codiscoverer of Ebola virus during the Yambuku outbreak, was harsher. "It's the regional office in Africa that's the front line," said Piot. "And they didn't do anything. That office is really not competent."

WHO's global role combined with its reluctance to share global health space heaped disproportionate blame on the agency. WHO's modest funding and limited autonomy contrast with the high expectations the world has of the organization, especially in times of crisis. WHO is managed by a secretariat reporting to member states, so, ultimately, member states should remember that they are responsible for WHO's funding, management, and functioning. Simply blaming WHO and its regional office in this saga is too easy and ignores committed and technically excellent work by many of its staff.

Of all the reports and recommendations emanating from the West Africa Ebola experience, perhaps the most powerful was that from the Harvard–London School of Hygiene and Tropical Medicine panel on the global response to Ebola, published in the *Lancet* in late 2015.[76] Ten overarching recommendations covered prevention, response, science and technology, and governance, providing a framework for epidemic and pandemic preparedness. Cynics might say that some of this was old wine in new bottles, that we had heard much of this before, and doubtless would again. Warnings of epidemic threats and emerging infectious diseases had been made loudly over many years.[77-79]

Parting Thoughts

I emphasized to colleagues I supervised that the control of Ebola was simple, but that simple was not the same as easy. In addition, unmeasured, and therefore unseen, were the secondary effects of the epidemic in health and beyond. Disruption of routine public health programs must have cost many lives, perhaps even more than from Ebola itself. On the other hand, Ebola offered opportunity for substantial strengthening of public health capacity in the heavily affected countries.[80] Two deficiencies evident early in the epidemic were gross underinvestment in data management and in real-time laboratory capacity.

Although the urgent priority was containment of the Ebola outbreak, it is essential that we learn as much as possible from these dire situations. This requires that research infrastructure and all that entails—from regulatory and ethical requirements, to investigators, commodities and logistics—be ready for immediate evaluation of therapeutic, prevention, and other interventions before the epidemic in question peaks.

Open-mindedness is required. "Common things occur commonly" is a maxim in clinical medicine, but when large numbers of cases of a disease occur, uncommon things may be uncovered. Subject matter experts may be especially reluctant to question "truths" that seemed inviolate in smaller epidemics. New observations about survivors, including persistent morbidity and potential later infectiousness, were cases in point. Another dogma to question is whether asymptomatic Ebola infections can occur and be a source of transmission.[81]

Sometimes specialized expertise leads to rigidity and difficulty accepting the need for broader involvement. I sensed frustration among hemorrhagic fever specialists at their loss of total control in West Africa, different from their absolute independence in smaller Ebola epidemics.[13] At the same time, the sorely needed expertise that characterizes groups like the CDC's VSPB is priceless and needs to be maintained and promoted. With greater visibility and funding for global health overall, specialized science needs to be better integrated into programmatic functioning. CDC's categorical funding and subject-organized structure too often lead to tension and competitiveness between groups, impeding a coordinated "one CDC" approach in international work.[82]

Especially jarring and incompletely resolved were issues related to inequity in access to care. Following the precedent of the Samaritan's Purse staff being evacuated from Liberia in August 2014, international responders who acquired Ebola were systematically repatriated. By contrast, African staff who became infected were treated locally.[83] WHO estimates that more than five hundred health care workers died during the epidemic.

To address, at least in part, this stark dichotomy, the US government constructed and staffed a temporary twenty-five-bed hospital in Monrovia (The Monrovia Medical Unit) to care for regional health care workers with Ebola.[84] As with research studies, the epidemic had largely subsided by the time the unit became operational. Therapeutic and technical advances years later have improved the quality of patient management in the field, lessening, if not eliminating, the inequities encountered.

The CDC's large field deployment forced the agency to reconsider organizational and logistic support. With the West African epidemic being discussed at the White House and by the National Security Council, the somewhat "gung-ho" approach of the EIS program of earlier years was challenged. Patricia ("Pattie") Simone oversaw EIS and highlighted need for greater attention to the health and security of deployers.[85] She recounted how she insisted on repatriating one EIS officer who had been exposed to a febrile WHO staff member who later died of Ebola. At the height of the epidemic, community exposure was always a possibility and scrupulous attention to distancing and avoiding physical contact was important. Ebola challenged the old paradigm that EIS officers should be able and allowed to deploy alone, anywhere, and just get the job done.

For me, Ebola in West Africa felt like coming full circle in my CDC career, because I had started as an EIS officer in VSPB. I emphasized to younger CDC colleagues that this Ebola epidemic and its demands were exceptional and historic. I mused on this, having met with the presidents of two countries to discuss their epidemic situations and having given numerous global press interviews, none of this typical in an outbreak response.

Responders were affected personally by their experiences in the West African Ebola epidemic. A rich resource, amply drawn upon in this narrative and to which I also contributed, [86] are oral histories captured by Samuel ("Sam") Robson in the Global Health Chronicles under the auspices of the CDC Museum and Emory University.[87] "You can leave Liberia, but Liberia cannot leave you," said one colleague. I had to agree.

CHAPTER 9

Ebola in the Democratic Republic of the Congo

Following the epidemic of Ebola in West Africa, numerous after-action commentaries, promises, and preparedness plans appeared, conveying the single message that such events should never happen again. An international effort initiated by the United States in 2014 just before the Ebola outbreak, the Global Health Security Agenda,[1] seemed ever more relevant. The initiative brought together some seventy countries to commit to epidemic preparedness under the rubric "prevent, detect, respond." So-called action packages targeted specific improvements in areas such as laboratory and surveillance capacity. The aims were laudable, but the situation on the ground in remote areas of Africa was little changed.

The Democratic Republic of the Congo and the Tenth Ebola Outbreak

Ebola has been irrevocably associated with the DRC. By end of 2022, 46 years after Ebola's first recognition in Yambuku in the Équateur Province,[2] a total of fifteen discrete outbreaks of Ebola had been described in this vast country that is the size of western Europe.[3] I had resumed my full-time position in Kenya after the Liberian deployments during 2014–2015 and had been asked to stay on beyond the usual maximum of 6 years as director in one country. In mid-2019, Rebecca Martin, incumbent in my former position as director of the Center for Global Health in Atlanta, asked me to take on the role of senior advisor from Kenya and engage in the now-year-old epidemic of Ebola in eastern DRC.

Whereas first contact in Liberia required the CDC's immediate hands-on engagement in the field, involvement in the DRC was wholly different. In this year-long epidemic, managing relationships, looking for opportunities, and seeking technical areas for useful engagement were the essentials of complex diplomacy. We were one agency among many. If the work in Liberia had been technical more than political, the reverse was often the case in the DRC.

This tenth Ebola outbreak in the DRC came to attention in early August 2018 with the report of cases from Mangina in North Kivu Province, in the eastern part of the country.[4] A year later, almost three thousand cases had been reported, with a case fatality rate of 64%, meaning this was the second largest and second longest-lasting outbreak of Ebola ever described, after the West African epidemic. In addition to North Kivu, the province of Ituri also had become affected, these areas approximating to the combined sizes of Liberia and Sierra Leone (Figure 9.1). The total population of these provinces amounted to more than thirteen million, exceeding that of Guinea.

The World Health Organization had watched the epidemic in the DRC but waited to declare it a Public Health Emergency of International Concern (PHEIC), believing it was unlikely to spread geographically. That changed on July 14, 2019, when a visiting priest from North Kivu was diagnosed with Ebola in the regional capital of Goma.[5] This densely populated city of about three-quarters of a million people lies on the shores of Lake Kivu, borders Rwanda, and has an international airport. WHO declared a PHEIC 3 days later. A second, unrelated Ebola death occurred in

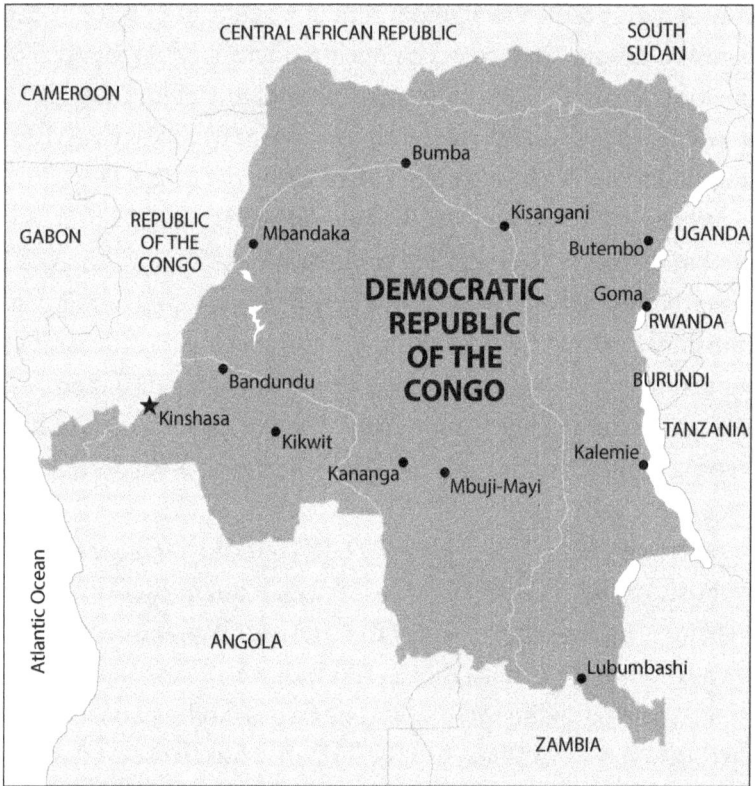

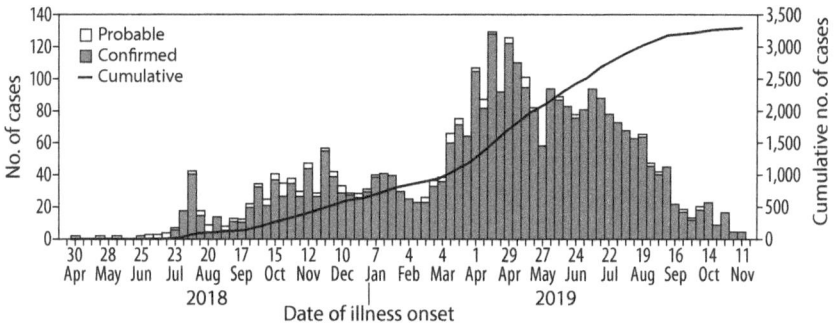

Figure 9.1 (a) Map of the Democratic Republic of the Congo.
(b) Epidemic curve of Ebola cases, Democratic Republic of the Congo,
April 2018–November 2019.

(MMWR 2019;68:1162-1165)

Goma later that month in an artisanal miner who had been work-ing hundreds of kilometers away in Ituri Province but who had traveled back by motorcycle when ill.

If logistics and travel were difficult in West Africa, the situation in the DRC proved even more challenging. The DRC is fabulously rich in natural resources and minerals but appallingly poor in infra-structure and development. This huge country has a population of about one hundred million people, shares land borders with nine other countries, but has only a few thousand kilometers of roads. The imposing River Congo stretches north and east from Kinshasa, offering a vital transport route that links the capital with Kisangani, almost certainly the unnamed town in V.S. Naipaul's classic book *A Bend in the River*.[6] Travel to much of the country must be by air.

The DRC's turbulent history following its independence from Belgium in 1960 was accentuated by massive population displace-ment from Rwanda into the eastern DRC after the genocide of 1993–1994.[7,8] Perpetrators of the genocide, as well as its victims, were among the displaced, and strife and tension within Rwanda, Burundi, and Uganda all spilled over into their giant neighbor. Militias sprung up, supported to greater or lesser degrees by these other countries. The undeclared wars that started in the 1990s eventually involved numerous regional powers and resulted in about six million deaths, with the eastern part of the country never regaining stability. Eastern Congo's natural resources, including gold, diamonds, cobalt, and coltan, provide a strong incentive for persistent engagement in the region by Uganda, Rwanda, and their militaries.

Kinshasa

While working in-country, US government employees, including CDC staff, are under the authority of the US ambassador, which, in 2019, was Michael (Mike) Hammer, a short, stout man with strong opinions. I had visited the embassy residence on the River Congo while conducting HIV research in 1986 and remembered an impressive house bordering the river. The residence and its environs now seemed drab, like much of the rest of the city.

Security of all official Americans is the responsibility of the regional security officer (RSO), and the absolute priority for all the RSO's staff is assuring nothing adverse happen to long- or short-term employees. In the DRC, this meant that much of the country was off-limits, especially in the troubled eastern region. Unfortunately, that was where the Ebola outbreak was occurring.

Reading material on the websites of Western embassies yielded similar advice about travel. Large parts of the DRC, especially eastern Congo, were to be avoided because of fighting, civil unrest, or risk of terrorism and kidnapping. Fighting between different militia groups, government forces, and, to a lesser extent, United Nations peacekeepers, was a constant in eastern Congo. As the epidemic worsened, WHO Director Tedros was quoted saying, "The world has never seen anything like this," referring to this Ebola outbreak in what resembled a war zone.[9]

The Ministry of Health held meetings in Kinshasa to discuss the epidemic, but health workers dealing with the outbreak in the field were thousands of kilometers away, and communications were poor. The strongest technical institute in the DRC is the Institut National de la Recherche Biomédicale (INRB), led by the internationally renowned microbiologist Jean-Jacques Muyembe-Tamfun. Muyembe was the first responder in the 1976 epidemic of Ebola in Yambuku,[2] has participated in every Congolese Ebola outbreak since then, and has played a leading role in all aspects of health and medical education throughout the country's turbulent history. If there were a Nobel Prize in public health, Muyembe would be a reputable contender.

Like every institution, INRB was rife with politics and rivalries, especially concerning the future direction of the agency and succession planning for Muyembe, then in his late 70s. These tensions were largely invisible from the outside, and I only gleaned them from different international colleagues who were long-term collaborators with the INRB. The institute was well resourced by international donors, and the staff were highly trained and competent. A large poster on the INRB wall showed Muyembe receiving one of his many international prizes, the Christophe Mérieux Prize, and an honorary doctorate.

As I started this deployment, the Ministry of Health put Muyembe in charge of controlling the epidemic. I had met him several times over the years, including during HIV meetings at WHO headquarters in Geneva. His senior staff knew Belgian and French colleagues with whom I had interacted, and they had quietly sounded me out. These personal contacts and the institutional weight of the CDC meant we had good access to senior Congolese colleagues. At the same time, however, the many competing interests from different countries and agencies meant that the prime position the CDC held in Liberia did not materialize here. Muyembe skillfully orchestrated his private and public benefactors and collaborators knocking at his door. Although he valued and respected longstanding relationships such as with the CDC's Inger Damon for monkeypox* work, he was his own man.

Ambassador Hammer courted Muyembe and pressured the CDC to place a technical advisor in the INRB. This was unrealistic because epidemic information was not concentrated at the institute, the role for such an advisor was not clear, and Muyembe and his staff did not want it. I argued with Hammer that what was needed was visibility on what was going on in eastern Congo, the beginning of an approval process for me to accompany a United Nations mission into the interior.

---

* In November 2022, WHO recommended that monkeypox be renamed mpox.

United Nations Politics

WHO had been heavily criticized, sometimes unfairly, for its delayed response to the earlier Ebola crisis in West Africa and was determined to escape the lingering skepticism about its capacity. WHO had been stung by the creation in September 2014 of UNMEER that resulted from discussions at the UN General Assembly and the Security Council.[10] The head of UNMEER was a special representative of the secretary general, and the initiative was designated as a new emergency health mission. UNMEER was closed at the end of July 2015. Whether it was successful is debatable, but what was clear was that UNMEER's creation was an expression by the UN's of lack of confidence in its own specialist health agency, WHO, to manage the West African Ebola crisis.

The ninth outbreak of Ebola in the DRC, earlier in 2018, in classic Ebola territory of Équateur Province on the other side of the country, was rapidly contained, with only fifty-four cases and thirty-three deaths.[11] This gave WHO a false sense of security that more of the same, with overwhelming resources, was all that was needed. The outbreak in eastern DRC, the tenth outbreak, was different.

After almost a year of epidemic activity and more than one thousand deaths, Ebola presented more than a health challenge. Instability and violence, displaced populations, lack of roads, inhospitable terrain, poor infrastructure, and difficult logistics characterized the environment. The possibility that Ebola would be exported across porous borders to Uganda and Rwanda was a constant concern.

In May 2019, the UNMEER scenario repeated itself. Recognizing that a multidisciplinary approach was needed to provide stronger humanitarian relief, political engagement, security, and overall coordination, the UN secretary general appointed an Emergency Ebola Response coordinator (EERC). He selected

David Gressly, a senior official from the UN peacekeeping operation.[12] Gressly was the deputy director of the Mission de l'Organisation des Nations Unies pour la stabilisation en République démocratique du Congo (MONUSCO), the UN stabilization mission focused on eastern DRC. Often criticized and controversial, MONUSCO had an operating budget of approximately US$1 billion per year, and had more than fifteen thousand military and police personnel. It was the biggest and most expensive peacekeeping intervention in the UN's history.

The DRC's Ministry of Health and international partners were now collaborating under the fourth version of a strategic response plan.[13] The plan aimed to integrate five response pillars: (1) public health, (2) political engagement and security, (3) support to communities, (4) financial planning and management, and (5) preparedness for surrounding countries. The proposed budget for the period July to December 2019 amounted to US$500 million. The novelty of the plan was integration of approaches across the various pillars and enhancement of community engagement and support, which were inadequately prioritized early on. The essentials of Ebola control such as rapid case isolation were unchanged, but one technical novelty was availability of a vaccine. Particularly important was to assure synergy between the public health pillar and provision of security and safety for response workers.

Just as with UNMEER, the authority and expectations of the EERC vis-à-vis the overall response, and specifically WHO, were imprecisely defined. WHO's lead in the field was the Assistant Director General for Emergency Response, the Senegalese Ibrahima Socé Fall, who was considered of equal rank to Gressly (Figure 9.2). WHO insisted it oversaw the health response and expected Gressly to solve everything else, especially security. Gressly felt his mandate concerned all aspects of Ebola. He considered it his prerogative to intervene in health sector work as

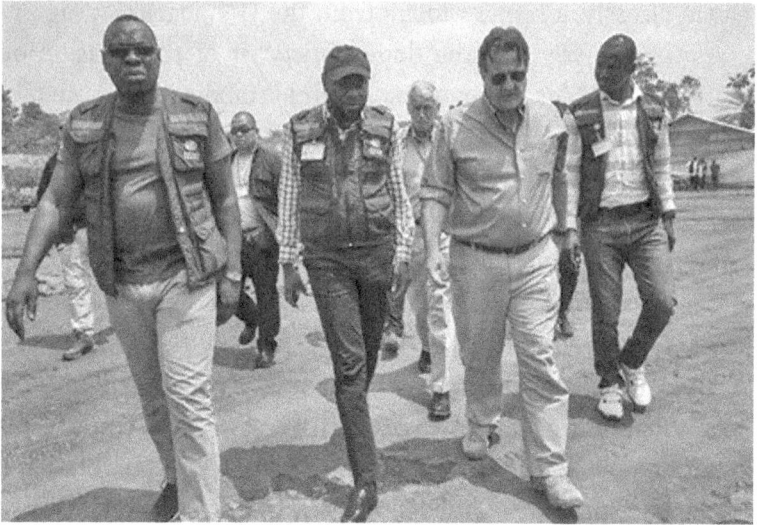

Figure 9.2   United Nations response: *Left to right, front*: Ibrahima Socé Fall, WHO; Michel Yao, WHO; David Gressly, Emergency Ebola Response coordinator.
(Kevin De Cock, personal collection)

necessary, including criticizing aspects of the health response he felt deficient. Tension between the EERC and WHO was palpable.

North Kivu

While political and diplomatic power was concentrated in Kinshasa, the epicenter for Ebola was far away. United Nations agencies, including WHO, UNICEF, the World Bank, and others, as well as different nongovernmental organizations (NGOs) such as MSF, had established their base in Goma. I felt it imperative to see the epidemic zone firsthand and strove to accompany David Gressly on a rapid tour of North Kivu Province.

I was astonished at the complexities of approval required—extensive discussions at the US embassy between the ambassador and the RSO, support from the State Department, and sign-off by the National Security Council in Washington. Ambassador

Hammer countered my objections by asking me to contemplate the consequences of an American official being kidnapped by a militia group, a remote but not completely impossible scenario.

Travel from Kinshasa to Goma was with UN charter flights crewed by Kenyan contractors, a journey of about 1,500 kilometers that took 2–3 hours. Goma exemplified the majesty, diversity, and chaos of the DRC. Solid lava was visible in parts of the town, remnants of the last major eruption of Mount Nyiragongo in 2002. Lake Kivu, a deep lake, is potentially at risk of a limnic eruption, in which the sudden release of gases such as carbon dioxide and methane could result in a suffocating cloud. North of Goma lies the Virunga National Park, home to endangered mountain gorillas and a sanctuary for rebel groups. In early 2021, the Italian ambassador, Luca Attanasio, was killed in an attempted kidnapping while traveling in convoy outside the park.[14] Within Goma, traffic is dense, dominated by predominantly Chinese-made motorcycles that can travel vast distances.

I accompanied Gressly on a 4-day tour of the Ebola-affected province, including visits to the towns of Beni, Mangina, and Butembo. The EERC had constant, armed personal protection, which was also accorded to me. My bodyguard was a Lebanese policeman with experience in security work. We traveled between towns by Mi-17 helicopter (Russian helicopters, with Ukrainian pilots on contract) and otherwise in a convoy of two armored four-wheel-drive vehicles. Embassy security personnel had scouted the environment and insisted I spend the night in the MONUSCO military base outside Beni rather than in a hotel in town. I slept on a camp bed in an office after being escorted from town by a military personnel carrier along a deserted road known for insurgent attacks. All in all, this was again not a typical CDC deployment.

My first realization was how geographically dispersed Ebola was, and second, that this was essentially an urban epidemic involving large conglomerations that outsiders like me had never heard of. Mangina, where the first Ebola cases had occurred, was a small town of a few tens of thousands, but Beni and Butembo were cities, the latter with a population of well over half a million people. Despite the poor roads, people traveled extensively, mainly by motorcycle taxis.

Gressly and I moved constantly, visiting Ebola Treatment Units (ETUs), transit centers housing suspect cases, Emergency Operations Centers (EOCs), living quarters of respondents in the field, and community groups. The ETUs and transit centers we visited in Beni, Mangina, and Katwa, near Butembo, were functioning well. Two of the units were participating in a well-run clinical trial funded by the NIH. Beni's general hospital was rundown, but valiant efforts were being made to triage patients and isolate those with symptoms possibly indicating Ebola.

Innovative modifications to assuage patients' fears in ETUs included isolation rooms that were transparent plastic bubbles from inside which patients could see their families and the outside world; use of immune Ebola survivors to act as "buddies" for sick patients, sitting in their rooms to reassure them; and a crèche (a nursery) for uninfected children of patients with Ebola.

Discussions about community perceptions and hostility were illuminating. When the Ebola outbreak was declared in August 2018, the community was initially cooperative with restrictions and intrusive requests for measures such compulsory handwashing. Subsequently, inadequate attention was paid to communication and information sharing. WHO entered the scene with a stated "no regrets" approach that included an influx of responders from elsewhere in the DRC as well as from francophone West Africa, and financial resources that greatly distorted the local economy.

The culture of North Kivu was one of self-reliance and reticence toward outsiders, not least because of years of neglect by the central government. A community perception arose that outsiders were there for personal gain; that Ebola was not real; or if real, that it was intentionally introduced; and that those associated with the response were involved for monetary or political profit. Political and religious leaders fostered or failed to combat these ideas. Community beliefs, suspicion, and resentment were enhanced by the government's decision to exclude the Ebola-affected area, a stronghold of opposition, from the presidential election on grounds of public health and safety.

"Ebola business" referred to the corruption and distortions to the local economy that the Ebola response created.[15] At the first meeting I attended at MONUSCO's headquarters in Goma, I was pulled aside by a senior worker for an international NGO whom I had met in Liberia. He said he had never seen corruption of the scale he was witnessing in this response, and he intimated it involved staff of multilateral organizations.

WHO was reportedly paying nine thousand people at an approximate cost of $70 million for the period July–December 2019. In Beni alone, more than two thousand people were paid under the auspices of the public health response. Overall, some twenty-three thousand people were employed in some fashion. Many responders were paid three to four times the local salary, and commerce and trade were intensely affected.

Corruption at different levels and in different organizations was enhanced, affecting employment and multiple aspects of logistics (e.g., procurement of commodities, accommodation, rental of vehicles). Some of the responders were security forces used additionally as escorts for protection or enforcement, deepening community hostility. Efforts to contain these unsustainable expenditures fostered resistance among those benefiting, leading to strikes, sabotage, and sometimes violence.

Some of the deaths of responders in earlier months are believed to have been related to money. The well-publicized murder of Richard Mouzoko, a Cameroonian doctor, in Butembo in 2019 may have resulted from his efforts to report or stop malfeasance.

Suggestions of corruption extended to international staff and included demands for sexual favors from women.

Some political leaders changed their opinion about Ebola, coming to believe it was indeed real, but then sometimes encountered hostility and suspicion of having been co-opted for personal benefit. Some religious leaders judged official guidance on Ebola credible, even asking to be vaccinated, but were unable or unwilling to spread the message to their congregations. Several clergy members knew the pastor who became the first Ebola case in Goma in July 2019 but declined to testify to having known him.

Adding to hostility was the perception that the international community previously ignored this region, and was only there now because of concern about the spread of Ebola beyond the DRC. Sometimes contradictory feelings were at play, community members hoping for employment and opportunity without their denialist attitudes necessarily having changed. Subtle undermining of the response sometimes occurred, such as by persons taking a salary but, for example, facilitating unsafe burials at night. And the perverse but understandable reaction emerged that Ebola needed to be stopped but that Ebola business was simply too good to let it end.

UNICEF had an innovative, active social science unit, including local researchers, that conducted studies of knowledge, attitudes, and practices, as well as other community research. Unfortunately, its findings and recommendations were sometimes communicated late, and they were rarely integrated effectively into the health response.

The need to highlight negative aspects of Ebola business and the overall control effort should be balanced by recognition of heroic work done by many responders of diverse levels and from diverse local and international organizations. The whole experience reiterated the need for much closer engagement of local communities and leaders from the beginning of the response.

Research

Cliff Lane was Anthony Fauci's deputy at the National Institute for Allergy and Infectious Diseases of the NIH. I had known Cliff a long time from work on HIV, but we had reconnected in 2014 over the West African Ebola epidemic. Therapeutic research was attempted late during the West African outbreak but was hampered by inadequate numbers of new cases to evaluate interventions. In the DRC, research started while large numbers of new cases were still occurring, with groundbreaking results.

There have been intense discussions over the years about the ethics of research in the context of epidemics. Some argued that it would be unethical to compare potentially useful compounds against placebos or simply standard of care for epidemic diseases of high lethality like Ebola. A highly influential group, including Muyembe, penned a letter to the *Lancet* during the Ebola epidemic in West Africa proposing that alternate trial designs should be used in evaluating interventions under these field conditions.[16] Others, including Lane, argued the opposite, that the only ethical approach in settings of uncertainty was to insist on placebo or standard of care as controls, or else a reliable conclusion about a drug's efficacy might never be reached. Lane's argument would seem supported by questions about use of convalescent blood or plasma from survivors, discussed as a potential intervention since Ebola was first recognized. Lack of evaluation against rigorously chosen comparison groups limits the certainty of conclusions about this therapeutic approach, even decades later.[17]

In eastern DRC, four different compounds were compared against each other. Placebos or standard of care were not used as control scenarios, because of suggested but unproven benefit from two compounds, the antiviral remdesivir and the monoclonal antibody cocktail ZMapp,[18] the agent that had been given to the Samaritan's Purse missionaries infected in Liberia.

The Congolese study was conducted under exceptionally difficult circumstances. The participating ETUs were mostly managed by nongovernmental organizations like MSF, the Alliance for International Medical Action (ALIMA), and others working with DRC officials. Two treatment units were attacked during the study, in at least one case requiring seriously ill patients to be urgently moved to another ETU. Despite the logistic challenges of poor supply chains, uncertain availability of electricity, and the social and political difficulties, the trial showed that the monoclonal antibody treatments Mab114 and REGN-EB3 provided significantly better survival than the comparison compounds.[19] Survival was better the earlier the patients were treated after symptom onset, emphasizing the need to persuade the community to access care early. Importantly, the trial showed the feasibility of conducting important therapeutic research during an active epidemic, even in such a harsh environment.

Two other scientific advances had practical applications. Genetic sequencing of Ebola specimens could show which infections were linked.[20] Combined with traditional field work, this gave insight into transmission chains and locations, allowing contact tracing to be more specifically targeted. Most importantly, research in Guinea had shown the high efficacy of rVSV-ZEBOV, a recombinant, replication-competent vesicular stomatitis virus–based vaccine that incorporated Ebola's surface glycoprotein.[21] The cluster randomized trial compared immediate vaccination of contacts of patients with Ebola, and contacts of contacts, with vaccination of similar individuals after 21 days, a way of addressing the aforementioned problems of valid but ethical comparators.

A second vaccine produced by Johnson & Johnson, a product based on two different viral vectors in a two-dose regimen given over 56 days, was proposed for evaluation in the DRC and neighboring countries. The two-dose requirement makes this unsuitable for situations requiring immediate protection as in an acute outbreak but can be envisaged for prophylactic use.[22]

Evolution of the Epidemic

By September 2019, the epidemic was stable but widespread. More than 3,000 Ebola cases and 2,000 deaths had occurred in three of the DRC's 26 provinces, affecting close to 30 of DRC's 516 health zones. North Kivu and Ituri Provinces remained the epicenters, but individual infections had been exported to locations far away, including Goma and into western Uganda. A total of about ten cases per day were being reported but over large distances. Clusters would be extinguished in one location only to have new cases erupt somewhere else.

The situation continued to cause international concern, and senior international dignitaries regularly passed through, such as WHO Director General Tedros, the director of WHO's Regional Office for Africa, Tshidi Moeti, and others. In mid-September, an unusually large and high-level delegation visited from the United States, led by the secretary for Health and Human Services (HHS), Alex Azar. The visiting team included the head of global health at HHS, Garrett Grigsby; NIH's Tony Fauci; CDC Director Robert ("Bob") Redfield; and senior officials from USAID.

At an opening meeting at the US embassy, I was asked to brief the delegation on the current situation. I had said about two sentences when Azar cut me off, saying: "I've read the briefing papers, just tell me what we should be doing differently." Reticence in such situations, I had learned, does not serve one well, so I skipped over what I had planned to say and made some recommendations. The epidemic was not in Kinshasa or Goma, it was in hard-to-reach, unsafe, interior parts of eastern Congo—responders had to go where the virus was. The epidemic response was fragmented and poorly coordinated. Drawing on experience from Liberia, an

Incident Management System was required, with an incident manager and clear lines of authority.

The latter suggestion was met with surprising enthusiasm, and Azar made this recommendation to President Tshisekedi during a meeting at the presidency later that day. I reflected that this was the third time I was meeting a head of state because of Ebola, having met the leaders of Liberia and Sierra Leone in 2014.

The delegation flew to Goma and was then ferried by helicopter for the 90-minute journey to Butembo. We toured an ETU and later met local leaders, community representatives, and Ebola survivors. Most of the visitors spoke only English and, as had happened so often over my years in Africa, I acted as translator between the francophones and anglophones for intense and poignant discussions. The discrimination against Ebola sufferers and survivors was vividly described, and Secretary Azar heard the community's concerns that extended beyond Ebola to issues such as access to clean water and basic medical services. Azar listened and engaged attentively, surprising me with the strength of his promises about assistance beyond Ebola. I left wondering to what extent the hopes that he raised could be fulfilled.

Ebola Denial

A week before the delegation's visit in September 2019, a Tanzanian doctoral student who had been conducting field research in Uganda and Tanzania died of apparent Ebola in Dar es Salaam, the capital of Tanzania. Rumors indicated that laboratory tests on the case patient were positive, but this was later denied by Tanzanian authorities.

As in many countries, laboratory facilities for Ebola testing were heavily supported by the CDC. A further two possible cases of Ebola occurred, and unofficial information suggested contacts of these cases were quarantined, sometimes in military facilities far away from the capital. All this was officially denied. WHO issued unusually critical public comments highlighting national responsibilities under the International Health Regulations to share information.[23,24] The CDC and the US State Department alluded to possible Ebola in Tanzania in their health advisories.[25]

I said goodbye to the visiting delegation on the tarmac of Goma airport in mid-September 2019. Secretary Azar ordered CDC Director Redfield to visit Tanzania to try to persuade openness about the situation, but he was stonewalled and obtained no new information. The highest levels of the Tanzanian government clamped down on all information sharing. The CDC country director, Kevin Cain, was a close colleague who had worked under my supervision in Kenya. He recounted how usually close Tanzanian collaborators were prevented from speaking, and access to laboratory facilities and records was denied. The official line was that there was no Ebola in Tanzania.[26]

The restriction on communicating data undoubtedly came from the Tanzanian president, John Magufuli. He maintained his denialist attitude, and when COVID-19 struck some months later, he was a leading skeptic of the virus and the pandemic, recommending prayers and herbs as remedies. Magufuli denied that Tanzania faced a health challenge, but he died after a short illness in March 2021 that was widely attributed to COVID-19.[27]

A Seat at the Table

To coordinate the Ebola response, the international community's multilateral agencies, the DRC's Ministry of Health, and selected NGOs based their leadership teams in the converted grounds of a resort hotel on the shores of Lake Kivu. The CDC joined the conglomeration, working out of a small office. The CDC teams were now strictly organized along disciplines such as IPC, contact tracing, laboratory, communications, vaccination, and so forth.

Administrative supervision was provided by logistics officers out of Atlanta, and CDC country offices often lent assistance. Eastern Congo is largely Swahili-speaking, so participation from our office in Kenya was especially welcome.

Despite all this investment, and despite a prominent seat at the regular meetings of the Incident Management System, the CDC was still remote from the epidemic. Data from the field came into the WHO office where we were welcomed somewhat warily. Only the most specialized staff with strong data and analytic skills, and particularly familiarity with the statistical and graphics computing program R, were integrated into the inner data sanctum. Regular interactions with Atlanta kept headquarters informed, but I was continuously struck at how different this experience was from what the CDC had witnessed and achieved in West Africa.

Our staff participated intensely in activities within Goma, but security restrictions prevented us from traveling to the epidemic zones. Our situation reminded me of the joke about the drunk man searching for his lost keys, not where he had lost them, but under the light where he could see. Working in Goma gave the impression of doing something, provided useful feedback to the CDC in Atlanta, strengthened the international presence, offered useful experience to younger colleagues, and kept the CDC flag flying. It was, nevertheless, a less than satisfactory situation for field staff eager to contribute to combating the second worse Ebola outbreak in history.

My underlying concern about our limited impact was reinforced by two experiences: a comment from a Congolese colleague and a 3-day scientific conference in Kinshasa in November 2019. Steve Ahuka, the INRB scientist who was acting as incident manager in Goma, said to my CDC colleague John Neatherlin, "Your help must be helpful." He spoke good English, and I remained uncertain whether this was a slightly clumsy translation from his native French, or whether a deeper message was intended.

At the INRB conference in Kinshasa, attended by about three hundred people, the authority and stature of INRB Director Muyembe was evident. INRB scientists gave excellent presentations on cutting-edge topics such as therapeutic trials and genetic sequencing of viruses. I was struck by the diversity and quality of INRB's partners attending, including the NIH and various other American academic groups. The CDC was not mentioned once during the conference.

Competition and distrust between agencies were never fully overcome. Pierre Rollin, a CDC Ebola world expert with immense experience, wrote a scathing commentary, focusing especially on lack of data sharing.[28] His criticisms were stinging because of his international stature and the prominent journal in which they were published, *The Lancet Infectious Diseases*. Problems he cited included poor leadership, lack of coordination, failure of agencies to share data, mistrust, emphasis on personal and institutional research and advantage, and denial on the part of communities as well as responders.

At least seven different databases existed, numerous reports were generated by individual organizations, and different numbers were regularly communicated. Harmonizing and streamlining the data process into one common database, with agreement on unique identifiers for cases, including for linkage of contact tracing and vaccination, controlled by the DRC Ministry of Health but accessible to all with legitimate need, were never achieved. Collaborating organizations might reasonably have performed analyses for their own purposes, but a single official report and one set of numbers would have enhanced communication and avoided confusion, including for the overall response, the media, and funders.

Some databases that would have been operationally important were not shared, including the laboratory line list of Ebola test results. Results from whole-genome sequencing of positive samples were not made widely available, suggesting this was viewed as research rather than a response activity. Line lists of vaccine recipients were not shared, even with those responsible for surveillance and contact tracing, ostensibly because vaccination was conducted under research protocols for unlicensed products subject to confidentiality stipulations. This restriction limited the ability to assess whether the right people had been vaccinated. Other analyses not possible included assessment of vaccine effectiveness in Ebola contacts and in health care workers, utility of vaccinating contacts of contacts, and the course of disease in vaccinated persons who nonetheless became infected. Discussions between the directors of WHO and the CDC about data access failed to resolve these challenges, indicative of fragmentation and distrust.

Security in a Waning Epidemic

As the epidemic continued to slowly decline, security challenges worsened. On November 27, 2019, the MONUSCO base in Beni was attacked, its outside wall destroyed, and buildings inside the compound and several vehicles burned.[29] Intense community anger toward MONUSCO resulted from its inability to prevent civilian killings by militias in the region. When UN peacekeeping chief Jean-Pierre Lacroix arrived in Goma during this period, his convoy was stoned in a well-prepared attack.

On November 27–28, 2019, about thirty assailants, five armed with automatic weapons and the rest with machetes and knives, attacked a WHO-supported compound in Biakato.[30,31] A female Congolese staff member with the Ministry of Health was sexually assaulted and killed, and two drivers also died. The assailants appeared to know the layout of the compound and identified the room in which the senior WHO doctor usually slept. They were eventually forced to flee by intervention of the Tanzanian MO-NUSCO contingent.

Dr. Annie Iko Abikaa, a graduate of the CDC-supported Field Epidemiology Training Program and a senior medical officer with the Ministry of Health, heroically commandeered response vehicles the next morning and organized a convoy to evacuate about one hundred response workers to Beni. The reasons behind this violence were uncertain but local explanations included resentment about money, interference with illegal activities such as gold mining and smuggling, personal feuds, and misinformation about Ebola.

As these appalling attacks were occurring during the night, WHO staff called EERC David Gressly. Calls went unanswered because Gressly was in the United Kingdom, holding discussions aimed at securing longer-term funding for the Ebola response and whatever came after. Senior WHO staff reacted with fury, considering that security was the responsibility of the EERC. I was debriefed by Abdou Salam Gueye, an outstanding WHO epidemiologist who had previously worked for the CDC. Stressed and exhausted, he almost dissolved in tears as he angrily described the experience.

Important indicators of the quality and impact of the response, other than absolute numbers of new cases, were the time between symptom onset and case isolation, whether new cases were linked to known transmission chains, and the number and proportion of Ebola deaths that occurred in the community without isolation. The latter could be detected by oral swabbing of dead bodies or testing them with rapid tests usually applied at point of care. By early December 2019, these indicators had all improved, and an average of only one new case was being reported per day. I left the DRC at the end of the first week of December 2019, making a

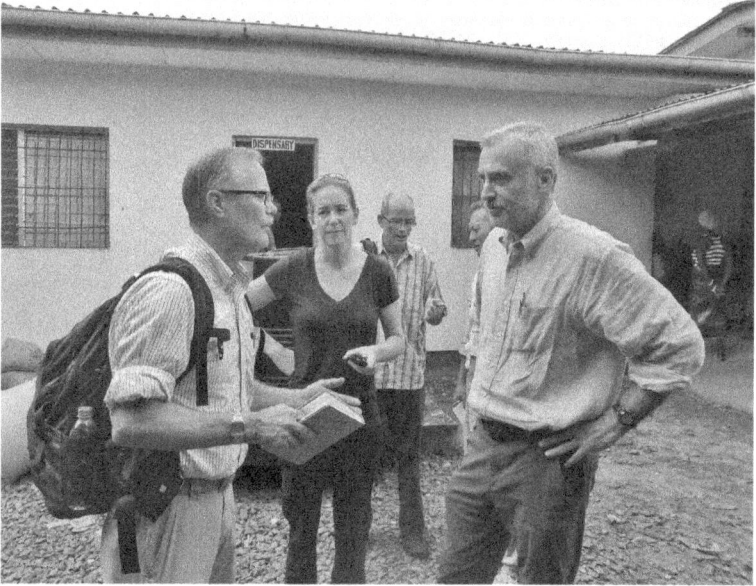

Figure 9.3 *Left to right, front*: Michael Beach, Athalia Christie, Larry Slutsker; Monrovia, Liberia, December 2019.
(Kevin De Cock, personal collection)

series of recommendations about optimal structure and size of the CDC team on the ground.

One recommendation was for a high-level visit from the CDC, which occurred in early January 2020. I joined senior epidemiologist Ray Arthur, Inger Damon, and Michael Beach, the latter two, respectively, the head of the division dealing with Ebola at the CDC and the current Atlanta-based incident manager. Beach, a water and sanitation expert, had worked in Monrovia in 2014 (Figure 9.3). My appreciation of the visit was somewhat diminished by a brewing tooth abscess, but it was important for these senior headquarters colleagues to review the situation on the ground, including the CDC's internal organizational challenges. The diverse difficulties faced never were all resolved, but Ebola slowly declined over subsequent weeks and months. On June 25,

2020, WHO declared the outbreak over, two incubation periods after the last known case.[32]

Ebola in the Modern Era

The DRC suffered a further five small outbreaks of Ebola over the period to 2022, and outbreaks also occurred in Guinea and Uganda, the latter with the Sudan strain of the virus. At least two outbreaks, in the DRC and Guinea, likely resulted from Ebola survivors with persistent infection.

Ebola epidemiology has changed since the days of its first recognition. Of the approximately thirty-five thousand cumulative cases reported to date, 95% or more have occurred since 2014. The large outbreaks in West Africa and the DRC covered huge areas, were largely urban, and involved large conglomerations and sometimes capital cities. The virus crossed borders and was transmitted internationally. Health care workers affected included international deployers, and the world saw medical evacuations to high-income countries, something previously unthinkable.

Reasons for this altered pattern are uncertain but must lie in the classic triad of infectious disease epidemiology: agent, host, and environment. Ebola is not a rapidly mutating virus and there is no evidence that its pathogenicity or infectiousness have increased. Extensive environmental and human behavioral changes have occurred in Central and West Africa with localized deforestation, urbanization, and population growth. Whether environmental degradation and these other factors have made it more likely for humans to encounter Ebola, either directly from its presumed bat host or an infected intermediary animal, is speculative. Once humans are infected, demographic changes, urbanization, and increased mobility, including by Africa's ubiquitous motorcycle taxis,[33] make dissemination more likely, sometimes over great distances. Ebola can no longer be considered simply as a remote, obscure, tropical infection.

In early January 2020, as Inger Damon, Ray Arthur, and I were in DRC, the world began to hear of unusual cases of pneumonia in Wuhan, the capital city of Hubei Province in the People's Republic of China. The genetic sequence of the causative novel coronavirus was released to the public domain over the course of our visit, and diagnostics became available shortly thereafter. Unbeknown to us as we left the DRC, the world was heading into the gravest acute health emergency since the influenza pandemic of 1918.

CHAPTER 10

The Pandemic

In late December 2019, as the DRC was slowly gaining control over its tenth outbreak of Ebola, cases of an unusual pneumonia were being recognized on the other side of the world, in the city of Wuhan, Hubei Province, China.[1] Home to more than eleven million people, Wuhan is the largest city in Central China and has an international airport with direct flights to Europe, the United States, Australia, and countries in Asia.[2] Wuhan also happens to house one of the world's leading high-security laboratories, the Wuhan Institute of Virology, known for studying bat viruses, including coronaviruses.[3]

I traveled home to Kenya in December 2019 after my second deployment to the eastern DRC, returning there a month later to meet with senior CDC colleagues to discuss our involvement in the declining Ebola epidemic. We read reports on the internet of cases of this severe but undiagnosed respiratory infection that was reminiscent of severe acute respiratory syndrome (SARS), the novel coronavirus infection that emerged in China in 2002, lasted almost 2 years, and killed close to eight hundred worldwide.[4]

On January 9, 2020, Chinese and WHO authorities announced that a new coronavirus, subsequently called SARS-CoV-2, had been identified as the cause of the unexplained pneumonia, and the full genome sequence of the virus was published on January 11.[5] The associated disease became known as COVID-19; as with Ebola, the same name began to be used for the disease and its agent in common parlance.

These bare facts might have been incidental trivia in global health history, or examples of praiseworthy international collaboration concerning a novel infection. Unfortunately, a global respiratory epidemic resulted that rivaled the great influenza pandemic of 1918, suspicions arose about a Chinese cover-up concerning the origin of the virus and its early spread,[3,6-8] and political fallout and recriminations continue to this day. And as far as pandemic performance was concerned, the world was found wanting.

The retrospectoscope is a powerful instrument, focusing images more clearly than those available to earlier observers. It is the tool of preference for the many experts in what might be called Advanced Hindsight. In actual fact, if addressed honestly, the question "What would *you* have done?" can be humbling. Analysis of past events with knowledge of the present is open to bias and misinterpretation, and cautious humility is always appropriate.

Treatises and books on COVID-19 have begun to appear, and others will follow. Broadly, they fall into three categories. First are the memoirs of people in positions of responsibility.[9,10] They mostly write about what happened but was not their fault, or what they advised but was not done. Second are the recollections of scientists proud of the advances made but clarifying that poor implementation was not their responsibility.[11] And, third, there are analyses by those who had no formal appointments or duties and are therefore free to castigate and comment.[12] All deserve to be heard but also interpreted with caution. It may take years to have analyses not influenced by institutional or personal interests and for COVID-19 to make its lasting lessons clear. Nonetheless, examination of what went right and wrong should not be delayed.

I lived outside of the United States throughout the tumultuous pandemic period, and I retired from the CDC at the end of 2020. From Kenya, colleagues and I watched events unfold in the United States, observed how the pandemic affected the CDC, and strove to support Kenya and its government in its response. The CDC was a trusted partner in Kenya, but the country had evolved technically, showed strong independence, and benefited from its own medical and scientific leadership. The pandemic of COVID-19 will be remembered as a critical event in the CDC's history, and a painful stimulus to the agency to reform to a changed world.

Early Assessment: Missed Opportunities

Exponential growth is a difficult concept to grasp. Exponential growth of an infection is often difficult to recognize until it is too late. A well-known student exercise concerns a water lily that doubles in size daily on a lake and will cover the whole surface in 28 days; when is the lake half covered? Many will answer instinctively that it will take 14 days. The correct answer, of course, is that half the lake will be covered after 27 days. Only 1 day then remains to recognize the impending catastrophe from the final doubling. To curb exponential growth, interventions must be instituted early, or else growth will quickly escape any control efforts. This logic is relevant to the early spread of COVID-19.

The first meeting of WHO's International Health Regulations (IHR) Emergency Committee to discuss COVID-19 was held on January 22, 2020.[13] The role of this committee is to assess whether outbreaks constitute a global threat and to advise WHO's director general whether to declare a Public Health Emergency of International Concern (PHEIC), the highest category for preparedness and response. WHO's IHR were revised in 2005 after SARS. Since then, a PHEIC had been declared seven times at the time of this writing: once for H1N1 influenza, once each for polio and Zika, twice for Ebola, and twice for mpox.

In addition to cases in China, by the time of the first IHR Committee meeting, infections with SARS-COV-2 had been reported from the Republic of Korea, Japan, Thailand, and Singapore. Almost six hundred cases had been recognized in China, which had imposed stringent internal travel restrictions. Person-to-person spread had been documented, with chains of transmission of several generations. WHO's committee declined to declare a PHEIC at its first meeting but did so at its second gathering, on January 30, 2020.

A statement from WHO on January 23 provided an estimate of the basic reproductive rate or number of the virus, the R0 estimate.[14] The basic reproductive number is the number of secondary transmissions from a primary case in a susceptible population. If each case generates more than one secondary case, an R0 of greater than 1, then the outbreak will expand. For an epidemic to decline, R0 must fall below 1. Over ensuing weeks and months, the term R0 entered the public lexicon as politicians, the media, and ordinary citizens began to debate epidemiologic trends. In this first statement, WHO estimated the R0 was in the region of 1.4–2.5, indicative of brisk spread.

The concept of susceptibility is important because it offers a natural limit to exponential growth. What goes up must come down, and exponential growth is not endless. In the example of the water lily, once the lake is full, further growth of the lily is not possible. If parts of the lake were protected by a chemical or other barrier, incomplete susceptibility would limit the lily's growth.

For some infections such as measles, once people have been infected, they develop permanent immunity and are no longer susceptible. A vaccine can also protect against infection. Natural and vaccine-induced immunity can provide "herd immunity," whereby a large enough proportion of the population is protected to prevent the infectious agent gaining or maintaining a foothold.

Susceptibility may be furthered, however, by the pathogen mutating to circumvent natural or vaccine-induced immunity, or if immunity is short-lived. With COVID-19, we learned over time that immunity was fragile. Just "letting it rip" in the quest for herd immunity, as some suggested, would have resulted in an even larger number of deaths.[15] Separate from susceptibility to infection, but relevant to COVID-19 discussions, is variation in disease expression. Some factors predispose to more severe illness, and we learned that disease severity may be blunted by vaccination, even when infection is not prevented.

Looking back, one must conclude that valuable time was lost early on. Experience with SARS earlier in the century, spread of COVID-19 in January 2020 to other countries in the region, evidence of person-to-person transmission, recognition of hundreds of cases in China, and a high estimated R0—all these should have raised an early and high-level alarm that exponential spread was occurring. Furthermore, two actions by Chinese authorities indicated the severity of the threat as they perceived it.

Extensive and severe travel restrictions had been imposed in Wuhan and beyond.[16] Most telling was the emergency construction of a one-thousand-bed hospital in Wuhan over 10 days in the second half of January 2020, an extraordinary feat of logistics.[17] That the Chinese government, recalling the impact of SARS, imposed an economically and socially damaging lockdown so early on, and that they so dramatically scaled up emergency medical care in Wuhan where the epidemic started—these were all indicators of their assessment of the gravity of the situation. More attention should have been paid early on to what the Chinese did as opposed to what they said. The Chinese were investing not in preparedness but in a full-scale response to a major infectious disease emergency.

Stumbles and Politics at the CDC

Over the years, the CDC has consistently had some of the most favorable ratings among all federal agencies.[18] Responding to epidemics was what the CDC was best known for, its history replete with investigations that have entered public health lore. The outbreak of Legionnaire's disease in 1976, or the response to AIDS after the first reports in 1981, contributed to the CDC's reputation as the leading public health agency in the world. Other countries emulated the CDC and even copied its name. Former directors Jeff Koplan and Tom Frieden often recounted that China called its national agency the China CDC, though the acronym CDC meant nothing in Chinese.

COVID-19 presented the CDC with the opportunity to prove its very *raison d'être*, but things went awry early on, and public trust in the agency suffered. By late 2022, more than half the US population felt the CDC was doing a poor or only fair job in its response to COVID-19.[19] Missteps by the CDC, public misunderstanding of the context and authorizations under which the agency works, the politics of the Trump administration, and polarization within the United States all contributed to the assessment of suboptimal performance. And this perception extended far and wide. I was saddened in mid-2020 to hear a public health professional in the Middle East lament in a National Public Radio interview that the CDC no longer was the reference she had always looked up to.

On January 21, 2020, the CDC announced that a traveler from Wuhan to Washington state had tested positive for COVID-19, the first recognized case in the United States.[20,21] Isolating those with infection before they can transmit to others is a traditional public health control measure. Symptoms of COVID-19 resembled those of other common respiratory infections such as influenza. The frequency and severity of complaints such as cough, nasal congestion, headache, shortness of breath, and fever varied, and none were specific for SARS-CoV-2 infection.[22] An unusual symptom more specific to COVID-19 was loss of smell, but this was present in only a small minority of cases. Having a diagnostic laboratory test, therefore, was of the utmost importance.

At this time, only the CDC was able to test for SARS-CoV-2 in the United States. Testing capacity was essential for public health as well as for clinical purposes. Testing was required to measure the extent to which the virus had penetrated the population and to understand its distribution. Testing was necessary to implement preventive measures such as case isolation, but it was also needed to accurately diagnose individuals with what was proving to be a potentially serious, sometimes fatal disease.

CDC accepted strictly selected specimens for in-house testing and, in early February 2020, began to distribute its own test kits to state health departments. Within a few days of receipt, peripheral laboratories reported that the tests were unreliable, putting the United States at a disadvantage compared with other high-income countries that had already initiated extensive testing.[23] The CDC test was a polymerase chain reaction (PCR) assay with different probes for detecting coronaviral genomic material. Test malfunction could have resulted from a design flaw, contamination during the preparation of the test kits, or inadequate quality control.[24]

Although the CDC has often produced tests for novel infectious agents, it is not in the business of manufacturing diagnostics at large scale. WHO and countries other than the United States had validated different tests for COVID-19 earlier in January 2020, and these might have been sourced were it not for complex regulatory requirements overseen by the FDA. It might have been possible to urgently involve private-sector companies whose manufacturing expertise concerned diagnostics. This was done effectively by the government of the Republic of Korea, which committed major funding to diverse companies that could produce tests, so that widespread testing was rapidly available (Anne Schuchat, personal communication).

As it was, the CDC soldiered on trying to rectify the situation, losing time in the face of exponential expansion of the infection. By the end of February, many tens of thousands or more Americans were likely to have been infected, but just over one thousand COVID-19 tests had been performed.

Responding to guidance from the congressional Labor and Health and Human Services Appropriations Committee, a laboratory work group was assembled in 2022 to investigate what went wrong. In a swipe at another later deficiency, timely collection and reporting of data, the group was also asked to review communications and electronic reporting with diverse laboratory systems in the country, covering both the private and public sector. The Senate's Homeland Security and Governmental Affairs Committee published a report on the early federal response, after almost 2 years of investigation. This also delved into the testing experience as well as other aspects. Both investigations highlighted major deficiencies and made wide-ranging recommendations.[24]

I was involved with organizing the annual Conference on Retroviruses and Opportunistic Infections that brings together leading infectious-disease scientists from around the world. The meeting was scheduled to be held in Boston in early March 2020. The meeting's leadership agonized over whether to proceed with the meeting, wisely deciding with just a few days to spare to cancel the gathering and hold it virtually. Unquestionably, a superspreading event was avoided.

For the CDC, the testing debacle became the original sin haunting subsequent history. Lack of testing lost the country precious weeks during which exponential viral spread was neither recognized nor prevented. Early and extensive testing could have clarified the importance of asymptomatic infection. Testing became more widely available once private sector companies were engaged in the manufacturing and delivery of kits.

It became apparent that asymptomatic transmission of SARS-CoV-2 was not only possible but accounted for a large proportion of cases.[25] This is a critical point, because with some other conditions such as SARS or Ebola, transmission essentially only occurs from people with symptoms, simplifying case isolation. For COVID-19, testing symptomatic cases alone would prove ineffective for isolating infectious sources.

Testing and contact tracing alone, therefore, would not have prevented epidemic spread. The sheer amplitude of the accelerating outbreak, combined with transmission from asymptomatic persons, precluded testing being the magic prevention bullet for this person-to-person pandemic virus. Nonetheless, the loss of credibility resulting from this early experience overshadowed the solid and hard work on COVID-19 that an increasing proportion of CDC staff were engaged in, and increased skepticism toward later CDC advice and initiatives.

Politics and personalities played their inevitable roles over the course of the pandemic, and no personality was bigger than President Trump. The fact that the CDC is based in Atlanta, outside of the Washington, DC, bubble, has long given staff a sense of isolation from the partisan politics of the far away capital. There was pride in the agency that its work and judgments were driven by science and evidence, not politics. The CDC leadership over the years defended the agency's evidence-based focus and decision-making.[26-28] This was to change; COVID-19 robbed the CDC of its relative independence and injected politics into the agency's technical work as no other crisis had done previously.

Clear and consistent communication about a health threat is essential, as captured under the risk communication rubric "be first, be right, be credible."[29] The Trump administration delivered mixed messages throughout 2020, initially about the severity of the threat. On January 31, 2020, Health and Human Services Secretary Alex Azar used his authority under the Public Health Services Act to declare a public health emergency in the whole United States.[30] The very term *public health emergency* conveys the gravity of the situation, but this contrasted with diverse and inconsistent comments from the administration about the country's situation.

High-level communications downplayed risk. CDC Director Robert Redfield, at the very time Azar declared a national emergency, said national risk was low. Someone who did accurately assess the threat some weeks later, and who communicated it clearly, was Nancy Messonnier, director of CDC's National Center for Immunization and Respiratory Diseases. At a press briefing on February 25, 2020, she warned, in words ordinary people could understand, that families should be prepared for major disruptions to their lives. And there was certainty: it was not "if," but "when." The message was widely reported, the stock market dropped, and President Trump was furious.[31]

National authority over the outbreak was transferred to Vice President Mike Pence who, 2 days later, selected Deborah ("Debi") Birx as White House Coronavirus Response coordinator.[32] Trump himself became a frequent public commentator. The CDC briefings were restricted and controlled so that the nation's public health agency was no longer the country's prime source of communications about COVID-19 and its implications. Messonnier largely disappeared, although her message had been correct. The CDC felt blamed for communicating the truth. Instead of leading the nation in a public health response to COVID-19, the CDC was buried in the hierarchy among other agencies, its public health work and guidance now overseen by political appointees.

Redfield and Birx were national figures in the 2020 COVID-19 response who influenced communications and the CDC's degraded stature. Redfield was appointed CDC director in March 2018 under inauspicious circumstances, replacing Brenda Fitzgerald, who resigned after it became known she had invested in tobacco stocks while in office.[33] Redfield, known as an HIV scientist and who had strong Catholic credentials, had long aspired to lead the CDC. He was perceived as a kind and caring man, but these attributes did not facilitate his taking on a large, unfamiliar bureaucracy constantly dealing with crises such as the opioid epidemic or Ebola.

Few thought that Redfield had the persona for the cut and thrust of Washington, let alone pandemic politics. He was not a natural communicator and was overshadowed by NIH's Anthony ("Tony") Fauci when both were speaking at media or congressional briefings. In his autobiography, Fauci describes often defending the CDC.[10] Morale at the CDC sank because staff felt Redfield yielded to pressures to put political gain before technical excellence and accuracy, including adapting communications and other guidance under instructions from the White House.[34]

Staff were shocked when President Trump announced in late May 2020 that the United States was withdrawing from WHO, where the CDC had many fruitful collaborations.[35] Only WHO had the authority to convene countries of the world around common pandemic aims, and the US absence would increase, not reduce, the influence of China that Trump railed against.

I was told that even global health staff in the Department of Health and Human Services were caught unawares by this impulsive decision. For several CDC staff detailed to WHO, important to the US government for their influence and information gathering, this was personally and professionally disruptive. Top American diplomats in Nairobi asked my opinion about leaving WHO, but when I expressed a dissenting view, I was firmly told this was the non-negotiable decision of the president of the United States.

Discussion about morale at the CDC came to a head with the leak of a letter from former CDC Director Bill Foege to Redfield in September 2020.[36,37] Foege urged Redfield to accept that the administration's pandemic response was a failure, that a federal plan was needed, and that coalitions needed to replace the divisiveness that Trump fostered. He called for greater international collaboration and for sound science and administration. Playing to Redfield's deep Catholic convictions, Foege urged Redfield to make a public statement, citing Martin Luther: "Here I stand, I cannot do otherwise." He described COVID-19 as "a slaughter and not just a political dispute."[37] It was an extraordinary intervention from one of the world's most respected public health leaders but resulted in no action other than passing media attention.

Birx was a physician and immunologist by training who, in earlier life, was in the military and conducted HIV research under both Fauci and Redfield.[9] She was widely respected for her role leading the President's Emergency Plan for AIDS Relief (PEPFAR) from 2014[38] before which she had spent nine productive years at the CDC directing the agency's international AIDS work. I was always grateful for the personal support she extended to me.

Committed and exceptionally hard-working, she was strategic, strong-minded, directive, and guarded in sharing her inner thoughts or political leanings. She had little patience for opinions different from her own. As described in her autobiography focusing on her time at the White House, she wanted to be known as driven by data and detail, and she strongly argued for expanded COVID-19 testing.[9]

Some felt Birx's interpretations of data and their nuances were sometimes unrealistic, as in insistence on completeness of data when partial coverage gave adequate understanding for public health action. Having come to the CDC as a senior appointee in 2005, she knew the agency well, though not its relationships with state and local health departments, and she had always kept strong links in Washington.

Several events contributed to the fraying of Birx's relationship with the CDC. In an interview with the Christian Broadcasting Network in March 2020, she praised President Trump effusively for his attention to scientific literature and data, attributing this to his long-standing business acumen.[39] Colleagues were dismayed because the President ignored scientific evidence, made inaccurate statements about the virus just disappearing, and promoted ineffective treatments like hydroxychloroquine.

Another episode was the televised press conference Trump gave in April 2020, when he speculated about injecting disinfectants, or use of heat and light as treatments for COVID-19.[40,41] Birx looked shocked but stayed silent, and the moment was captured for posterity in widely disseminated images. Public health colleagues noted the contrast with Tony Fauci, who walked the fine line between not openly disrespecting the president but ensuring messages were scientifically valid. "You should never destroy your own credibility. And you don't want to go to war with a president. . . . But you got to walk the fine balance of making sure you continue to tell the truth," Fauci said in an interview.[42] Birx was in a more difficult position in the White House, expected to coordinate people who resisted coordination.

Frustrated with what she considered incomplete hospital data collected by the CDC through a long-standing program, Birx unilaterally canceled reliance on CDC information and arranged a private sector contract to conduct the same work. A comment she made at a White House Task Force meeting in May 2020 was particularly stinging: "There is nothing from the CDC that I can trust."[43] These words reverberated around the world; the American ambassador in Kenya cited them to me, asking me to justify the advice we gave him. Foege referred to her remarks about the CDC in the previously mentioned letter to Redfield.[36] Her comments that PEPFAR data from Africa were better than what the CDC collected in the United States caught attention but were not a meaningful comparison for a respiratory pandemic.

Combined with pressures from the intensity of work, the perception of being under constant attack, lack of confidence in its leadership, and the loss of staff camaraderie with people now working from home, the CDC was reeling in a way it had never done before. Trust and reputation are essential for a public health agency, and the CDC finished 2020 on the backfoot.[44] Stumbles and criticism eclipsed the solid, committed work the agency conducted, not only on COVID-19 but on all the other public health challenges the nation faced. Advances in vaccine science raised hopes at the agency for a brighter 2021, but the optimism of vaccines becoming available was overshadowed by events surrounding the 2020 presidential election, the transition, and the attack on the Capitol on January 6, 2021.

COVID-19 in Kenya, 2020

Those of us working overseas were protected from the discouragement prevalent at the CDC's headquarters, even as we worried about our domestic colleagues. In early 2019, Kyle McCarter had taken over as US ambassador to Kenya from the career diplomat Robert Godec. McCarter, a political appointee, was a staunch Christian and Trump supporter from Illinois. He had had strong connections with Kenya, where his father had set up a religious charity many years before, and which, as ambassador, he and his wife continued to support.

The CDC was well regarded at the embassy and McCarter and I, as CDC Kenya director, struck up a respectful relationship. He was strongly committed to addressing corruption, including in that most lucrative areas of development assistance, the procurement of AIDS and other commodities. In the middle of 2019, having been in Kenya longer than the usual time allowed, I transitioned from the directorship to working on the Ebola response in the DRC.

On March 13, 2020, Kenya's President Kenyatta announced the first known case of COVID-19, diagnosed at the National Influenza Center's laboratory, which had long received major funding and technical assistance from the CDC. This was about a month after diagnosis of the first case on the continent, in Egypt, and 2 weeks after the first case below the Sahara, in Nigeria. It was evident that the infection would reach everywhere, and every country had to be prepared.

By the end of March 2020, almost half a million cases had been reported to WHO. The agency had declared COVID-19 a pandemic on March 11,[45] a statement that attracted a lot of attention but had long been evident and made no practical difference. Derived from the Greek word for "all," applying *pan* to describe the outbreak simply meant it was a global epidemic. Indeed it was, and it had been developing as such for many weeks.

Two important events influenced the CDC's work in Kenya over ensuing months. First, the State Department instituted a global authorized departure on March 14, 2020, meaning that US government staff and dependents in diplomatic posts around the world could leave for the United States if they wished.[46] Complex regulations apply to this voluntary situation as well as to ordered departures, when staff are instructed to leave posts considered unsafe. We had twenty-seven American staff in country; to my surprise, two-thirds elected to depart, and I stepped back into the role of director.

I understood that many had family responsibilities back home, and it was unknown whether travel restrictions would be imposed more widely or for how long. It was easy for me to stay, because my immediate family was Kenyan. Nonetheless, combating infectious diseases domestically and around the world was core to the

CDC mission, and I subsequently heard expressions of surprise from numerous quarters at our depleted team.

A second experience showed me how roles and relationships had changed. In my earlier work on large or sensitive outbreaks, the CDC had always been invited to work with the highest levels of the Kenya Ministry of Health. I attempted to use my connections to get us a place in the inner circle of Kenyan government deliberations on COVID-19, thinking that the CDC's long-standing history in Kenya, our strong technical group, and the opportunity for collaboration with CDC headquarters in Atlanta would be considered useful. I was politely but firmly rebuffed, and the CDC took its place in regular meetings along with other national, bilateral, and multilateral partners.

Initially disappointed, I came to see this as a positive development. Kenya was now much stronger in laboratory and epidemiologic capacity than it had been. The CDC could take credit for some of that improvement because of longstanding support through efforts such as the Field Epidemiology Training Program and PEPFAR.

Our nine remaining Americans and about fifty of our Kenyan staff, close to one-third of the workforce, now worked closely with the Ministry of Health on COVID-19, aligned with the Ministry's response structure (Figure 10.1).[47] Specialist areas included laboratory, infection prevention and control, epidemiology and surveillance, clinical management, and border screening. The CDC had supported the health ministry some years before to develop an Emergency Operations Center (EOC) and had trained staff in the implementation of an Incident Management System. Activating these elements contributed to better organization of the Kenyan response, and similar approaches were later emulated at the level of some individual counties.

Initially, testing for COVID-19 attracted the greatest attention. International partners were essential in expanding access to

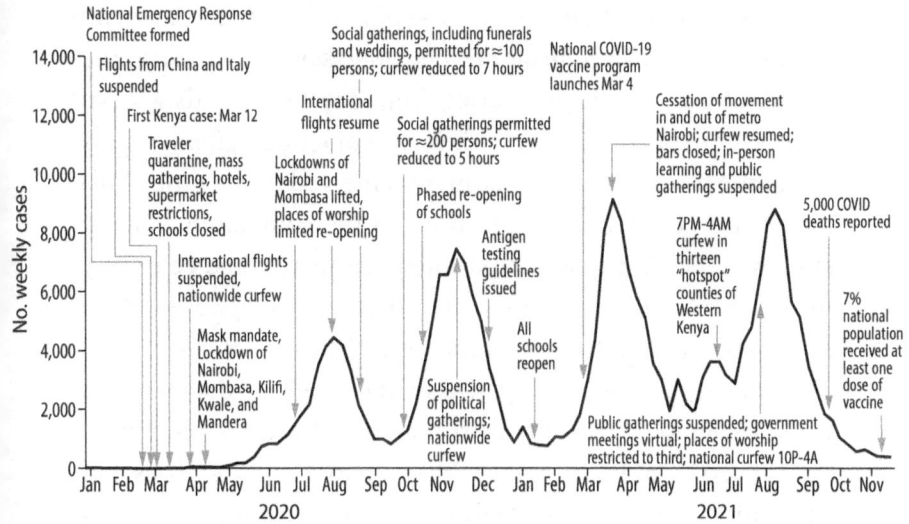

Figure 10.1   Interventions applied by the Kenya government and weekly reported COVID-19 cases, February 2020–November 2021 inclusive.
(From: Herman-Roloff A, et al. Emerg Infect Dis. 2022;28:S159–S167)

testing and included organizations such as the CDC, the US army's research group, and the strong technical research collaboration supported by the United Kingdom's Wellcome Trust. Global approaches to SARS-CoV-2 testing were similar across the world, relying on PCR technology to detect genomic material of the virus. Rapid point-of-care tests for viral antigen detection or antibody testing for epidemiologic studies were to come later.

Testing was grossly inadequate for the potential demand, and prioritization was never fully resolved, a criticism that could be applied in most countries. Scarce tests were needed for testing of patients, but there was also need for screening of contacts of known cases. International travel requirements resulted in a global industry of COVD-19 testing for travel certificates showing absence of infection.[48] Testing was insufficient virtually everywhere in the world, and who was being tested was heterogeneous, so it was not possible to derive meaningful estimates of the prevalence of infection. Instead, the proportion of test positivity became used as an indicator of epidemic severity. Because the nature of who was tested varied from day to day, this was an imperfect measure. Later, with more epidemiologically rigorous approaches to testing, estimates emerged of the ratio of diagnosed cases to overall infections in the community.[49] Early studies in the United States indicated that there could be twenty times more unrecognized infections than cases diagnosed,[50] but in low-income countries, the ratio would be even greater.

University groups also began to synthesize global data, and the world began to rely on outputs from Johns Hopkins University,[51] the University of Washington's Institute for Health Metrics and Evaluation,[52] and Oxford University's Our World in Data[53] as much as on WHO's dashboard.[54] In his famous letter to CDC Director Redfield, Bill Foege alluded to this entry of academia into what previously were strictly public health functions.[36] Elements of the media such as *The Economist*[55] contributed powerful analyses, suggesting the true burden of cases and deaths were two to three times greater than officially reported numbers.

As descriptions spread around the world of disease and death overwhelming facilities in New York[56] and Lombardy, Italy,[57] there was grave concern that Africa's health infrastructure would be devastated. Papers describing the natural history of the infection and pattern of disease were published, and many groups undertook mathematical modeling to project the future of the epidemic and the impact of interventions.[58,59] The outputs and opinions of academic modelers had great influence over different national policies.

Based on published data from China and Europe, we made some crude calculations in March 2020 of what Kenya might expect. We assumed the R0 of 2–3 observed in China, and outcomes described of 80% asymptomatic infections, 14% severe, and 6% critical illness, with no interventions implemented,[58] and taking no account of variations in outcome by age. These scenarios for Kenya's population of approximately 50 million suggested ranges of adult infections of 9 million–18 million. Among these, we expected 1.3 million–2.5 million seriously ill patients; 540,000–1.1 million critically ill patients; and 27,000–360,000 deaths. No African country would have the capacity to deliver care to such numbers of seriously ill patients, and the outlook seemed grim.

At our suggestion, a consortium of academic and research institutions in Kenya was formed to give unified modeling advice to the Ministry of Health. The different institutions used different approaches but intended to provide a synthesis of their different estimates and projections based on more sophisticated models that took account of the age structure and social characteristics of the population.[60] Estimates were still wide ranging but indicated that, even with interventions, Kenya might suffer more than eighty thousand deaths.

The Kenya government was aggressive in early implementation of nonpharmaceutical interventions, including isolation of cases; quarantine of contacts; compulsory masking; a ban on mass gatherings; closure of bars, schools, and universities; a nationwide curfew; and travel restrictions that included suspension of international flights and prevention of movement into and out of Nairobi and Mombasa, the country's two largest cities. "Stay at home" orders were not given, understandably, because a large proportion of the population depended on daily wages for subsistence. The words of a taxi driver in Nairobi summarized the challenge: "If the virus does not kill us, it will starve us." As in many countries, controversy and concern surrounded the safety of health care and health workers, with personal protective equipment (PPE) in short supply.

The dire predictions of the models did not come to pass, or not fully and not immediately. Ambassador McCarter walked the line between repeating some of President Trump's assertions that the pandemic was overblown and listening to cautionary voices such as ours at CDC Kenya. I dissuaded him from repeating his incorrect and potentially offensive jest that Kenyans were likely protected by high concentrations of chloroquine in their blood from antimalarial treatment.

We remained on good terms, and I was regularly at the ambassador's side to brief the embassy community. I joked with him that models were imperfect, their reliability somewhere between weather forecasting and astrology. Joking aside, I explained to him that models should not be viewed as predictions but as tools to understand the present and, importantly, to change the future.

Yet, with time, the pandemic did make itself felt. The US embassy lost several Kenyan members of staff to COVID-19. Nurses and doctors died. Hospitals were stretched, beds were full, and people recounted having to drive around with ill relatives looking for a health facility able to accept them. Several prominent politicians across the continent died, including President Magufuli of Tanzania, who succumbed in early 2021 after ridiculing public health guidance around the pandemic. The pandemic was real, but Kenya fared better than we had feared.

When data were scrutinized, COVID-19 in Kenya behaved as elsewhere. More than three-fourths of infections were without symptoms. Overall, by mid-late 2021, most of the Kenyan population were likely to have been infected.[60] In cases reported, however, outcomes replicated experience in other countries. Most striking was the relationship between adverse outcome and age and sex. Kenyans ill with COVID-19 who were older than 50 years were ten times more likely to die than those younger. Men were about three times as likely to die as women. And these risks persisted when older men were compared with younger men, or men were compared with women of the same age. We did not have information other than anecdotally on the adverse effects of comorbidities, such as diabetes and hypertension, but they likely were substantial.

Several waves of COVID-19 occurred over ensuing months.[47,60] Laboratory capacity did not allow genomic sequencing in real time to track SARS-CoV-2 variants. Later in 2020, the US State Department rescinded the authorized departure order, and American CDC staff returned. I stepped back from the front line and prepared for my retirement from the CDC, effective at the end of 2020.

Kenyan Lessons

Kenya is a lower-middle-income country whose gross domestic product (GDP) per capita is just over $2000. The GDP per capita in the United States is about thirty-five times higher. Yet, the American death rate per million from COVID-19 was more than thirty times higher than the Kenyan rate.[54] What should we conclude from this counterintuitive observation of a poor country doing so much better with COVID-19 than the world's richest country? How can such a discrepancy be explained?

The impact of COVID-19 in Africa was certainly underestimated. Testing was more limited than in wealthier countries, so reported cases undoubtedly misrepresented the true burden. Causes of death are difficult to ascertain accurately in low-income settings, and reporting of mortality, both all-cause mortality and cause-specific mortality, is weak. One of the ways that deaths due to COVID-19 were estimated in different countries was to look at excess mortality, the increased number of deaths over what would have been expected in a typical year. We tried such approaches in Kenya but found that systems were simply not robust enough to draw meaningful data.

A study in Lusaka, Zambia, reported on postmortem nasal swabs for SARS-CoV-2 infection in 2020 and found that 16% of cadavers tested positive.[61] Most of the decedents with clinical information available had symptoms compatible with COVID-19. Most deaths occurred in the community and very few decedents, including those hospitalized, had been tested while alive. The authors concluded that COVID-19 deaths were occurring at a high rate but were not being recognized because of lack of testing capacity.

The only African country with strong testing and reporting capability was South Africa, which, by late April 2023, had reported just over four million cases and one hundred thousand COVID-19 deaths.[54] South Africa's population-based mortality rate was half that of the United States. The same comorbidities were relevant as elsewhere in the world, especially obesity, diabetes, and cardiovascular disease, but HIV was an additional risk for adverse outcome in East and southern Africa.

We must accept uncertainty about the true extent of COVID-19's impact in Africa. There was undoubtedly substantial under-recognition and under-reporting. On the other hand, despite periods of stress on urban hospitals, Kenya did not see scenes of clinical facilities and mortuaries filled beyond capacity with critically ill and dying patients. Although official WHO reports must be an underestimate of the true situation, the mortality burden on the continent was unquestionably lower than in Europe or North America. The most likely reasons for this are the differences in the age structure of the population, lower rates of comorbidities, and shielding of the elderly.

I was always surprised by the strength of association between age and death rates from COVID-19, as well as by the paucity of discussion of relevant mechanisms. As stated earlier, outcomes in reported, mainly hospitalized COVID-19 cases in Kenya mirrored those described elsewhere, especially in relation to age. Serologic studies examining antibody prevalence showed large proportions of the population to have been infected.[47,48] CDC Kenya had been supporting a surveillance platform in Kibera, a large informal settlement in Nairobi, famous for having featured in the movie *The Constant Gardener*. Two-thirds of the population there showed evidence of prior infection, but disease had been relatively rare.[47] The great majority of reported infections in Kenya were asymptomatic.

The median age of the population of Kenya is 20 years; of South Africa's, 27; whereas that of the US population is 38. In Italy, the scene of gruesome images in hospitals and mortuaries early in the pandemic, the population has a median age of 47 years. Other countries in Africa where fertility has not declined to the extent it has in Kenya or South Africa have median ages even lower. These differences in median age mean that much lower proportions of African country populations are elderly, which is the group at highest risk of adverse outcomes from COVID-19. Age must be the most important factor that protected the African continent against the extreme devastation from COVID-19 that was first feared. Infection with SARS-CoV-2 was rife in Africa, but severe disease and death were less common because the population is young.

A contributing factor may have been how African societies deal with the elderly. Older people often leave urban centers upon retirement to return to their ancestral home areas. Care homes concentrating older people are a rarity if they exist at all. In this way, the elderly may have been protected to some extent against exposure to SARS-CoV-2. Although noncommunicable diseases such as obesity, diabetes, and cardiovascular disease are increasing, they are still less common than in high-income countries with older populations. It is likely that lower rates of comorbidities and different patterns of SARS-CoV-2 exposure contributed to lower death rates.

South Africa deserves special mention for several reasons. It offered a model of transparency in data sharing and demonstrated an extraordinarily high quality of science. In addition to its severe

HIV epidemic, the largest in the world, South Africa also has a burgeoning problem with noncommunicable diseases. Greater than 40% of women and close to one-fifth of men in South Africa are obese, rates that are about double the regional average. These factors could help explain the country's severe COVID-19 outbreak, which also, it must be remembered, was better measured than elsewhere on the continent.

South Africa's scientific contributions were noteworthy, especially its leadership in molecular epidemiology.[62] Dispiritingly, instead of receiving plaudits for recognition of the Omicron variant of SARS-CoV-2 in late 2021, the country promptly had travel restrictions imposed by the outside world. South Africa's openness about its epidemic contrasted with the attitudes of many other countries, and the nation deserves great credit.

Age and comorbidities were clearly important, but other factors, albeit more intangible, were also likely relevant. Public health action requires technical expertise, but implementation depends on leadership and management.[26,36] Although individual leaders failed their countries, such as President Magufuli in Tanzania, broadly speaking, the extreme politicization that occurred in the United States was not seen in Africa. Quarantines, social distancing, masking guidance, vaccine recommendations, and the like were not popular anywhere, but in most African countries they were accepted as necessary social adaptations.

In the United States, by contrast, behavior related to masks and vaccines came to represent political choices and affiliations. Attitudes and beliefs about treatments ignored scientific evidence, so advice that drugs like chloroquine and ivermectin were ineffective was dismissed by certain groups as false. Medical and public health leaders offering evidence-based scientific advice were pilloried and even threatened with violence.

The quality of leadership is difficult to measure. If my preferred definition of leadership applies—the ability to get others to do what needs to be done—then the United States was lacking in leadership. The American population was not united in how it addressed the pandemic, vaccine hesitancy flourished,[63] and alternative truths were fostered. Leadership matters; ultimately, the divisiveness and lack of social cohesion in the United States that leadership should have prevented cost lives.

The CDC and the Postpandemic Future

In December 2020, Rochelle Walensky was nominated by incoming President Joe Biden to take over leadership of the CDC.[44] Every new director will want to make organizational changes, but for Walensky, a respected infectious diseases physician from Boston, the changes to consider were profound. The combination of the CDC's self-inflicted wounds, undermining by the Trump administration, inadequate legal authorities, and the vagaries of the pandemic itself posed an unprecedented and existential challenge to the CDC.

Collective humility is required as we review what might have been done differently overall, or what the CDC could have done better. The severity of the threat from COVID-19 was widely underestimated, and the importance of person-to-person spread and predominance of transmission from asymptomatically infectious persons took too long to be acknowledged. In addition to the catastrophic error concerning the CDC's early tests, testing was inefficient, inadequate, and poorly planned. Infection prevention and control in health care settings, including the adequacy and positioning of PPE, was insufficiently prioritized. Acknowledgment that the virus could be airborne was delayed by prolonged, almost theological discussions about the relative sizes of infectious particles and droplets.

Communications were sometimes unclear, best exemplified by inconsistent advice about the protective benefit of masks, a subject that focused science could have resolved earlier. Non-pharmaceutical interventions such as avoidance of mass gatherings and social distancing could have been implemented more consistently and the practice and politics of lockdowns better managed. Dissecting out the relative prevention benefit of the different nonpharmaceutical interventions is difficult. It has been speculated that early and widespread mask wearing in Asia, along with trust in public health advice and leadership, contributed to limiting pandemic impact in that region.

An astonishing achievement was the delivery of vaccines in less than one year of the first cases of COVID-19 being reported.[64,65] Here, bowing to right wing antivaccine pressure, President Trump and his political followers missed opportunities for taking credit for and simultaneously ensuring public health success. The development of COVID-19 vaccines was built on years of government support for basic science and implementation of public health vaccination programs. Operation Warp Speed, a government-funded, public-private partnership, invested more than $10 billion in the quest for COVID-19 vaccines and therapeutics.[65,66] It is perplexing that this success was allowed to morph into conspiracy views, vaccine hesitancy, and, ultimately, higher death rates from COVID-19 in Trump-supporting states.[67,68]

Walensky, an HIV researcher earlier in her career, delivered a speech to young investigators at the 2023 Conference on Retroviruses and Opportunistic Infections, encouraging them to look to public health as a calling.[69] She outlined in detail, in words some might have perceived as discouraging, the constraints the CDC faces in collecting national public health data. Listening to her, I recalled unsuccessful CDC efforts in the late 1990s to streamline and harmonize the dozens of surveillance systems that exist for different infectious diseases in the United States.

Walensky painstakingly described how data flow to the CDC from state health department as well as local, tribal, and territorial jurisdictions. All in all, there are more than three thousand reporting entities. No overarching data legislation exists, so the CDC must deal with innumerable individual data-sharing agreements, and each entity can decide what data to share, how, and when. The technical capacity of reporting sites varies widely, from use of the most modern electronic systems to outdated technologies such as fax and paper-based spreadsheets. Data transmission to the CDC is fragmented, incomplete, and slow.

Walensky reminded critics that, before complaining about lack of access to CDC data, they should ask whether the CDC itself has been provided the data or has authority to seek them. She emphasized the need for legislation to implement standardized approaches to data collection, with appropriate privacy protections, on a national basis.

As criticisms and recommendations rained down from different quarters, agency reviews were conducted. Walensky acknowledged that the CDC had stumbled, that its COVID-19 response had been slow and confusing, and that corrective action was needed. In 2021, she announced the creation of the Center for Forecasting and Outbreak Analytics, a new organizational entity to focus on public health data gathering, mathematical modeling, emergency response, and communications.[70] She emphasized the need for greater agility on the part of the agency, clearer communications, and a more practical, less academic approach. Rather than waiting for peer review, preprint information should be made available, acknowledging that scientific communications might have to be modified based on further experience.

Political commentaries called for increased congressional control over the CDC and for requiring confirmation by the Senate of the CDC director.* Other recommended fixes included

---

* As of January 2025, Senate confirmation is required for incoming CDC directors. Previously, the director of CDC was appointed by the president.

oversight boards, increased funding, organizational restructuring, and enhanced technology. A paper in the influential journal *Health Affairs* argued for the agency to go back to basics, meaning limiting itself to communicable disease control.[71] By trying to cover all public health, the argument went, bureaucracy increased while core capacity diminished. The authors deemed public health impact from funding on problems such as obesity and diabetes, or on surveillance capacity, negligible. They argued for major strengthening of the uniformed Public Health Service and the EIS program, and for increased recruitment of informatics specialists.

Former CDC Director Frieden countered strongly that the CDC should maintain a broad public health mandate.[72] He admitted the CDC was slow, impractical, and not strategic, but pointed out the restrictions under which the agency works, such as its many dozens of individual funding lines. He called for an increase in CDC field staff, observing that many professionals at the CDC had little experience in public health implementation across the country. Fundamental was the need to regain the trust of the American people as well as of international colleagues. These arguments were later expanded in a joint op-ed by eight former CDC Directors highlighting the importance of the agency keeping a broad public health mandate.[73]

As discussions about the CDC played out and global discourse promised better pandemic preparedness, COVID-19 began to recede into the distance. On May 5, 2023, the WHO director general declared COVID-19 over as a global health emergency, though emphasizing to the World Health Assembly that it remained a global health threat.[74,75] In the United States, May 11, 2023, marked the end of the federal COVID-19 Public Health Emergency Declaration.[76]

The world was moving on, although the virus was not necessarily of the same mind. WHO reported almost 2.3 million cases and 15,000 COVID-19 deaths over the month spanning these events.[77] In the United States, there were almost 1,500 COVID-19 deaths the week the emergency was considered over.[78] On the same day that WHO declared the end of the pandemic, Walensky announced she was resigning as CDC director.[79] She had been forthright in criticism of the agency and in defining some of the needs for reform.[80] Rather quickly, a new CDC director was announced, Mandy Cohen, who among other influential roles, had served as the health secretary of the North Carolina Department of Health and Human Services. These rotating chairs caused inevitable speculation. For the loyal staff of the beleaguered agency, they communicated a sense of uncertainty and undermined the cohesiveness and mutual support that characterized the CDC at its best. People were waiting for yet another shoe to drop.

Parting Thoughts

COVID-19 has presented the CDC with its greatest existential challenge since it was established in 1946. Reasons for suboptimal performance were technical as well as social and political. The United States has some characteristics as a society that sets it apart from other countries. For a nation so rich, unequal access to health care, poor health outcomes, and health disparities are astonishing. Rates of obesity, diabetes, and other noncommunicable diseases are high. National public health infrastructure is degraded and staffing inadequate. When things go wrong, somebody must be blamed. The CDC made mistakes during the pandemic but was not unique among government entities or representatives in that regard, any more than the United States was the only country in the world that should have done better. The blame does not lie solely with the CDC, despite the agency's avoidable missteps.

My time at WHO as HIV/AIDS director from 2006 to 2009 gave me insight into the high expectations of that organization, expectations that contrast with the inadequate support and flexibility accorded to it. All too often, blame for adverse health events was laid at WHO's door, amid calls for reform. Reflecting on my WHO service, I drew comparisons between WHO and the CDC,[81] believing the latter operated more freely and was less encumbered by budgetary, political, and regulatory constraints. The COVID-19 experience suggests that challenges faced by the two organizations are more similar than I realized. These observations, however, do not dismiss the need for critical self-examination on the part of the CDC.

The crisis of COVID-19 offers opportunity to re-examine and find consensus on core and realistic expectations of the CDC. Public health is inherently political, and protection of the nation's health is a political responsibility of the government. Former CDC Director William ("Bill") Roper articulated what is needed but was lacking during COVID-19: "We need the best of science to guide the decisions that are made by political leaders to implement effective public health programs. We need a constructive working together of science and the political process."[82]

To provide objective, evidence-based guidance, a national public health institute needs a certain level of independence and room to maneuver.[25-27] The CDC lost its independence during COVID-19. Government and agencies need to ensure decisive leadership and effective organizational structure for decision-making, implementation, and communication. Leadership and organization during COVID-19 were chaotic, inconsistent, and weak.

Jim Curran, former head of AIDS at the CDC and former dean of Emory University's public health school, advised me for one of my positions that surveillance was the CDC's most important responsibility. Surveillance, in his words, is the conscience of any epidemic and provides epidemics their milestones. COVID-19 has shown that for future surveillance and public health reporting to be fit for purpose, strategic thinking is required about necessary adaptations and investments.

What is required is not only funding but extensive revamping of systems, increased personnel, investment in technology of the future such as artificial intelligence and informatics, and regulatory reform. Innovative approaches to environmental sampling and data collection closer to the community will be required. The CDC should not be expected to deliver twenty-first century results with twentieth century technology and systems, nor with regulatory impediments conflicting with the performance demanded.

Delivery of health care and public health services to a federated country is complex. States' rights and responsibilities are seen differently across the nation. To what extent the CDC is a data and normative agency, like WHO, and to what degree it should be involved in program implementation at the local level needs clarity. To reduce the CDC's responsibilities from broad public health to only communicable diseases would restrict the agency's impact. Not only would this ignore the leading causes of morbidity and mortality in the American population, noncommunicable diseases, it would restrict the breadth of response capacity.

The criticisms of the CDC's COVID-19 response need careful addressing, but it is important to protect long-standing strengths. Rapidity of data gathering and provision of advice are essential, but so is accuracy. I recall former CDC Director Julie Gerberding at the time of SARS saying to me, in relation to competition to prove its viral etiology, "It's good to be first, but it's important to be right." That science is an evolutionary process needs to be considered as public health guidance is issued. The public must understand that rapid guidance may need subsequent modification based on new information.

At a geopolitical level, major crises such as COVID-19 or Ebola in West Africa stimulate calls for reform and new initiatives. Everyone agrees that performance next time must be better and that the same deficiencies and mistakes must not be tolerated. Negotiations through WHO have been ongoing since 2021 to formulate an instrument committing countries to strengthen pandemic prevention, preparedness, and response. A funding mechanism, the Pandemic Fund, was launched in 2022.

These efforts deserve support but will not change local field realities quickly. And countries must live up to their commitments to transparency and adherence to the IHR, without which pandemic agreements are ineffective. China was not open about SARS nor about early COVID-19, and Tanzania was a COVID-19 and Ebola denier. We will not do better without attention and commitment to basics—scientific openness and transparency, data and specimen sharing, leadership, and getting simple things right at the field level. Ultimately, it is operational effectiveness at the local level that determines much of epidemic outcomes.

In early interviews, the CDC's latest director, Mandy Cohen, emphasized the need for public trust. Therein lies the future—ensuring the population's trust in the quest for health equity. The CDC's strongest asset is, and always has been, its dedicated workforce. As my own time at the CDC closed and I now look back, I support the words of former CDC Director David Sencer, commenting on his years at the agency: "I think my favorite memory is the fact that this was an organization made up of people. It was the finest group of people you can imagine."[83]

PART III

BUREAUCRAT

The career of an EIS officer who remains at the CDC typically falls into three phases. The 2-year EIS program and subsequent early years are devoted to technical work and projects, protected time to hone epidemiologic, public health, and communication skills. Supervisory and other responsibilities are scant. After a while, mid-level positions are sought, such as chief of a branch, heading a group that may encompass several dozen people in different sections.

Several branches together make up a division, which number many more employees. The highest organizational units at the CDC are centers, institutes, or offices. Centers employ many hundreds of people or more. The third and final phase of a CDC career may involve a senior leadership position or another post providing high-level support in the running of the organization that in total numbers about fifteen thousand personnel. Whatever this later assignment, it is likely to be more remote from day-to-day scientific investigation, and more supervisory, advisory, or regulatory.

Immediately after my EIS period, I was assigned overseas to Cote d'Ivoire in West Africa, to conduct research into HIV-2.[1] We modeled the establishment of this research site, what became known as Projet RETRO-CI, on earlier CDC experience of HIV research at Projet SIDA in the Democratic Republic of the Congo. My subsequent senior positions included directorship of a division (HIV/AIDS Prevention—Surveillance and Epidemiology) and a new center (Center for Global Health). I also served as director of the Department of HIV/AIDS at WHO in Geneva, and, repeatedly, director of CDC work in Kenya. Scientific and technical aspects of HIV/AIDS work are largely captured in an earlier book describing the CDC's response to AIDS, written in conjunction with Harold Jaffe and Jim Curran.[1]

The final section of this book offers observations and perspectives on more supervisory, less directly technical experiences that still offer lessons. The term "bureaucrat" is often used pejoratively, especially by technical specialists and academics. Yet, sound administration and organization are essential for smooth functioning of any group or institute. I have commented on expansion of CDC work in Cote d'Ivoire and Kenya, and experiences at WHO, focusing as much on the "soft" aspects of work as on the purely scientific that are recorded in the literature. One chapter discusses leadership and management, topics I regret not having been formally trained in or exposed to earlier in life.

Although my later CDC positions were supervisory, it was possible and important to remain scientifically involved. Over the years, I have been drawn into research and programmatic work on tuberculosis, the subject of one chapter in this section. This ancient disease remains frustratingly difficult to control despite the availability of effective tools. It is emblematic of the social, political, and practical challenges we face in global as well as domestic health, challenges that are not simply scientific. It is because of these "soft" barriers that it is included in this section. Although I principally focused on other infectious diseases, I have dealt with tuberculosis throughout my medical career. It cries out for involvement by the best and the brightest.

Section III of this book is less directly scientific and links technical with other essentials of health work, activities, and collaborations. As I look back, I realize that the lessons from human interactions are as relevant as clinical trials, perhaps often even more, to success in global health. I wish I had learned those lessons earlier.

CHAPTER 11

More Than Just a Disease: Tuberculosis

Some infections represent more than just medical pathology. Syphilis, cholera, tuberculosis—these are not simply disease states but indicators that all is not well in society. They point to structural deficiencies for which these ancient conditions are markers. All three infections have long been preventable and treatable.

John Snow demonstrated that cholera was transmitted through contaminated water more than a century and a half ago. Yet, we continue to see cholera epidemics in low- and middle-income countries,[1] including in capital cities. More pregnancies worldwide are affected by congenital syphilis than by HIV.[2] Tuberculosis is the world's leading cause of death from a single infection.[3] These three diseases are measures as meaningful as any economic or social indicator of our precarious commitment to health, development, equity, and social justice.

Missing a diagnosis of tuberculosis should haunt medical practitioners, but it still occurs. When I was a medical student, I was affected by two siblings from an impoverished Irish family admitted to Bristol's pediatric hospital with undiagnosed fever, one going on to die of undiagnosed tuberculous meningitis. In the mid-1990s, while working in one of London's prime university hospitals, I witnessed a delayed diagnosis (despite my recommendation she be treated presumptively) of tuberculosis in a Nigerian cleaner working in this same facility. Results of a bone marrow examination showing a heavy mycobacterial load were too late to prevent her from dying.

I became interested in tuberculosis because of clinical experience, that it was a problem disproportionately affecting the Global South, and through personal involvement in research, especially concerning the relationship of tuberculosis with HIV. Tuberculosis bridges clinical care for individuals with programmatic requirements for a public health approach. For a clinician interested in epidemiology and public health, it is a disease impossible to ignore. Tuberculosis should be seen as an individual injustice as well as a global priority. Innumerable vignettes shaped my understanding and perception of the disease, a dominant but still under-resourced and under-researched entity in global health.

Tuberculosis and HIV: Historical Aspects

More than 40 years into the recognized pandemic of AIDS, older physicians are often struck by how the early history of the disease seems to have been forgotten. The pretreatment era, before the advent of effective antiretroviral therapy (ART) around 1996,[4] is now essentially ignored by medical workers as well as affected communities. So it is with tuberculosis, which, in earlier times, just as when AIDS was untreatable, was a dominant topic of discussion and a potent social force.

Tuberculosis occupies a special place in history.[5-8]. In the nineteenth century, it was the leading cause of death in the United States and Europe, its main victims adolescents and young adults. Diseases of the lung were responsible for up to one-fourth of all deaths. Two centuries earlier, John Bunyon had personified tuberculosis as "the captain of all these men of death."

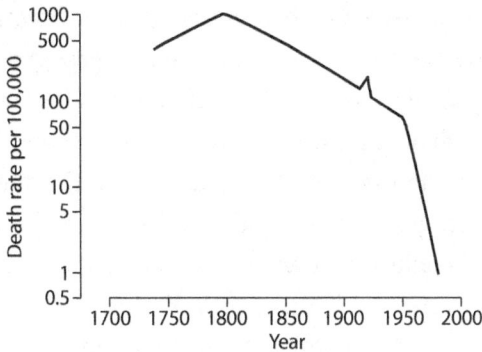

Figure 11.1   Tuberculosis mortality rate, western Europe, 1740–1985.
(From: Murray JF. A century of tuberculosis. Am J Respir Crit Care Med. 2004;169:1181–1186)

Just as with AIDS, fear of tuberculosis was extreme, leading to prejudices that Robert Koch's discovery in 1882 of the causative organism, the tubercle bacillus or *Mycobacterium tuberculosis*, never fully dispelled. Recognition of the tuberculosis microbe was one of the scientific highlights of the late nineteenth century that, along with the work of Louis Pasteur and others, founded modern microbiology. In analogous fashion, research on AIDS has been central to advances in modern virology and immunology.

Previously, individual and family vulnerability were considered to lead to consumption, the favored term for tuberculosis. Although the germ theory of disease refuted such a blanket explanation, later understanding clarified increased susceptibility from conditions such as malnutrition, alcohol dependence, diabetes, or immunosuppression. Indicative of the role of social factors, especially poverty and deprivation, were the declining rates of tuberculosis that accompanied improved nutrition and living standards over many decades, long before the advent of effective chemotherapy (Figure 11.1).

The evolution of tuberculosis, socially and biologically, mirrored some of the later history of the early AIDS epidemic. Art and literature focused on tuberculosis as they subsequently would on AIDS. The extreme wasting that characterized both diseases was striking. One of the best-known fatalities from tuberculosis was the English poet John Keats, whose mother and brother also likely died of the disease. "The weariness, the fever, and the fret. . . . Where youth grows pale, and spectre-thin, and dies," wrote Keats,[9] conjuring up images of end-stage tuberculosis that could equally refer to advanced HIV disease.

The violinist and composer Paganini wasted away, Chopin died of tuberculosis, and numerous English writers were casualties. A certain romanticism accompanied the despair engendered by tuberculosis and HIV when both were untreatable. Although tuberculosis is transmitted through the air and HIV through bodily fluids, these modes of spread result in both diseases clustering in groups with close contact. Untreated, they disproportionately affected and killed family members or people in relationships, each erased cluster a little civilization lost.

Other attributes shared between the two diseases across almost a century were the stuttering advances in therapy, interest in the use of preventive therapy, and lack of an effective vaccine. The first drugs to show efficacy against tuberculosis were para-aminosalicylate and streptomycin, discovered in the mid-1940s, and then followed by thiacetazone and isoniazid.[10-12]

It took some years to recognize that treatment with individual drugs led to resistance and that they needed to be given in combination. A series of international clinical trials laid the foundations for modern chemotherapy that cures tuberculosis in 6 months.[11,12] History repeated itself in the experience with zidovudine monotherapy for HIV/AIDS, licensed in the United States in 1987 but later shown not to prolong life on its own, and only effective when combined with two other drugs.[4]

It is surprising, in retrospect, that multidrug therapy, standard in tuberculosis as well as in cancer chemotherapy, took so long to be adopted in HIV medicine. Combination therapy consisting of three drugs only became standard practice in 1996 when their spectacular impact on reversing advanced immunodeficiency was highlighted at that year's international conference on AIDS in Vancouver, Canada.[4] In similar vein, the long road to immediate rather than deferred therapy in HIV disease seems one of lost opportunities.[4] By contrast, debate in tuberculosis has been about what constitutes a minimum duration for curative therapy, not when to start it.

Analogies exist for the prevention of both diseases. Isoniazid for 6 to 9 months can prevent tuberculosis disease in persons with latent infection.[11] Exhaustive research among people with HIV, as well as realization that about one-fourth of the world's population has latent tuberculosis infection, have increased attention to use of this intervention. In the world of HIV, pre-exposure prophylaxis has emerged as an important prevention tool, its use highest among men who have sex with men.[4] Despite intense research, no effective vaccine has been developed for HIV. For tuberculosis, bacillus Calmette-Guérin has been used for decades, but its efficacy in preventing tuberculosis is questionable.[11,12]

One of the most inspiring aspects of our struggle against AIDS has been the role of activism and civil society.[4] Fighting for their lives, gay men in the 1980s organized to demand change as well as to provide support to those afflicted. Organizations such as Act-Up and Gay Men's Health Crisis influenced research agendas, treatment access, and public health programs, their aims then emulated by other affected groups around the world. Social movements were important a century ago to combat tuberculosis, but the advent of effective chemotherapy lessened emphasis on these efforts, and tuberculosis became viewed almost exclusively as a medical issue. Despite attempts to stimulate such support, community responses to tuberculosis have been limited in recent times.

Prior to the advent of antituberculous chemotherapy there were diverse initiatives to assist the wealthy as well as the poor with "consumption," principally through the sanatorium movement that began in the late nineteenth century. Sunlight, fresh air, nutrition, and high altitude were believed to contribute to remission of tuberculosis and stimulated expansion of sanatoria, institutions where patients were isolated and provided good food and bedrest.

The nature of such facilities was famously captured by Thomas Mann in his epic *The Magic Mountain*.[13] The best friends of my parents in Belgium sent their young adult daughter to Switzerland just before World War II, to die, nonetheless, of tuberculosis. Most sanatoria closed after curative medicines for tuberculosis became available, just as AIDS hospice beds disappeared after the advent of treatment.

Tuberculosis was known to be contagious, and early attempts at infection control included separating children from households with active case patients. Hermann Biggs, later State Commissioner of Health for New York, designed a program around the turn of the twentieth century that included case diagnosis and reporting, hospitalization for indigent patients, and advice on prevention of transmission.[14] He is remembered by many in public health for his oft-cited dictum that public health is purchasable, and every society can determine its own death rate. His rigorous approach had long-lasting influence on tuberculosis control programs that contrasted with the subsequent individual and rights-based approach to HIV.

Despite medical mobilization, such as with creation of the International Union Against Tuberculosis and Lung Disease (IUATLD) in 1920,[15] tuberculosis, like syphilis, has remained bereft of the broad societal response we have seen to AIDS. AMFAR, the American Foundation for AIDS Research, is a powerful AIDS advocacy and research funding organization that benefited from having the actress Elizabeth Taylor as its first national chairperson.[16] A well-endowed, influential organization, the Elizabeth Glazer Pediatric AIDS Foundation, exists to end mother-to-child transmission of HIV.[17] No such groups advocate for the infant with congenital syphilis or to support the single young man or unhoused woman with tuberculosis.

Tuberculosis and Health Care Settings

We too easily forget that health care work can be dangerous, that work in medicine can lead to exposure to diverse infectious agents. A balance is required between duty of care for patients and prioritizing prevention of infection in health care staff. However, inherent risks of acquiring a serious infectious disease have always existed and must be acknowledged.

Prior to the introduction of antimicrobial therapy, a period covering more than half of my surgeon father's career, an infected cut to the finger could be fatal. Contact with blood can expose staff to hepatitis viruses. For a presentation I gave at the Los Angeles County Hospital–University of Southern California Medical Center in the mid-1980s on the newly developed hepatitis B vaccine, I reviewed a decade of staff records and found three of interest, described in Chapter 4. One medical resident had died of fulminant hepatitis B, another became a chronic hepatitis B carrier, and a third (whom I looked after clinically) had an uncomplicated but significant illness. All three were infected with hepatitis B in the course of their work.

Years before, I met up with my colleague Paul Finan to wish him well as he was leaving Bristol but observed that he was jaundiced. If he had not subsequently cleared his acute hepatitis B infection, his surgical career would have stopped before it had even started—hepatitis B–positive surgeons were not allowed to operate because of the risk of transmission to patients. Today, hepatitis B vaccine is recommended or required for all health care personnel.

When giving talks on the 2014–2016 epidemic of Ebola in West Africa, I always remind listeners that several hundred health care workers likely died during that outbreak, most of them infected in the course of their professional duties.[18] For COVID-19, the toll has been much higher, WHO estimating that well more than one hundred thousand caregivers may have died.[19] Health care workers are the backbone of any health system, and much more needs to be done to ensure their safety. One infection that is greatly increased in this population is tuberculosis.

A medical resident with whom I worked in Los Angeles in the mid-1980s recounted to me how the year before he had become very tired, attributing his increasing exhaustion to a heavy clinical workload. When he began losing weight, he put this down to lack of time and inadequate attention to cooking. When he started coughing, he finally sought care and was astonished by his own chest X-ray, which showed extensive cavities in his lungs from tuberculosis.

My pathology colleague Sebastian Lucas underwent a tuberculin skin test (a test to detect prior infection with *Mycobacterium tuberculosis*) after performing hundreds of autopsies on patients who died of AIDS in Abidjan, Cote d'Ivoire, in whom the leading cause of death was tuberculosis.[4] He developed a large ulcerating nodule on his forearm, indicative of a brisk immune response to a heavy infection. Several mortuary staff with whom we worked at Abidjan's university hospital died at a young age of tuberculosis likely acquired in the course of their work. Whether they were infected with HIV was unknown.

Lessons learned by personal experience are often the most powerful. Around 2005, working in Kenya, I read accounts in the newspapers of exceptionally high rates of tuberculosis in staff at Kenyatta National Hospital, where my career in global health had started. Working with the Ministry of Health, CDC headquarters, and the Field Epidemiology Training Program, we arranged for an epidemiologic investigation.[20]

There was ample evidence that health care workers were, indeed, becoming infected with tuberculosis through their work. The annual incidence of tuberculosis in staff ranged from 645 to 1,115 per 100,000 population, more than 100–200 or so times greater than in the general population of the United States at the time. Health care workers deployed to areas where patients with tuberculosis were congregated had twice the risk for acquiring the disease compared to other colleagues. Nonetheless, other social factors were also relevant, such as living in a slum (five times increased risk) and HIV infection (twenty-nine times increased risk). None of these findings were novel in themselves but did indicate how much still had to be done to protect health care personnel.

Although low- and middle-income facilities do not have the resources available in more privileged environments, the CDC's prioritized, three-tiered approach to tuberculosis prevention in health care settings is still applicable.[21] Intervention measures are categorized as administrative, environmental, and based on use of respiratory equipment. Preventive measures should be part of an overall infection prevention and control plan, with written guidance and clearly defined supervision to ensure rapid detection of active cases of tuberculosis, reduction of exposures, monitoring of health care workers, and education of patients, visitors, and staff, including about cough etiquette. Environmental measures should assure ventilation and airflow, which, in under-resourced settings, may simply be opening windows. Respiratory measures can include provision of personal protective equipment (PPE) such as high-quality masks in areas of potential exposure.

Lack of PPE for health care staff, suggestions of corruption in procurement of PPE, and uncertain advice about masks were some of the complexities that handicapped the global response to COVID-19. An under-recognized opportunity from the COVID-19 experience is the possibility of greater collaboration and coordination on how we address diverse respiratory pathogens, including tuberculosis and influenza.

Tuberculosis and HIV

It took the better part of a decade after 1981, the year that AIDS was first described,[4] to recognize how devastating the impact of HIV was on global tuberculosis epidemiology. Evidence that tuberculosis was an opportunistic disease complicating HIV infection came from clinical observations, data from tuberculosis and AIDS surveillance, HIV seroprevalence studies in tuberculosis patients, the results of observational cohort studies, and the effect of antiretroviral therapy (ART).[22,23]

Initial clues in the early 1980s were frequent diagnoses of tuberculosis, often disseminated or extrapulmonary, in patients from low-income settings with AIDS-defining illnesses. Many Haitians with AIDS in the United States and many African patients presenting in Europe exemplified this. The large autopsy study led by Lucas in Abidjan, Cote d'Ivoire, in 1991 showed that tuberculosis was the cause of death in about one-third of patients dying with HIV disease.[24] I mentioned this last observation to Michael (Mike) Merson and Arata Kochi, the respective heads of the HIV and tuberculosis programs at WHO in Geneva,[4] while on a visit there later that same year. Their look of shock and disbelief was memorable.

Surveillance data from the United States showed that the long-standing annual decline in tuberculosis cases ceased in the mid-1980s and was then followed by an increase (Figure 11.2).[12] Trends were most marked in geographic areas with the most AIDS cases and in the populations with the highest rates of AIDS. Research-

Progress towards TB elimination, United States, 1982–2022

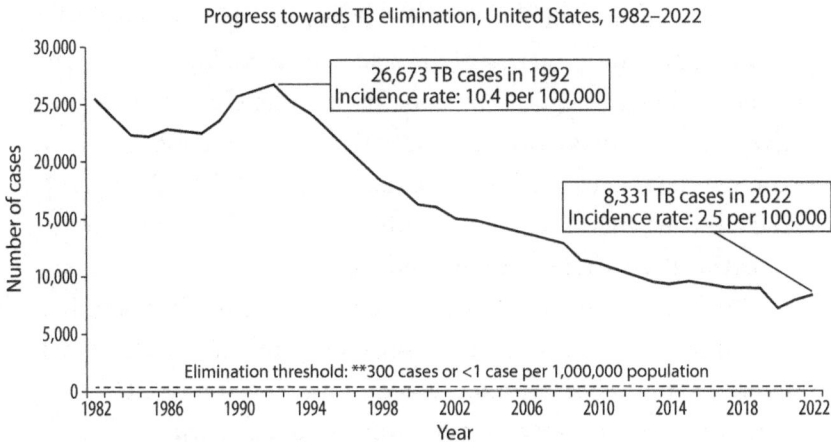

Figure 11.2   Progress toward tuberculosis elimination, United States, 1982–2022.

(https://www.cdc.gov/tb/statistics/reports/2022/default.htm)

ers at Projet SIDA in the Democratic Republic of the Congo in 1986 showed there was an increased prevalence of HIV infection in patients with tuberculosis.[4,25] A subsequent avalanche of reports from around the world then showed similar findings, that patients with tuberculosis had an elevated frequency of HIV infection compared with the general population. This was true for HIV-1 as well as HIV-2.[4,26]

Extrapulmonary tuberculosis is associated with more extreme immunodeficiency than pulmonary disease. A global review in the early 2000s that focused strongly on Africa showed that as general population HIV prevalence increased, so HIV prevalence in patients with tuberculosis was elevated also, anywhere from three to six times higher.[27] National tuberculosis incidence was correlated with the prevalence of HIV in the general population: the higher the HIV prevalence, the higher the incidence of tuberculosis.

Two final pieces of evidence, perhaps the strongest, were the results of cohort studies comparing HIV-infected and uninfected persons over time, and the impact of ART in reducing HIV-associated immunodeficiency. HIV infection converts the generally accepted lifetime risk of disease from reactivation of latent infection in HIV-negative persons, approximately 10%, to a relatively similar *annual* risk in those with HIV.[28] Infection with HIV compresses the natural history of tuberculosis in time, "speeds up the tape," as well as leaving the infected person vulnerable to reinfection even after treatment and cure.[29]

The introduction of ART greatly changed this situation, but not entirely.[30,31] The first demonstration of public health impact came from analysis of experience in an eleven-city CDC surveillance cohort. Between 1996 and 1998, the period covering the introduction of ART on a large scale, tuberculosis declined by 80% in those patients who received ART.[23] Nonetheless, despite such important reductions in tuberculosis incidence, later work has shown that even with treatment, persons with HIV in high-burden countries retain an elevated incidence of tuberculosis, as high as 2%–3% per year. Such an incidence in HIV-positive persons undergoing ART approximates the rates of tuberculosis seen in Europe or North America in the early 1900s, heydays of the "white plague." ART is a tremendous advance for all people with HIV, but on its own will not solve the problem of tuberculosis.

Tuberculosis Control, Including in HIV Infection

Compared with the treatment of HIV, which requires life-long adherence to therapy and does not lead to cure, the treatment of tuberculosis seems simple. Nevertheless, early identification of persons with the disease, instituting treatment, and assuring adherence and completion of the required 6 months of therapy are challenging. Long-standing research aspirations have been the development of simple diagnostics and shorter, simpler treatment regimens. Early diagnosis and treatment of patients with pulmonary tuberculosis, the source of transmission, have been the basis of tuberculosis control at the population level.

Training in internal medicine in the United Kingdom in the 1970s, I rarely saw cases of tuberculosis. In preparing for specialist exams, I was advised to update myself on the recently introduced drug rifampicin (called rifampin in the United States), considered an important advance because of its potency and tolerability. When I started work in Kenya in 1979, tuberculosis was a frequent diagnosis. Patients were treated with a daunting 12-month regimen that required hospitalization for the first month for daily injections of streptomycin combined with two oral drugs taken over the whole treatment period (isoniazid and thiacetazone). A special facility separate from the main hospital housed such patients who, unsurprisingly, found adherence to this punishing schedule difficult.

At the end of the 1980s, I found myself in Cote d'Ivoire studying HIV-1 and HIV-2 infections.[4] We immediately established strong links with the national tuberculosis program—we had included patients with tuberculosis in a pilot study of overall HIV prevalence in Abidjan in 1987. The director of the national program was Raymond Bretton, a small, wiry Frenchman with an intense stare accentuated by his bushy eyebrows and large spectacles. Because we offered HIV testing for all patients attending Abidjan's two large *Centres Antituberculeux* (tuberculosis centers), Bretton was only too pleased to collaborate.

A review of African data at the time showed HIV prevalence in patients with tuberculosis ranged from 20% to 67%.[32] In southern Africa, it later increased even further so that the great majority of patients with tuberculosis also had HIV. In essence, African tuberculosis facilities became AIDS centers, and AIDS clinics had to address tuberculosis.[33] Bretton focused on the tuberculosis program rather than on individual patients. Much of his time was spent searching for funds and assuring an adequate supply of drugs. He taught himself computer skills and the use of spreadsheets to manage commodities and forecast requirements.

As tuberculosis worsened, its programmatic rigidity was increasingly contrasted with the evolving rights-based, individual approach to HIV. Fresh from leading Projet SIDA in the Democratic Republic of the Congo, Jonathan Mann had joined WHO in 1986 to lead the agency's response to the rapidly escalating pandemic of HIV.[4] With effective HIV treatment a decade away, initial prevention efforts were based on behavior change. Mann grounded his program in countering stigma and discrimination, protecting human rights, and involving civil society. These approaches, as well as the nature of key populations affected by HIV—men who have sex with men, sex workers, people who inject drugs—were alien to the conservative tuberculosis establishment.

As HIV-associated tuberculosis increased in Africa and some other parts of the world, attention in the early 1990s was drawn to New York City.[12] Outbreaks of tuberculosis were occurring in different institutional settings, including hospitals and prisons. These outbreaks disproportionately affected HIV-infected persons and some involved multidrug-resistant disease that had a high fatality rate.

This all represented a coming together of different, apparently intractable problems: high rates of HIV; drug-resistant tuberculosis from lack of adherence to therapy; poorly ventilated, overcrowded, and unsafe facilities promoting airborne infections; high rates of incarceration, much of it for drug offenses; racial disparities, with African Americans and Hispanics disproportionately affected; and large numbers of immigrants from countries with high tuberculosis incidence. And all of this was occurring on a background of localized poverty, drug use, homelessness, and long-standing erosion of tuberculosis control infrastructure. Outbreaks in prisons were enhanced by regular movement of prisoners between facilities to prevent the emergence of gangs, which inadvertently disseminated tuberculosis throughout New York State's large prison system. Concern was greatly heightened by tuberculosis cases among prison guards, some multidrug resistant and fatal.

Alarmed by global trends and the North American experience, WHO declared tuberculosis a global emergency in 1993.[34] Its tuberculosis program was directed by the hard-driving Japanese insider, Arata Kochi, and was heavily influenced by Karel Styblo, a Czech-born citizen of the Netherlands who had survived imprisonment and tuberculosis during World War II in the concentration camp of Mauthausen in Austria. Styblo, who at one time was head of the IUATLD, made seminal contributions to understanding the epidemiology of tuberculosis and designing effective but simple control programs.[35,36]

Styblo drew attention to the association between the risk of tuberculosis infection in a population, the prevalence of active pulmonary disease at one point in time, and the annual incidence of new active cases. He showed that standardized programs could function effectively even in the poorest countries, such as Tanzania, and emphasized measuring specific outcomes: cure; treatment failure; death; loss to follow-up; or transfer out.

Drawing heavily on Styblo's contributions, WHO rebranded its approach under the slogan DOTS—directly observed therapy (DOT), short course.[37] DOT referred to observation by a health care worker that a patient swallowed his or her therapy, and short course indicated the shorter regimens now used throughout the world—shorter than the 12-month, injection-containing regimen, but still not uniform. Therapeutic research had advanced and rifampicin-containing regimens (four drugs for 2 months, and then two drugs for the final 4 months) were used in high-income countries. In low-income settings, longer regimens were given because rifampicin and some other compounds were prohibitively expensive. The actual direct observation of therapy also was variable.

A new problem emerged with the drug thiacetazone. This medicine was cheap and continued to be used in low-income countries, including throughout Africa. In persons with HIV, however, there was a high rate of adverse drug reactions, including Stevens-Johnson syndrome, a painful and disfiguring, sometimes fatal, blistering condition of the skin and mucous membranes, often involving the eyes and mouth.[38]

The beauty of DOTS was its simplicity, affordability, and standardization. It could be applied everywhere, based on its principles of political commitment, diagnosis through microscopy of sputum, a secure drug supply, outcome evaluations, and direct observation. Unfortunately, several awkward findings and events interfered with smooth implementation, acceptance, and impact. These related to program performance, even without HIV; feasibility in the face of rising cases; and philosophic differences and conflicts between the world's HIV and tuberculosis communities. Most importantly, tuberculosis associated with HIV did not obey Styblo's epidemiologic rules.

DOTS was not just standardized, it was rigid, and its proponents tended to be also. Bretton in Abidjan frequently told me that 80% of tuberculosis control was organization, not medicine—an indication there was not much room in his efficient but poorly funded program for individual patient concerns. The requirement for sputum microscopy during treatment and at its completion rapidly outstripped capacity in African countries, but neither WHO nor Styblo accepted this reality. A colleague in South Africa and I suggested documenting completion of therapy might replace universal sputum examination as a more realistic option,[39-41] but this was considered heretical.

Thiacetazone caused much debate. AIDS activists demanded this drug be withdrawn because of its toxicity in persons with HIV, whereas tuberculosis experts such as Hans Rieder, formerly with the CDC and now with the IUATLD, defended its important role in tuberculosis control. Eventually, but after much pathology and suffering, funding increased, drug costs diminished, thiacetazone was abandoned, and short-course, rifampicin-containing regimens became essentially universal.

Most striking, however, were trends even in countries with respected and previously effective tuberculosis programs but high rates of HIV, such as Botswana. Despite rigorous implementation of DOTS, tuberculosis cases and deaths continued to increase.[42] Styblo was deeply disheartened by the HIV experience, taking it as an affront to his life's work.

At a conference of the IUATLD in 1996, I asked him about potential modification of DOTS in the face of HIV. His reluctant, inflexible answer was that we might have to wait decades for the HIV epidemic to pass and, in the meantime, rely more on chest X-rays than sputum examination for diagnosis in heavily affected cities. However, that DOTS alone was insufficient was not countenanced, and that patients required attention to other HIV-related disease was considered not the responsibility of tuberculosis programs.

Richard ("Dick") Chaisson, a tuberculosis expert from Johns Hopkins University, and I wrote an opinion piece entitled "Will DOTS do it?" arguing that tuberculosis programs needed to adapt to the realities and needs of the HIV epidemic.[43] I had wanted to use the title "DOTS don't do it" but thought that was provocative. To our surprise, this became one of the most widely cited papers in the history of *The International Journal of Tuberculosis and Lung Disease*.

In New York City, Tom Frieden—former EIS officer, later New York City Commissioner for Health, and later still CDC director—led his program to contain the epidemic of drug-resistant tuberculosis, describing the experience in an eloquent article in the *New*

England Journal of Medicine entitled "Turning the tide."[44] Frieden's experience with tuberculosis in New York and later in India profoundly affected his overall public health outlook, leading to wry comments from others that the prism of tuberculosis, India, and New York did not always provide an adequate life view.

Frieden, often inspiring, recounted that Styblo galvanized him with one question when the expert was visiting New York in the early 1990s. Frieden had given Styblo an extensive overview of his innovative program but was blindsided when asked "How many patients did you cure?" Expressing shame at his inability to answer, Frieden realized his program had concentrated on process indicators such as numbers of diagnoses and treatments, not outcomes. He aggressively reformed his practice, and his insight led to suggestions that a similar approach was needed for HIV treatment programs: cohort analysis with documentation of standard outcomes, providing accountability to every individual patient.[45]

Much later I heard Frieden talk to a group at the CDC concerning our work in global health. He emphasized that tuberculosis programming was hard, boring, and yielded few quick results. "Well," I thought, "I am not sure that's the way to recruit the best and the brightest," but it captured a sense of mission, hard work, and rigidity that had been rather consistent in the tuberculosis community.

Central to this conflict between approaches is the fact that HIV-positive and HIV-negative tuberculosis are fundamentally different conditions. HIV-associated tuberculosis represents a failing immune system of which tuberculosis is but a symptom and that antituberculous therapy alone cannot correct. We showed in Abidjan, prior to the advent of antiretroviral therapy, that 2-year mortality in HIV-positive persons treated for tuberculosis was about 20%–25%, very much higher than in those without HIV.[46]

Bretton in Abidjan often observed that he did not understand why the overall tuberculosis case load did not increase in a city with such a severe HIV epidemic, where 40% of his patients were HIV infected. An elegant analysis of tuberculosis trends by Sonia Richards, an EIS officer assisted by Michael ("Mike") St. Louis, gave insight. Bretton's well-functioning program succeeded in reducing the incidence of tuberculosis in the HIV-negative population, but this was compensated for by increased cases in HIV-positive persons, the net result being a stable case load overall.[47]

What persons with HIV require is ART, the only currently effective way of preventing and correcting the immune deficiency that predisposes HIV-infected persons to develop tuberculosis. Different country analyses have shown how ART scale-up abruptly reduced tuberculosis incidence, but only in HIV-positive persons.[23,48-51] To understand tuberculosis trends, the two populations need to be analyzed separately.

A final divergence in attitudes and program implementation concerned drug-resistant tuberculosis. Drug resistance results from lack of adherence to therapy or erratic drug administration, leading to selection pressure and emergence of resistant mutants. Multidrug resistance in the context of tuberculosis was defined as resistance to at least rifampicin and isoniazid.[52] More complex resistance involving additional classes of drugs became known as extensively drug-resistant disease, which threatened to render tuberculosis incurable.[53] Older regimens for drug-resistant disease were extremely demanding in time (often longer than 1 year) and acceptance (drugs administered by painful injections or with severe side effects), cure rates were low, and the mortality rate was high. Fortunately, there has been progress in developing shorter regimens requiring only drugs taken by mouth, and for less than 1 year.[54]

Traditional dogma was that well-functioning programs cured patients, and that drug resistance represented program failure. This was best addressed, then, by correcting program performance, rather than focusing on individual patients with drug-resistant, often fatal disease. And because resistance is driven by lack of adherence (formerly referred to as "compliance"), patients were often considered at fault for not taking their medicines. High rates of tuberculosis and drug resistance in minority populations and people who inject drugs compounded such attitudes. Frieden's energetic leadership in New York City showed that the challenge of drug resistance could be lessened or contained by program strengthening, strong supervision, and prioritizing and measuring outcomes at the individual patient level.[44]

New York may have been an exception, however, and to HIV and other activists, traditional tuberculosis views exemplified the chasm in outlook. Individuals with drug-resistant tuberculosis, advocates argued, had the right to the best treatment.[55] Moreover, for biological as well as social reasons, persons with HIV were especially at risk, so not prioritizing patients with drug-resistant tuberculosis was doubly discriminatory. And with high levels of drug resistance, dangerous strains could be transmitted to others just like drug-sensitive strains, so, surely, they should be treated to prevent further spread. Civil society groups such as Partners in Health lobbied strongly for drug-resistant tuberculosis to be considered a priority.[55]

Fortunately, with time and research, differences in opinion and practice have lessened. Advances have been made in treatment of multidrug-resistant tuberculosis with all-oral regimens taken for less than 1 year, with high cure rates.[54] WHO, in its annual report on tuberculosis, now recognizes what are three very different scenarios: "old-style" HIV-negative tuberculosis, HIV-associated tuberculosis, and drug-resistant tuberculosis.[3] Silos and frictions still exist, including in measurement—do persons dying of HIV-associated tuberculosis count as AIDS deaths, tuberculosis deaths, or both? Such questions illustrate that a person can only die once but be counted many times. Nonetheless, HIV and tuberculosis programs now collaborate better, and although complete program integration is rare,[56] the need to coordinate efforts is universally accepted.

The South African Gold Mines

I was teaching at the London School of Hygiene and Tropical Medicine in the mid-1990s, writing up research work from 5 years in Cote d'Ivoire,[4] and still focusing on HIV and tuberculosis in sub-Saharan Africa. I was asked to meet with Gavin Churchyard, a physician working for the mining consortium Anglo-American in South Africa. Churchyard directed medical services for the company in the gold-mining town of Welkom and was visiting to seek collaboration.

He was adept at computer graphics and toured the School with bar charts and histograms describing health trends, including for tuberculosis, in the mining community. He sought out academics interested in tuberculosis, but when he appeared in my office he was worn down, dejected from the dismissive reception shown by leading experts. It took me only a short while to realize that his setting was, literally, a gold mine for research.

Welkom in its heyday was a booming town with several mining companies employing well more than one hundred thousand miners.[57] Churchyard oversaw health services for Free Gold, a gold-mining subsidiary of Anglo American, and its associated Ernest Oppenheimer Hospital that hosted the tuberculosis control program. Health care was free for miners, medical records and investigations were linked through unique identifiers, work histories were documented, annual chest X-rays were performed, and an electronic medical records system was in place.[58] It was an ideal environment to support different epidemiologic investigations on the interactions between HIV and tuberculosis.

Gold mining is a dangerous, curious business. Gold, a nontoxic, malleable metal resistant to rust and with high electrical conductivity, has few practical uses. It is prized in jewelry and used to a limited extent in medicine, dentistry, and electronics. Its greatest role, of course, is in finance, where bullion serves as a security and asset of wealth, exchangeable for other commodities or financial entities. And therein lies the strangeness: a multitude of people laboring dangerously under the earth or in artisanal pits to extract ore that yields a metal that, when purified, is used for vanity products or again rendered inaccessible in underground or locked vaults.

As South Africa's gold seams became progressively depleted, the mining shafts went ever deeper, as much as 3 kilometers down. Temperatures were extreme, working space was often not more than 1 meter high, and injuries were a constant risk. Gold mining is inextricably linked to the history of apartheid and its dependence on migrant labor.[59,60] The recruitment of men from surrounding countries to work in the mines is hauntingly captured in the 1974 song "Stimela" by the late South African trumpeter, Hugh Masekela.[61] The single-sex hostels in which miners lived promoted excessive alcohol use, an industry of commercial sex, high rates of sexually transmitted infections, and then an epidemic of HIV.

Prior to the spread of HIV, which began in southern Africa several years later than in East Africa, the leading cause of death in miners was work-related injuries, and these remained the main killer of HIV-negative workers.[62] Tuberculosis and disease from other mycobacterial agents ("nontuberculous mycobacteria" [NTM]) were common, predisposed to by crowded living conditions but especially exposure to silica-containing dust underground.[63] Inhalation of dust led to the occupational lung disease silicosis, which can result in progressive loss of lung function and respiratory failure. It also predisposed to tuberculosis. Environmental and occupational measures were supposed to be in place to limit dust exposure. Miners underwent regular chest X-rays, which served to diagnose tuberculosis or NTM disease and grade the severity of silicosis.

Like many, I had refrained from ever visiting South Africa in the apartheid era. The release of Nelson Mandela from prison and his ascent to the presidency changed attitudes, and a delegation from the London School visited South Africa in late 1994. We met with senior representatives of the Chamber of Mines as well as mining unions and were struck by the denial expressed by representatives from all sides, employers and workers, of the severity and implications of the expanding HIV epidemic. South Africa seemed far ahead of other African nations in infrastructure and development, but behind in addressing AIDS, and post-apartheid inequities and racial disparities continued to blight all discussions.

Studies in the Gold Mines

One of the advantages of working in London was the quality of junior medical staff and postgraduate students. I oversaw three outstanding individuals, Julia del Amo, Alison Grant, and Elizabeth ("Liz") Corbett, who obtained grants for their PhD research. Del Amo conducted a large review of the natural history and spectrum of HIV disease in Africans in London, showing the different opportunistic infections, including tuberculosis, in this population, and their similar survival to non-Africans when medical care was available.[64-66] The latter observation indicated that different HIV subtypes (subtype B predominant in Europeans, and subtypes A or C in Africans) did not have major influence on overall outcomes. Grant went to Projet RETRO-CI in Cote d'Ivoire to further clarify disease manifestations of HIV in this West African setting.[4,67-69]

It was Liz Corbett who furthered the collaboration with Gavin Churchyard. Having finished her clinical training in internal medicine and rejecting my advice to enroll for a 1-year master's degree program in epidemiology, she threw herself into work in Welkom and taught herself sophisticated data analysis and mathematical modeling. Another key individual was Brian Williams, whom I first met during the London School's exploratory visit in 1994 when he headed science and public health for the Chamber of Mines. Williams, a cheerful, informal individual, was the right man in the wrong job. A mathematician by background, his strengths were in analysis, not organization or implementation. When aspects of program or scientific management came up, he looked forlorn. When discussion turned to theoretical questions potentially addressed by mathematical modeling, his eyes lit up.

My experience at the London School impressed on me the importance of surrounding oneself with the right people. The PhD students have all gone on to have stellar careers. Gavin Churchyard later obtained a PhD himself, became internationally renowned in tuberculosis circles, and now heads a health implementation and research organization in South Africa, the Aurum Institute, that brings in tens of millions of dollars of funding annually.[70] Williams has had major influence as one of the world's most incisive mathematical modelers in HIV and tuberculosis. Corbett has had a productive research career on these topics in southern Africa. I was heartened when my nomination of her for the prestigious Annual Scientific Prize of the International Union Against Tuberculosis and Lung Disease in 2003 was successful. "You are who you hire" has been a constant maxim for me, and scientific and medical achievements today are never individual accomplishments.

Our first descriptive paper laid the scene[71]; tuberculosis rates in miners more than doubled over the period of 1990–1996 from already high rates (>1,000/100,000 per year) to almost 2,500/100,000 per year, among the highest incidence in any population in the world. HIV prevalence in patients with tuberculosis increased from 15% to 45%. Patients with tuberculosis and HIV were more likely to present for medical care than those without HIV, who were more frequently diagnosed through routine X-ray screening. NTM disease was also frequent, with HIV infection and lung scarring from silicosis or prior tuberculosis as risk factors. In this way a vicious cycle could be envisaged: rising rates of HIV on a background of continuous exposure to silica dust predisposed to both tuberculosis and NTM disease, and the latter then was further encouraged by increased tuberculosis incidence and its associated lung damage.

Numerous separate studies considered drug resistance; NTM biology; diagnosis and utility of chest X-ray screening; increased risk of recurrence of tuberculosis; risk factors for disease and death; the spectrum and natural history of HIV-associated disease; and implementation of tuberculosis preventive therapy.[62,72-89] Miners with HIV infection were nine times more likely to die than those without HIV. The leading cause of death in HIV-negative miners was trauma, which was responsible for 60% of their deaths, compared with 6% for miners with HIV. The dominant profile of the tertiary-level mining hospital changed from a specialized trauma service to one providing AIDS care in the era prior to availability of ART.

Several studies gave sharp insight into the disturbing disease trends. Silicosis was a traditional accompaniment to a miner's career, and often its terminating factor. Autopsies were routinely conducted on miners who died, prioritizing examination of the heart and lungs. If silicosis or tuberculosis from industrial exposure were to blame, compensation would be paid. Miners unable to work also were compensated. Corbett became an expert in grading the severity of silicosis by personally reading about ten thousand chest X-rays.

A later report showed that silicosis rates among autopsied miners escalated from 3% in 1975 to 32% in 2007,[90] likely related to longer employment and, therefore, greater cumulative silica exposure. Although regulatory systems had long been in place to compensate miners and their families for occupational lung disease, a large proportion of compensation remained unclaimed or unpaid to miners and dependents in countries far away.[90,91]

Welkom's rich databases provided opportunity for retrospective analyses of exposures and outcomes over time, technically referred to as retrospective cohort studies. Such studies are efficient because they offer longitudinal observation of what has already occurred, obviating need for long follow-up into the future. Prior to the advent of HIV, silicosis was the strongest known risk factor for tuberculosis. Corbett showed that HIV and silicosis interacted, not independently, but in a multiplicative way.[84] In miners with HIV and severe silicosis, tuberculosis occurred with an extraordinary annual incidence of 16%.

By the year 2000, HIV prevalence in all miners had reached 30% and the annual rate of tuberculosis was greater than 4,000 per 100,000 miners, a fourfold increase over the rate a decade earlier. Corbett was able to dissect tuberculosis trends in HIV-positive and HIV-negative miners, yielding understanding of local epidemiology.[87] In those without HIV, the incidence of tuberculosis was high and increased with age (possibly because of increasing silicosis related to duration of exposure), but overall was stable, whereas it increased overall in the HIV infected.

The prevalence of a disease (the proportion of cases in a population) is determined by its incidence (the rate of new cases) and duration. At any incidence, the prevalence at one moment in time will be higher for a disease of long duration than for one that is short-lived. Corbett demonstrated that the incidence of tuberculosis was higher in miners with HIV than in those without, but prevalence was lower or the same. Most prevalent cases of tuberculosis were HIV negative. The unifying explanation was that

HIV-positive miners came to medical attention significantly earlier than HIV-negative miners. The HIV-negative miners lived with infectious tuberculosis much longer before detection and were thus the predominant source of transmission. Miners with HIV infection were the proverbial canaries in the mine, highly vulnerable to tuberculosis, susceptibles more than transmitters despite their high rates of disease.*

Conclusions from the Gold Mines

Experience in the gold mines of South Africa resembled a natural experiment of how to generate the worst possible tuberculosis epidemic by mixing relevant social, biological, occupational, and medical factors. Silicosis rates among miners increased over the years to high levels because of inadequate dust control, despite regulations being in place, and reduction in rotating employment. Miners stayed longer in the mines, thus increasing their cumulative dust exposure. HIV was layered onto this troubled occupational environment, already plagued by single-sex, crowded living conditions that promoted excessive alcohol consumption, unsafe sexual behavior, and contact with sex workers with high rates of HIV.

There was inherent inconsistency between laudatory evaluations of occupational measures to control dust in the mines and the observed high rates of silicosis in miners. Inadequate or incorrect application of safety standards, poor supervision and implementation of preventive measures, and nonadherence by workers who were paid for productivity rather than safety are possible explanations. Without control of the two most important risk

---

* HIV-positive patients with tuberculosis tend to have less cavities in their lungs than HIV-negative patients, so there is also a biological reason for lesser infectiousness.

factors, silicosis and HIV, tuberculosis rates in miners rose and will remain high.

Aggressive tuberculosis control by early case detection and treatment, especially for the predominantly HIV-negative case patients who are the main source of transmission, is essential. Churchyard's program succeeded in preventing the emergence of large-scale antituberculous drug resistance, though this remained a substantial risk.[72,92] For HIV-positive miners, rapid diagnosis and treatment also are required, but most important is what was not available at the time that Corbett was in Welkom: ART. Both HIV-positive and -negative miners would be expected to benefit from preventive therapy to prevent reactivation of prior tuberculous ("latent") infection. Unfortunately, a large randomized trial was unable to show benefit of what would seem a necessary intervention, probably because of tuberculosis reinfection after completion of the preventive therapy course.[93]

Although this body of work at Welkom was directly relevant to the local populations affected, its pertinence to understanding national or regional trends needs to be viewed in the context of South Africa and its history. It is tempting to attribute South Africa's extraordinarily severe national HIV and tuberculosis epidemics to the grim situation in the gold mines. As recently as 2010, former minister of health Aaron Motsoaledi likened HIV and tuberculosis to a snake, its head in the mines, and its tail extending into neighboring countries.[94]

Mathematical modeling, however, suggests a more complex situation. Miners are disproportionately affected by tuberculosis and contribute greatly to transmission in their own local communities, but their contribution to the overall tuberculosis situation in South Africa is small.[95] This is not to diminish the tragedy of the situation, the importance of local spread that can occur when migrant laborers return to villages and countries of origin,[96] or the injustice of ill or dead migrants never able to access treatment for

HIV or compensation for occupationally acquired silicosis and tuberculosis.

Unintended Consequences

Gold mining in South Africa has been an industry in decline, challenged by depleted seams, lower quality ore, the greater depth of remaining deposits, and escalating labor and energy costs. Between 1985 and 2020, South Africa's gold output reduced by approximately 80%, and the country has been overtaken by Ghana as Africa's leading producer.[97] The workforce in Welkom fell from a high of close to two hundred thousand miners in 1987 to well under fifty thousand in 2010.[57] But if gold mining does not drive today's twin epidemics of HIV and tuberculosis in South Africa as a whole, because the genie is well out of the bottle in the general population, the historical roots of these infectious diseases and the role of regional migration deserve further study.[98]

Tuberculosis and HIV in the gold mines powerfully show the role of social determinants ("the causes of the causes") of disease.[99] Cecil Rhodes initiated the political and economic systems to extract minerals from southern Africa in the nineteenth century, and roads and railways ensured subsequent recruitment and migration of single men in apartheid and colonial environments. Many millions of men migrated from neighboring countries to South Africa after the development of gold mining in the late nineteenth century.[60] Epidemic levels of sexually transmitted infections, tuberculosis, and, latterly, HIV were generated by the occupational and social conditions under which the Black workforce labored. Over the decades, infectious pathogens were carried back and forth throughout the region, and mining has indisputably affected the regional distribution of the diseases in question. Elegant epidemiology and first-class clinical care have not been adequate to overcome this force of infection that is driven by history as much as by biology.

Welkom itself is now a decaying town, following the closure over the 1990s of the majority of its fifty or so active shafts.[57] A new phenomenon emerged, *zama-zama* miners, illegal workers mining informally in the abandoned infrastructure for remaining, hard-to-reach seams.[59] The investigative journalist Kimon de Greef described a criminal industry overseeing this large-scale informal enterprise that has men working in shafts with none of the safety or support provided through the formal sector, sometimes staying underground for weeks or months on end. Thousands of *zama-zamas*, mostly undocumented immigrants from neighboring countries, have likely died from injuries, disease, or violence. The *zama-zama* phenomenon is widespread throughout the country, recalcitrant to official efforts to eradicate it. As much as 10% of South African gold sold internationally may be from the illegal sector.

The problems associated with gold mining that are well described in formal occupational evaluations surely apply to the infinitely more dangerous informal and illegal sectors. Systematic evaluations, of course, are lacking and problems only come to attention when they are so severe that they cannot be ignored. Outside of formal or *zama-zama* mining, there is also artisanal mining that involves little or no machinery or technology and is practiced in many countries.

Artisanal gold mining involves rudimentary methods of extracting gold from natural rock formations or derivatives. Such methods often involve use of mercury to form a mercury-gold amalgam. Some gold-containing ore is rich in lead. A CDC-supported investigation in 2010 documented perhaps the worst experience of lead poisoning in modern history, related to artisanal gold mining in northwestern Nigeria. In some of the villages we visited, up to 25% of children younger than 5 years old had died.[100] Gold mining offers a case study of the role of historical, social, political, and economic factors driving infectious and non-infectious disease epidemiology. It is another illustration of how social determinants of health are not contained by medicine or public health interventions alone.*

The Future of Tuberculosis

Over the course of this long experience with tuberculosis, colleagues and I wrote diverse commentaries, reviews, or other papers that together documented evolution of knowledge, available tools, opinions, and policies.[101-115] Yet, much remains the same and the problem of tuberculosis, in principle, is simple.

Of the 10.6 million new cases of tuberculosis estimated by WHO to have occurred in 2021, approximately 40% went undiagnosed and unreported.[3] Persons with active pulmonary tuberculosis are the source of infection for others. Transmission is more likely with close and prolonged exposure. Reducing transmission requires rapid identification of active pulmonary cases and

---

* Another industrial condition is Black Lung Disease (coal workers' pneumoconiosis, CWP), resulting from inhalation of coal dust. As with silicosis, progressive lung scarring can be complicated by respiratory and cardiac failure, as well as increased risk for tuberculosis. The prevalence of CWP in miners with 25 years or more of work in the United States has increased over past decades. The national prevalence of CWP in long-term miners in 2017 was over 10%, and in Central Appalachia 21%. Coal has increasingly come from mines rich in silica, which is more damaging to lungs than coal dust alone. (Blackley DJ, Halldin CH, Laney AS; Continued increase in prevalence of Coal Workers' Pneumoconiosis in the United States, 1970–2017: AJPH 2018,108, 1220–1222.)

The Coal Workers' Health Surveillance Program monitoring respiratory health of the approximately 50,000 coal workers in the US was directed by CDC's National Institute of Occupational Safety and Health (NIOSH). On April 1, 2025, staff implementing this program were initially fired under the administration's drive to reduce the workforce at CDC and other health agencies.

provision and supervision of treatment that eliminates infectiousness and cures disease. Congregate settings need to implement measures for infection prevention and control, such as education, administrative measures, ventilation, and protective equipment for staff.

The traditional approach of "passive case finding" (i.e., waiting for people with tuberculosis to self-present) fails to diagnose all active cases and allows prolonged circulation of infectious persons. There is now renewed interest in active case finding, such as through targeted screening of groups at special risk or community-wide screening. Research in Vietnam showed that bringing diagnosis and treatment closer to people, by use of point-of-care testing and screening of patient contacts and whole communities, almost doubled the detection of new cases.[116,117] There is an element of "back to the future" about this, recognizing that widespread screening for tuberculosis was a common activity earlier in the twentieth century. Nevertheless, the need to focus on early case detection for interruption of transmission is now widely acknowledged.[118,119]

A second issue is that about one-fourth of the world is latently infected with *Mycobacterium tuberculosis*.[120] Classic thinking* is that people with latent infection have an approximate 10% lifetime risk of developing active disease, more in certain groups such as those with diabetes or the immunosuppressed. Persons with latent tuberculosis can benefit from preventive therapy, which, in low transmission settings, can be limited in time, whereas in high-transmission environments it may need to be prolonged or lifelong because of the risk of reinfection. Because of the huge numbers of people affected, preventive therapy is

---

* Debate continues about the relative importance of reactivation of latent tuberculous infection versus reinfection as a cause of relapse and new cases (e.g., Dale KD, et al. Lancet Infect Dis. 2021;21:e303–e317).

necessarily used as a targeted intervention for those at highest risk. WHO recommends preventive therapy for persons living with HIV, household contacts of people with active tuberculosis, and other selected groups at special risk such as individuals with diabetes or other predisposing factors.

Tuberculosis epidemiology changes slowly. Implementing effective control measures in high-transmission environments such as southern Africa will require policy changes and resources.[118] The observation that much transmission of SARS-CoV-2 was from asymptomatic individuals applies to many respiratory pathogens, and asymptomatic transmission of tuberculosis may be more frequent than we realized. The experience with COVID-19 could give impetus to a more holistic approach to respiratory health in general, as well as protection of health care workers. Interruption of tuberculosis transmission will still leave a large population of latently infected persons whose risk for reactivation will stretch into the future. And attention is needed to the problem of drug-resistant disease, to save the lives of those affected and prevent onward transmission.

This summary provides a basis for defining research as well as programmatic priorities. Understanding of pathogenesis and epidemiology is vital. Basic science needs to clarify correlates of protection if immunology and vaccine research are to yield new tools. Transmission dynamics and the question of who infects whom, where, and how are relevant to targeting preventive interventions. Preventive measures, diagnostics, and treatment need to be democratized, expanded in communities rather than restricted to hard-to-access health facilities. Point-of-care diagnostics, tests applied at the bedside, and self-testing are important advances in diverse infectious diseases and need expansion in tuberculosis.

A duration of treatment of 6 months, the standard for drug-sensitive tuberculosis, seems short compared with life-long ART, but is still challenging. Therapeutic research focuses on shortening and simplifying treatment required, as is also the case for preventive therapy, including in persons with HIV. Implementation science should focus on expanding and facilitating access to tools currently available and incorporating new developments for communities at risk.

The world has agreed on ambitious targets for both tuberculosis and HIV: ending HIV as a public health threat by 2030[121], a 90% reduction in tuberculosis deaths, and an 80% reduction in the rate of new tuberculosis cases compared with those in 2015.[3] Although more could be hoped for, political attention to tuberculosis has increased in recent years. The field cries out for the best and brightest to apply their ambition, vigor, and careers to this ancient disease and its complex scientific, social, and epidemiologic interactions.

CHAPTER 12

Health Diplomacy

What Doesn't Get into "Materials and Methods"

The term "health diplomacy" has featured increasingly in global health parlance over the past three decades.[1] Greater funding for global health since the early 2000s, increased recognition of emerging infectious diseases, and concern about health security are some of the reasons. Health diplomacy concerns international relations for health, governance, funding, agreements in global public health, and responses to global health emergencies. At a more mundane level, health research and program implementation require local and interpersonal diplomacy to achieve results.

There is inadequate attention to these "soft" experiences that do not get into the Materials and Methods section of a paper. Career advancement and recognition often depend on scientific publications and grant income. Yet, moving research and public health agendas forward, let alone garnering personal respect, depends as much on emotional intelligence and environmental awareness as on technical competence. Jim Curran, then dean of Emory University's Rollins School of Public Health, observed that we always think science and technology will save us, but in the end, human relations are what matter most. This chapter describes some of the more nontechnical aspects and personal experiences behind technical and programmatic global health work.

HIV Origins

Scientific advances and time have relegated the early history of AIDS to a largely forgotten past. Older physicians and AIDS survivors are struck by the widespread obliviousness to the suffering and uncertainty that characterized the early days of AIDS. Some of this history is captured in a book describing the CDC's early work on AIDS, written with Harold Jaffe and Jim Curran.[2] Some of the lessons from early AIDS history remain relevant to global health today.

AIDS was different from other emerging infections because it presented as a syndrome, a constellation of different manifestations, rather than as a single-system disease such as from a novel respiratory agent. Once it was accepted that AIDS was an infectious condition, the race was on to identify the causative agent. When HIV was identified, obvious questions concerned where it had come from and when it had first affected humans. Controversy and sensitivity surrounded early discussions about the origin of AIDS.

In the United States, AIDS in Haitians was initially unexplained and posed a challenge to public health surveillance. Labeling Haitians as a risk group for AIDS caused stigmatization and discrimination. On the other hand, no diagnostic tests for the still-unidentified AIDS agent existed, and it was essential to track the epidemic. The CDC was in an awkward position, having to decide between following the disease or ignoring trends in a particular population. When scientific advances clarified the cause of AIDS and modes of transmission of HIV, and diagnostic tests became available, Haitians were no longer designated as an individual risk category. CDC staff believed there was no alternative at the time, but the earlier surveillance practice of considering Haitians as an individual group at risk was heavily criticized.

Sensitivity also surrounded AIDS in Africa. Having worked in East Africa and being knowledgeable about recent emerging infections such as Lassa fever and Ebola, it seemed to me that the AIDS agent could not be a novel infection. Much more likely was that it had long existed but gone undetected. In the early 1980s, increasing numbers of African patients with AIDS-like illnesses were being seen in Europe. An African origin seemed the only plausible explanation, and, in 1984, I published a paper entitled "AIDS—an old disease from Africa" in the *British Medical Journal*.[3] I was surprised by the interest aroused as well as the controversy, reminiscent of discussions about AIDS in Haiti. Subsequent multidisciplinary science clarified that HIV originated in nonhuman primates in West-Central Africa and that HIV jumped from the island of Hispaniola to the United States.[2]

The broad tenet of my original paper, an African origin for AIDS, was correct, even if some of the reasoning was wrong. More importantly, the experience was educational. First, science must be objective and cannot ignore questions because they may raise controversy. Where HIV came from was obviously important for deeper understanding of infectious disease emergence and would have public health implications. AIDS was a disease and should not have been seen as a disgrace. At the same time, underestimating sensitivities and likelihood of discrimination was a mistake.

An interesting contrast exists between the CDC's early approach to AIDS in Haitians, and, indeed, to surveillance in general, regarding stratification of disease trends by race or ethnicity, and practice in France. With consideration that all citizens are equal members of the Republic, France specifically does not collect health data on race or ethnicity. Although this may seem admirably egalitarian, it can render health disparities invisible. Nicola Low, a British epidemiologist, and I examined the incidence of AIDS, tuberculosis, and gonorrhea in the

United Kingdom, and found remarkable differences in these diseases by racial groups.[4] Such data are important for targeting interventions and services for where they are most needed. Without such data, disparities can persist or even grow.

Epidemiology is, by nature, a discipline that highlights differences, and such differences may amplify stigma and discrimination. Yet, science and public health must tell the truth. The CDC's initial communications on the outbreak of mpox in the United States seemed somewhat reticent in telling how it was—the epidemic was essentially restricted to men who have sex with men, infection resulted from close and sexual contact,[5] and the infection did not spread in the general population or by casual contact. Listening to a senior CDC official at the International Conference on AIDS in Montreal in 2022, I was left wondering whether people without medical knowledge would have understood the essence of the problem. The message was so cautious in avoiding sensitive topics that it almost suggested everyone was at equal risk.

I learned from the AIDS origins discussions, and from the Haiti experience, that sensitivity and diplomacy are necessary, but that science and public health must prioritize the truth above all else. How to do that is one of the arts of public health. Communication must convey essential truths but is about more than being right. Messaging must prevent, to the extent possible, adverse outcomes such as harm to marginalized and vulnerable groups.

HIV in West Africa

My EIS supervisor, Joe McCormick, and Jim Curran, the head of all AIDS work at the CDC, had a respectful relationship. McCormick, branch chief for the Special Pathogens Branch that addressed viral hemorrhagic fevers, had played an instrumental role in the CDC's entry into AIDS investigations in Africa.[2] He recognized that the CDC's expanding AIDS portfolio was overseen by Curran's organizational unit but maintained an interest in AIDS work in Africa.

One afternoon in May 1987, sitting in my gloomy, windowless office in the sub-sub-basement of a soon-to-be-demolished building at CDC headquarters, I took a phone call that was intended for McCormick. He was invited to a restricted meeting on AIDS research in Africa sponsored by the National Institutes of Health, prior to the large international AIDS conference in Washington, DC. After learning of the reason for the misplaced call, I obtained an invitation for myself. Serendipity was at play, for if I had not fielded that phone call, Projet RETRO-CI might never have been established and years of CDC work on AIDS in West Africa might never have happened.[2]

The meeting at the NIH in Bethesda, MD, convened groups working in Africa in these early days of AIDS, including CDC's Projet SIDA in the Democratic Republic of the Congo (then Zaire),[2] Susan Allen (then at the University of California, San Francisco) and her colleagues working in Rwanda, and Swedish, Danish, French, and American investigators focusing on West Africa. Technical aspects of the West African experience are described elsewhere,[2] the important point being uncertainty at that time about another human retrovirus circulating in the western part of the continent.

Harvard workers and their French colleagues had shown that sex workers in Senegal were infected with a retrovirus distinct from HIV-1 but emphasized that their study participants were healthy. Luc Montagnier's group in Paris had isolated a virus from West African patients with AIDS that the group called lymphadenopathy virus type 2, later renamed HIV-2. Swedish workers in Guinea Bissau described patients with AIDS who were infected with a non-HIV-1 virus. My eureka moment amidst this confusion was to propose to McCormick that we should set up a Projet

SIDA–like site in West Africa to reconcile the diverse science and clarify public health implications.

The large international conference was memorable for a plenary presentation by Curran on the central role that injection drug use played in the heterosexual and pediatric epidemics of HIV in the United States, and the disproportionate impact on communities of color. I recall Antwerp's Peter Piot, later the founding director of UNAIDS, turning to me and saying how completely unaware he was of these epidemiologic and social data, indicative of the incomplete understanding of AIDS at the time.

A controversial study from South Africa—controversial because of the continued system of apartheid and HIV testing in employment—examined HIV in gold miners by their country of origin. Workers from Malawi in Central Africa had higher rates of infection, almost 4%, than those from further south, whose HIV prevalence was well under 1%. Approximately one in ten miners acquired a sexually transmitted infection (STI) over the course of one year, and HIV prevalence in Malawian miners with an STI was 15%. Within a few years, however, South Africa was to suffer the world's worst HIV epidemic. At the conference, Jonathan Mann, now director of WHO's HIV program, came into his own with spellbinding oratory.[2]

I made extensive West African contacts at the meeting and sought opinions from senior American colleagues about the concept of a West African field site. Being able to speak French was important, because few francophone African colleagues spoke English. The colleagues I met were uniformly willing to engage, an indication of the high regard held for the CDC as well as positive opinions of the collaborative work ongoing at Projet SIDA in Kinshasa.[2]

The next piece of diplomacy that McCormick and I had to undertake was to persuade Curran. Because the CDC is a domestic agency whose prime function is protection of the health of the American people, a foray into West Africa was no small matter. Curran was supportive but with caution, and he agreed to fund an exploratory visit to three countries (Guinea, Burkina Faso, and Cote d'Ivoire), advising pilot studies in each for rapid assessment of local epidemiology.

My enthusiasm exceeded my good judgment, and I received more than one message over ensuing months instructing me to cease and desist and to let the senior decision-making process take its course. I never told my supervisors that after the international AIDS meeting I had called the US ambassador in Burkina Faso to ask if he would be supportive of the CDC establishing a research site (he was gracious and positive). This was behavior outside of normal protocol for an EIS officer. As US government employees, we had to get permission from the local US embassies for what were unusual visits. Everything we requested was approved, and the embassies could not have been more helpful.

In early September 1987, McCormick, William ("Bill") Heyward; John Krebs, a laboratorian; and I set off with boxes of laboratory equipment, flying from Atlanta to Paris and on to Guinea, Cote d'Ivoire, and Burkina Faso. Striking memories were the odor of cigarettes in the Paris airport, and the stop in Mauretania on the way to Guinea. Looking out of the plane's window, all one could see was desert, so I was surprised that so many men disembarked. These were Asian workers recruited to the international fishing industry that over subsequent years has depleted fish stocks off the West African coast, a later contributor to local unemployment and migration.

The skyline of Abidjan, Cote d'Ivoire's major city, its roads, the boats on the lagoon, and the restaurants and cafes illustrated why this city was referred to as "the Paris of West Africa." In comparison, Conakry, the capital of Guinea, and Ouagadougou, the capital of Burkina Faso, seemed drab and poor. Discussions in Guinea gave insight into the kinds of obstacles we might expect. Although technical counterparts such as K. Kourouma were keen to support a serosurvey, the official responsible for external relations expected a gift, repeatedly citing need for us to leave the CDC's testing equipment behind. McCormick grew increasingly impatient with our counterpart's refusal to accept that it was not in our purview to donate equipment belonging to the US government. Guinea was not an appropriate site for this collaboration for other reasons, but this official's tone deafness facilitated the decision.

Guinea was euphemistically described to us as "one of the more difficult countries to work in" by a US embassy staff member, an observation confirmed almost three decades later during West Africa's Ebola epidemic. Our dejection on leaving Guinea, which anyway was epidemiologically unsuitable for HIV-2 investigations, was lifted by early observations in Abidjan, Cote d'Ivoire. Our reception by Ivorian colleagues such as Koudou Odehouri, head of the country's National AIDS Control Program, was warm, and provision of space in the infectious diseases unit of Treichville's university hospital was the basis for long-term successful collaboration. Ambassador Dennis Kux, a career diplomat, was unfailingly supportive.

McCormick and Heyward returned to the United States, and Krebs and I began to organize a survey to measure HIV-1 and HIV-2 infections in different population groups.[6] I later went on to conduct a similar, smaller survey in Ouagadougou, the dusty capital of Burkina Faso. My principal memory of the Burkina Faso study was being surprised in the hospital at the large number of patients with forearm fractures. When I left at the end of the day, I understood: exiting the hospital, I had to wait to cross the road amidst a swarm of *mobilettes*, motorized bicycles, whizzing by. Over subsequent years, my assessment that road traffic injuries in Africa are a greatly neglected public health problem has only increased.

For the study in Abidjan, Cote d'Ivoire, I recruited some medical students in Abidjan to assist. This decision had long-lasting repercussions; several stayed with our group over the longer term and benefited from further academic training in public health. Another, Serge Eholie, became an internationally recognized HIV clinical expert and researcher. René Ekpini was as much a poet and philosopher as medic and became spokesperson for the students. They were proud; when M'Boye, one of the five, and I were walking from the hospital to the nearby Public Health Institute carrying our study supplies, he transferred the boxes to me, explaining it was unseemly for an Ivorian doctor to be seen in public this way. My collaborators' friends teased them about blood collection, a task usually performed by nurses. I had little pride and readily accepted to undertake any function necessary, no matter how menial, provided it furthered the cause of the study.

Extensive negotiations were required to take this whole enterprise forward. I returned to Atlanta in October 1987 and spent the following weeks entering data from our pilot studies, preparing a preliminary report on results, coordinating logistic discussions about how a field project would be set up, and learning about State Department requirements for long-term deployments. Curran gave definitive approval for establishing the project in early 1998, and Heyward and I traveled to Abidjan in March to sign a memorandum of understanding with the Ministry of Health.

I had met Alphonse Djédjé Mady, Minister of Health, some months before. Odehouri had been trying to arrange a meeting and one day came to fetch me unexpectedly for this long-awaited appointment. I had been working on the wards and in the laboratory, was sweaty and dusty, and wearing jeans. We were received in his large office by one of the most elegantly dressed men I had ever met, the minister going on to treat me with utmost courtesy while ignoring my dress, all the while leaving no doubt about his authority.

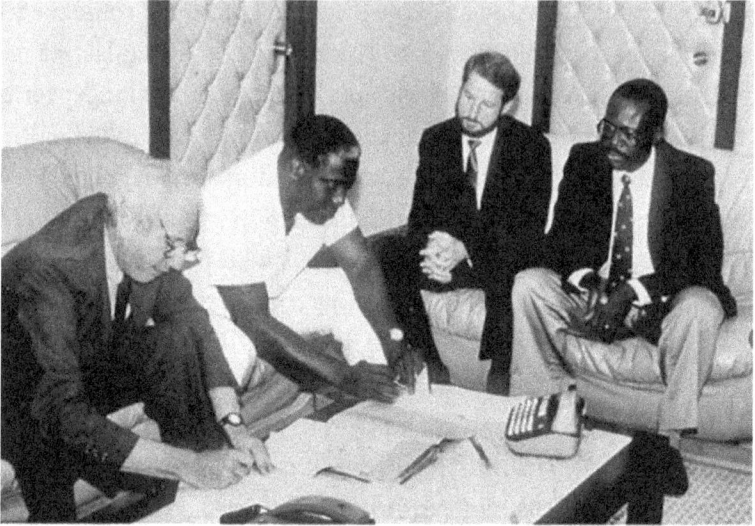

Figure 12.1   Signing of the RETRO-CI agreement. *Left to right*: US Ambassador Dennis Kux; Minister of Health Djédjé Mady; Bill Heyward, CDC; Koudo Odehouri, director, Cote d'Ivoire National AIDS Control Program.
(Kevin De Cock, personal collection)

This was to be repeated in March 1988, when we met with the minister and Ambassador Kux to sign our memorandum of understanding. I had drafted it with the help of a francophone employee at the embassy. Djédjé Mady glanced at it, pulled out a gold-plated fountain pen, and began to correct my French grammar like a schoolteacher. I expected a dressing down, but Ambassador Kux was utterly gracious, and we returned a few days later for a successful signing (Figure 12.1).

A further illustration of the minister's stylishness occurred when senior Atlanta colleagues traveled to Abidjan for their first site visit in early 1989. He eloquently discussed his aspiration that the project would emphasize capacity building and ultimately contribute to care for patients with AIDS. He received a call during the meeting, pulling out a small portable cell phone shaped like an oyster shell, a novelty at the time, leaving Curran duly impressed.

I moved to Abidjan full time in May 1988, still an EIS officer, for what would be a 5-year assignment.[2] Political and scientific challenges caused frequent sleepless nights. There was skepticism among other research groups that an American effort would be able to operate in this francophone, African environment. Some researchers felt their protected turf was being encroached upon, especially concerning laboratory testing for HIV. Our French collaborator, Jacques Moreau, an infectious disease clinician who suggested the name RETRO-CI (retro for retrovirus, CI for Cote d'Ivoire), informed the French embassy about our work, warning diplomats that France was missing an opportunity and emphasizing the rapidity of our progress.

Over time, fruitful collaborations were established with diverse colleagues and groups, but it required ceaseless attention and outreach. France guarded its sphere of influence, a policy referred to somewhat critically as *Françafrique,* and had advisors in every ministry. I ensured friendly communications with the Minister of Health's senior French advisor who reassuringly described me to his colleagues as "convincing." I exerted some personal diplomacy by frequently acting as interpreter between French- and English-speaking technical colleagues and dignitaries.

I learned that the best approach in moments of challenge was to put my head down and work harder, focusing on CDC expectations: scientific output relevant to the public health significance of HIV-1 and HIV-2. Presentations at international conferences drew visibility, and we promoted our African staff to give scientific presentations; younger colleagues were understandably awed by giving talks at such meetings. I advised RETRO-CI staff to be generous in allowing others to present, reminding them that long-lasting influence came from written rather than verbal communications. Trade-offs were often necessary about authorship and order of names, even as we strove to ensure credit was given where it was due. Staff recruitment and organization took much time, capacity and leadership having to be assured in different technical areas such as laboratory, informatics, medical epidemiology, and management.

Projet RETRO-CI's technical contributions were extensive.[2] Not captured in the scientific literature are the intense emotions associated with the work in Abidjan, including on leaving the city and country, and the deep and long-lasting friendships established. Activities and connections outside of work left enduring impressions, some tragic and others joyful. I had great respect for Alain Ekra, minister of Health from 1989 to 1992, who supported our work. He had a son who lost his way in drugs and criminality and was killed in a police shoot-out. Going to Ekra's house to express condolences on behalf of all RETRO-CI staff was a difficult obligation.

The country's generosity and friendship toward the CDC collaboration was demonstrated by my receiving a high-level decoration prior to departure. I refrained from drinking alcohol until after the speeches at the well-attended ceremony at the US embassy, then had a large gin. Ambassador Hume Horan, Kux's successor, unexpectedly invited my wife, Sopiato, and me to stay on, leading to consumption of two bottles of champagne and a hangover.

Horan's career illustrated the unpredictability of foreign service. A distinguished Arabist, he reached the pinnacle of diplomacy in that sphere with his appointment as ambassador to Saudi Arabia. Instructed to deliver a message of American displeasure to King Fahd concerning the Saudi acceptance of Chinese weapons, Horan was declared unacceptable and his ambassadorial career in the Arab world was finished. I always wondered what this intelligent, cultured man felt with assignment in a country of West Africa that, at that time, was of limited strategic relevance to the United States.

I recall him wryly saying to Professor Kadio, one of our Ivorian patrons, at a reception at my house, comparing their respective roles: *"Moi, je bouffe pour mon pays"* (Me, I eat for my country"). Our scientific success depended on bridging the different worlds of traditional diplomacy and health, conveying to the different communities the importance of these relationships.

The Atlantic coast outside of Abidjan has beautiful beaches that offered a respite from grueling weeks of work. I took on a concession for a *paillote*, a wooden beach shack worth less than $US100 but with a priceless view of the beach and ocean. The tides threatened the foundation of these structures, and we were regularly invited by neighbors on a Sunday to celebrate the last week of their *paillotes'* existence with drinks. The structures always survived.

Alan Greenberg succeeded me as Projet RETRO-CI director and we reflected on our broad experiences in interviews that formed part of an oral history project of the CDC's early AIDS work.[7,8] Abidjan drew diverse workers—cooks, guards, taxi drivers, gardeners, and others—from the whole sub-region. This heterogeneity influenced AIDS epidemiology because the large population of unaccompanied men were clients of a thriving sex industry, and the sex workers were mostly from other countries, especially Ghana.[2,9]

Alan's and my household benefited from the dedicated service of our Burkinabe cook, Gouba. His quiet dignity belied a *joie de vivre* that my wife Sopiato unwittingly discovered when she saw him, unnoticed, dancing down the road in town with a transistor radio pressed to his ear. He personified the warmth of our relations in Abidjan. Gouba comforted Greenberg's pregnant wife, Michele, who was suffering from morning sickness: *"ça va, Madame, ça va passer,"* he would say soothingly (it's alright, Madame, it will pass). But Gouba's own health declined and his cough worsened. He and his little new family in Abidjan, his principal family having been left in Burkina Faso, died of AIDS.

Numerous RETRO-CI publications have been cited hundreds of times. The two most frequently referenced papers have been

Sebastian Lucas's report on the pathology of patients dying from HIV-1 and HIV-2 disease,[10] and a review on HIV-associated tuberculosis in Africa.[11] Especially pleasing was the recognition of a paper drawing together understanding of HIV-2 epidemiology and trends, discussing why HIV-2 has not caused a global epidemic similar to HIV-1.[12] With that paper, I felt that RETRO-CI had fulfilled its core function, understanding the relevance of HIV-2, though potential for further important work remained great.[2,13]

AIDS in London

I left Abidjan in late March 1993. I drove to our *paillotte* to see the beach one last time, then stayed up all night to clear papers from my office, but more to experience the smell and atmosphere of the RETRO-CI building. I wept as I left to drive home and then depart for the airport.

I took a teaching position at the London School of Hygiene and Tropical Medicine, knowing that sooner or later I would rejoin the CDC, which had come to feel like a technical home. I underestimated the difficulty of reintegrating into this British, high-income work setting after intense West African field work. From directing a group of fifty or more people, I had to readjust to an unpleasant and empty office. Academic colleagues were kind but busy with their own concerns in a competitive environment of grant applications.

I remembered a comment by a CDC colleague, Nancy Binkin, that she valued work at the CDC because discussions generally started with "we," rather than "I." At the School, several groups worked on similar topics, such as HIV-associated tuberculosis, but collaboration was limited. Unlike at RETRO-CI, projects and applications were not designed for their own public health merit as much as responding to calls for competitive proposals and funding. I became friends with Daan Mulder, a Dutch academic who returned after several productive years in Uganda.[14] Seeing his low-grade depression gave me insight into the melancholy I also had suffered and that I have seen in others returning from intense field work.

My position in London included responsibility for the in-patient service at the Middlesex Hospital, then the city's second largest AIDS unit, for 3 months of the year. At the School, my main teaching responsibility was organizing an AIDS study unit that I arranged to cover basic science, epidemiology, clinical, and social aspects of AIDS. I introduced the unit with a showing of the movie *And the Band Played On*, taken from Randy Shilts's book of the same name on the early AIDS epidemic.[15] The movie ensured the students were gripped, and the study unit garnered the highest evaluation from the students within the School.

The international AIDS conference in mid-1993 was held in Berlin, Germany. Three memories have stayed with me from that meeting. First, I had been invited to give a plenary presentation on tuberculosis and HIV, the first time I had spoken to such a large audience. Second, the results of the Anglo-French Concorde trial were presented, showing that early zidovudine monotherapy conferred no survival benefit for persons living with HIV. This represented a nadir in global attitudes toward AIDS, engendering widespread feelings of hopelessness. And finally, I was housed in an East Berlin hotel, whose thin walls transmitted sleep-preventing noise of vigorous lovemaking in the adjoining room. It was all very disconcerting.

The contrasts between the university hospitals in Abidjan and London were extreme and troubling. Patients with AIDS in West Africa struggled alone and had to pay for the meager services provided under harsh physical conditions. More than one-third of hospitalized patients with AIDS died, generally within 1 week. In London, sophisticated care was provided free by the National Health Service. Every ounce of meaningful life was squeezed out of failing immune systems. Judicious use was made of the intensive care unit, and multidisciplinary teams provided medical as well as social advice and support. When further intervention yielded no benefit, aggressive therapy would be switched to palliative care, literally with the snap of a finger, reminiscent more of cancer care than management of an infectious disease.

The AIDS unit at the Middlesex, the first dedicated facility in the United Kingdom, had been opened in 1987 by Princess Diana, who contributed to combating stigma by shaking hands with a patient with AIDS, considered exceptional at the time. Years later, she was shown hugging an HIV-infected child. The unit was diverse in both its staff, many of them gay men, and patients. Gay men with AIDS occupied beds next to ill African women, cultural differences and opinions sometimes extreme. Some patients tried to cling to secrecy about their diagnosis, but as their disease progressed, this was impossible to maintain. It was possible to live anonymously with early HIV infection, but AIDS was physically evident. We tried to ensure confidentiality, but patients could not hide their visibly progressive disease. This distinction between confidentiality and secrecy was important and useful in later discussions about HIV testing and surveillance practices.[2]

Anne Johnson, a senior epidemiologist working on HIV and STIs, and I became interested in HIV testing policies. From earliest days, HIV testing had been treated differently from other medical investigations. At the first international conference on AIDS, held in Atlanta in 1985, I was handed a sticker by an AIDS activist that said "No test is best." To prevent mandatory testing and associated discriminatory actions, extensive pretest counseling and informed consent were required, and these conditions were extended to clinical settings. Unintentionally, these requirements could act as impediments to necessary medical diagnosis. A female colleague at the London School recounted how, when asked during antenatal care if she wanted an HIV test, her midwife responded to her affirmative answer by asking: "Are you sure?"

It was a clinical encounter in late 1996 that conveyed to us the inherent contradictions between HIV testing policies and provision of care for AIDS. A 37-year-old British man, married and with children, presented with life-threatening pneumonia. He was diabetic and his medical records were thick as telephone books. He had seen prominent specialists for more than a year for investigation of diverse conditions, including anemia. A resident specializing in respiratory medicine saw his chest X-ray and correctly suggested a possible diagnosis of *Pneumocystis* pneumonia, the commonest AIDS-defining illness locally, subsequently confirmed by bronchoscopy.

Retrospective review of his records revealed multiple clues to his HIV infection, whose diagnosis was delayed because he denied any risk factors, he had complicated diabetes, but above all, because of reluctance to broach HIV testing or even think of it for a married man with children. Routine testing for all manner of infectious and other conditions, including syphilis, had been performed, but not for HIV.

This clinical encounter had several memorable repercussions. The need for clinical humility was reinforced for me after I advised the patient's wife against his receiving mechanical ventilation in view of his end-stage immune deficiency. She, however, insisted that all possible measures be taken, and she was proven right. He underwent weeks of stormy intensive care but survived. My colleague Ian Williams informed me that the patient lived for almost another decade on antiretroviral therapy (ART), eventually dying of cardiovascular disease related to his diabetes.

Johnson and I published a discussion paper in the *British Medical Journal* calling for normalization of HIV testing in the context of clinical care.[16] It took almost another decade for diverse discussions to play out, with several papers with CDC colleagues

contributing to the debate.[17-20] Not only was there need to ratio-
nalize HIV testing in clinical settings but public health guidance
also needed to focus on prevention of transmission as well as ac-
quisition of infection.[17] HIV was transmitted from people living
with HIV, who were far less numerous than HIV-negative persons.
Providing targeted prevention and care services for people with
HIV was likely to be more effective than prevention efforts that
took no account of HIV serostatus. Publication by WHO and UN-
AIDS of guidance on HIV testing within health facilities in 2007
was an important step forward,[21] as well as guidance on "prevention for positives." Evolving science confirmed the validity of this
approach; large-scale studies showed that persons with HIV
whose infection was virologically suppressed with ART did not
transmit the virus.[22] "Undetectable = Untransmittable" became
the slogan.[23] For HIV/AIDS, treatment is prevention, but it has to
start with testing.

HIV/AIDS Surveillance in the United States

I used to say that the most extraordinary experience in my career
was witnessing the emergence and impact of AIDS around the
world. I later modified that to add that the second most impressive experience was seeing the introduction of effective ART. The
world of HIV was revolutionized in 1996 by recognition that a
triple combination of antiretroviral drugs could halt and reverse
immune deficiency.

The international AIDS conferences have served as milestones
in the history of the pandemic, and the 1996 conference in Vancouver, Canada, was iconic, a before-and-after moment in the
history of AIDS. I was stunned seeing posters that described re-
versal of previously lethal conditions such as progressive multi-
focal leukoencephalopathy, a demyelinating disease of the brain
due to a human polyomavirus (John Cunningham virus, com-

monly called JCV) that we saw in some of our patients with AIDS in London. Suddenly, AIDS did not have to be a fatal condition.

I wistfully thought of a patient I looked after for whom these advances were too late. I had regularly assessed his mental orientation on our ward by asking standard questions, including the names of political leaders. One day he asked to see me, saying he had a question. "Who is the prime minister?" he asked. I never knew whether this was a manifestation of his dementia or a practical joke.

Henceforth, discussions were focused on increasing access to therapy worldwide and ensuring that patients with advanced HIV received treatment. Research and technical advances reduced the pill burden and rendered drug regimens more tolerable. Drug prices for low- and middle-income countries decreased because of the introduction of generic preparations.

An immediate requirement was modification of surveillance practices because of the remarkable effects of ART. Because the relentless and predictable progression of HIV infection was interrupted by therapy, AIDS case surveillance no longer gave a reliable window through which evolution of the epidemic could be described. The urgent need was to focus on the reporting of HIV infections, though this was controversial.

I returned to the CDC in 1997 as head of one the agency's two AIDS divisions, mine responsible for surveillance and epidemiology in the United States. Frequent meetings were held with different civil society organizations to discuss HIV surveillance and the best way of reporting cases. AIDS surveillance involved reporting cases by name, and the CDC's recommendation that the same methodology be used for reporting HIV infections was highly controversial.

With time, the CDC's recommendation that HIV reporting be conducted by name became collectively accepted.[2,24] The methodical approach to this subject by surveillance staff, especially

Branch Chiefs John Ward and Pattie Simone, was instructive. Advocacy was combined with science in a series of studies and publications that sequentially addressed community concerns such as potential deterrence to testing or lack of confidentiality, as well as assessing validity of data. The experience provided a lesson in logical, sequential, and comprehensive scientific application; community engagement; and communications in achieving a public health objective.

HIV/AIDS at WHO

I had been working in Kenya for 6 years, from 2000 to 2006, longer than usually allowed for one assignment. I searched unsuccessfully for a senior AIDS position at the CDC but then was offered the position of head of HIV/AIDS at WHO in Geneva. WHO's role in the pandemic was a troubled one—dominant in the late 1980s under the late Jonathan Mann, performing well under Mike Merson's subsequent direction despite an unpopular director general (Hiroshi Nakajima), but then dysfunctional for almost a decade until the "3 by 5" initiative under Lee Jong-wook ("JW Lee").[2]

I was the twelfth HIV director over the 15 years that had elapsed since Mann's abrupt resignation in 1991. Positions of this level at WHO are never just technical, and to this day I do not know what discussions happened behind the scenes to appoint me to this post without competition. Because the United States was WHO's largest donor, I imagine some pressure was applied, but I do not know who my benefactors were. My tenure at WHO had an unusual and challenging start with the unexpected death of JW Lee, who had appointed me.[2,25] The Lancet generously described Lee's selection of me as "discerning and wise,"[25] though I found this position the most challenging of my whole career.

WHO is an indispensable organization in global health architecture; there is simply no other organization with a comparable mandate, global representativeness, or convening authority. Expectations of the organization are immense, yet support provided to it by member states is often lukewarm, and financial support also is limited—WHO's budget for its worldwide activities has been about one-fourth of the CDC annual budget.

WHO has lost ground and prestige over recent decades in the global health space. Global health has become more complex, civil society and philanthropy have more influence, and money inevitably talks. In this way, the United States had enormous influence, as did the Bill and Melinda Gates Foundation. The Foundation has been WHO's second largest donor after the United States, accounting for about 10% of the overall budget and dwarfing contributions from other nonstate actors.

In addition to the inevitable leverage that is derived from such large funding streams, a substantial proportion of monies ("voluntary contributions") are earmarked to varying degrees for specific priorities defined by donors. When I was HIV director, generous funds from Canada were allocated with a "soft earmark," a term I found difficult to define. It could be frustrating at times to speak with donor representatives who advocated for their positions but seemed insensitive to or misunderstood our technical knowledge and the administrative and other constraints under which we worked.

Like other arms of the United Nations, WHO has had its share of scandals, including mismanagement of funds, corruption, nepotism, and sexual abuse. WHO's system for investigating complaints is slow and protective of the organization's reputation. Yet, much criticism is unfair, especially in relation to the stresses under which WHO works. Inadequate responses or outcomes in global health crises are often laid at WHO's door,

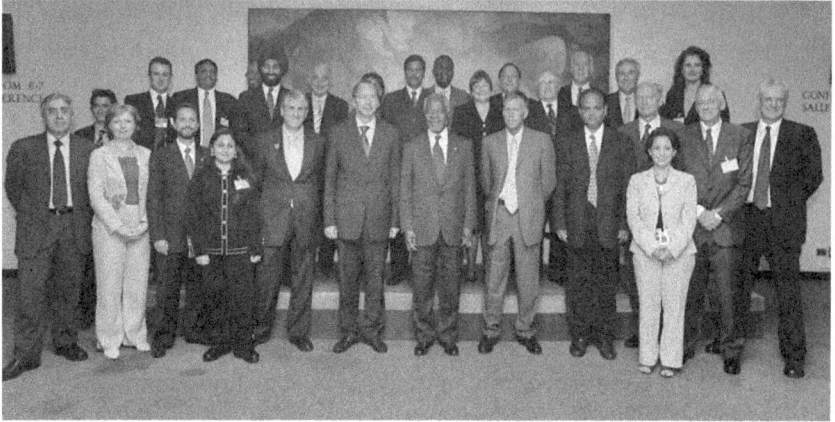

Figure 12.2   Meeting at UN Headquarters, New York, 2006, discussing access to HIV drugs and diagnostics. *Center three, Left to right*: Peter Piot, executive director, UNAIDS; Kofi Anan, UN secretary-general; Anders Nordström, acting director-general, World Health Organization.
(Kevin De Cock, personal collection)

whereas individual country performance or responsibilities too often go undiscussed.

The HIV director's position combined political, policy, technical, advocacy, and representational aspects (Figure 12.2), with exposure to the highest levels of international relations as well as the most disadvantaged of situations. Like in any large organization, it took about a year to learn which way was up or down, and although long-term insiders had enormous advantage in understanding and being able to manipulate the system, there was always benefit in having new ideas from outside.

Protocol and hierarchy were potent forces at WHO, and an uneasy, ill-defined relationship existed between headquarters in Geneva, the six regional offices, and WHO country offices. Assistant directors general reported to the director general, the head of WHO, and were politically appointed. Some were capable and respected technically, others less so.

Despite the challenges, serving at WHO remains a major opportunity and privilege. Six core functions describe the agency's role in global health: leadership; defining knowledge and gaps in knowledge; norm and standard setting; providing health policy; technical support; and monitoring of trends. Other entities have encroached on each of these elements, and WHO strives to manage transition from prime position to a more collaborative role with diverse global health players. Rather than criticizing WHO, a more constructive approach would be to discuss what its unique contributions are and how to strengthen them.

I would advise younger colleagues to consider time at WHO if offered the opportunity, but with eyes wide open. Nontechnical considerations will inevitably influence work and promotions. If seconded from member states rather than directly appointed, such staff will weather predictable suspicions and constraints. Bureaucracy will be onerous, but much can be achieved. However, I remember the advice I cited earlier from Edwin Beausoleil from WHO's Regional Office for Africa. "Do not go to WHO as a young man," he said, "you will become a nincompoop." Nothing can replace the credibility that can only be earned through field work prior to bureaucratic appointments in the corridors of power.

CDC Kenya: From Bed Nets to Breastfeeding

In early 2000, I took over leadership of the CDC's work in Kenya, deploying there three times for a total of 15 years before retirement from the CDC at the end of 2020. Much had changed since I had left Kenyatta National Hospital and the University of Nairobi in 1982, including the government becoming increasingly autocratic under President Moi, doubling of the population to thirty-two million*, and the visible emergence of the AIDS epidemic. The

---

* The population of Kenya in 2025 approached 60 million.

CDC's central activity in Kenya was malaria research in collaboration with the Kenya Medical Research Institute (KEMRI), the legacy of Harrison Spencer's work that had started in 1979 when we first met.

Of the five species of *Plasmodium* that cause disease in humans, *P. falciparum* is the most prevalent in Africa and the cause of most disease and death. More than eight hundred thousand global deaths annually were attributed to malaria at this time, most in children in sub-Saharan Africa. Two large expatriate groups dominated collaboration with KEMRI, the Wellcome Trust funded group from Oxford University that was based in Kilifi on the Kenya coast; and our own group that worked around Kisumu near Lake Victoria. Both groups illustrated commitment to long-terms studies and the importance of "being there." This type of collaboration yielded scientific and public health impact that was unachievable through any number of short-term visits.

Malaria epidemiology is different in the two study locations. Malaria around Lake Victoria stubbornly remains a leading cause of ill health and death in children, with about 40% of children younger than 5 years carrying the parasite in their blood despite extensive interventions. Every year, it was estimated, a child received about three hundred infectious mosquito bites, and it is impossible to grow up in rural areas around Lake Victoria and escape malaria exposure. The coast has also been an area of stable and predictable transmission, but at a much lower intensity.

When I arrived in 2000, the CDC had been involved for some years in a large, randomized controlled trial of insecticide-impregnated bed nets in the rural areas of western Kenya. Another focus of research was prevention and management of malaria in pregnancy, which can lead to maternal anemia, premature delivery, intrauterine growth retardation, low birthweight, and an increase in infant mortality. The work was scientifically important but also of direct importance to the CDC. Fieldwork offered training and experience for staff, many of whom went on to other positions of responsibility in domestic and global public health. It also provided opportunities for research and master's and doctoral theses for legions of Kenyan and other students.

I made some rapid observations on arrival in 2000. My predecessor, Bernard Nahlen, had skillfully directed the work with limited support and funding. The CDC's Division of Parasitic Diseases lived under constant poverty, expected to achieve much but with little support. The CDC infrastructure in Kenya was appalling. At the KEMRI campus outside of Kisumu, laboratory floors were coming up, roofs leaked, and the earthen road leading into the facility was impassable in the rain. The road often exposed sharp stones that slashed the tires of our vehicles.

The bed net trial had collected vast amounts of data, but decisions were required about optimizing management and analysis of the information, and when and how to terminate the study. There was also urgent need to focus on HIV as well as malaria, because rates of HIV around the Lake were as high as in southern Africa, twice as high as the average in the rest of Kenya, but little talked about.

The American community was still coming to terms with the 1998 bombing of its embassy in Nairobi, in which Louise Martin, former EIS officer and wife of the CDC's Doug Klaucke, had died. We also lost a driver, Josiah Owuor, along with his vehicle. Other than me, we had just two other direct CDC hire staff in Kenya, an administratively oriented public health advisor and an entomologist (Christi Murray and William Hawley, respectively). In Nairobi, we had two small offices at the KEMRI headquarters. Overall, we were understaffed, had poor facilities, and had to give thought to the longer-term future.

I arranged assessment visits by senior technical and administrative colleagues from CDC headquarters in Atlanta to seek advice but also to encourage a broader feeling of ownership at headquarters over this field presence. The dire need for investment was convincingly communicated to a visiting CDC administrator when he saw the poor state of one of our two vehicles, the covering of the steering wheel so worn out that the underlying metal was visible. The car then broke down as he was on his way to the airport to return to the United States.

We encouraged more collaboration across different disciplines and requested HIV expertise from headquarters to help with the laborious task of data cleaning for the bed net studies. Dan Rosen, a statistician from my old HIV/AIDS Division in Atlanta, spent months assisting in Kisumu, cleaning and extracting essential data relevant to the study's critical questions. Rosen obtained more than he anticipated, ending up marrying Annemieke Van Eijk, a Dutch malariologist completing her PhD in Kisumu. Her work and that of others contributed to understanding the complex interrelationships among malaria, HIV, pregnancy, and anemia as risk factors for adverse outcomes on maternal and child health.

Feiko ter Kuile and Penny Phillips-Howard were a husband-and-wife team working for several years with the CDC in the field; both now hold senior positions at the Liverpool School of Tropical Medicine. Ter Kuile characterized my role as a professional research manager, a description I realized illustrated that my work henceforth was supervisory rather than conducting or initiating research. I nonetheless attached importance to remaining technically up to date for the rest of my career.

The results of the bed net studies were published as a full supplement of the *American Journal of Tropical Medicine and Hygiene*,[26] a credit to the numerous Kenyan and other researchers involved. The KEMRI and CDC study was not the first to demonstrate the protective efficacy of insecticide-impregnated nets, but it was the first and most extensive community study in an area of such intense malaria transmission. The demonstration of approximately 25% reduction in all-cause mortality in children influenced global policy about scale-up of this intervention.

Another long-term outcome for the CDC and KEMRI was commitment to use the area where the bed net study was conducted as a formal demographic surveillance site (DSS). Such sites implement regular monitoring of births, deaths, and migration for overall measurement of health trends. Larry Slutsker, the field director in western Kenya, invested much work in this enterprise, aided by the newly hired demographer, Kubaje Adazu from Ghana.[27]

For a public health agency like the CDC, criticism could ensue if all that were done was watching without intervening for preventable and treatable conditions like HIV and malaria. Programmatic funding for malaria and HIV increased, and, separately, the DSS supported a wide variety of innovative evaluations in child mortality; adolescent health; noncommunicable diseases, including injuries; and trends in HIV incidence and mortality after introduction of interventions.[28-31]

The early 2000s were a time of increased investment in global health. Major programs were launched such as the Global Fund to Fight AIDS, Tuberculosis, and Malaria ("the Fund"), and the President's Emergency Plan for AIDS Relief (PEPFAR), the American program announced by President George W. Bush that provided treatment and was to change the face of AIDS in Africa.[2,32] Increased funding to the CDC placed stress on the agency's administrative systems and highlighted its limited regulatory authority for large-scale international activities. The CDC was established as a domestic agency and the regulations under which it operated were simply not adapted to international operations and expenditures.

CDC field work to date had been successfully supported on "can do" attitudes and creative interpretation of guidance and regulations. CDC pioneers in global health who had worked on issues such as smallpox eradication and Lassa fever in faraway places focused on getting their work done, with limited official administrative support. That this approach could not sustain international expansion was made clear at a conference organized with the State Department in Durban, South Africa, in the early 2000s. We were witnessing a rapid evolution from limited, individual technical efforts to a greater CDC presence and visibility internationally.

In a packed meeting a senior, very flamboyant administrative official from Washington, DC, expanded on a litany of approaches used by the CDC that were inappropriate or in breach of regulations. He finished his somewhat theatrical presentation with a callout to our work in Cote d'Ivoire that he said epitomized all the irregularities described. I laughed; if this was intended as criticism, I did not feel it because RETRO-CI had conduced important work in an era of limited guidance. We had managed funds responsibly, but this retrospective analysis indicated the CDC's international work frequently was not adherent to strict domestic rules. It was evident that the CDC would have to invest much more in management and operations if its global role was to expand.

Robert ("Rob") Janssen, my deputy from my prior position as director for AIDS Surveillance and Epidemiology, was strongly supportive of plans to increase HIV work in Kenya. We invested almost $US10 million in renovation, building and physical enhancements, rendering our site one of the strongest physical research infrastructures in East Africa. We also increased staffing from Atlanta, and the Kenya CDC presence became the largest outside of the United States, transitioning from a focus restricted to malaria to a broader and multidisciplinary agenda.[33]

These developments required intense interaction with and support from the US embassy in Nairobi, the largest on the subcontinent; only Embassy Cairo was larger. My time in Cote d'Ivoire had given me understanding of how embassies work, but Nairobi was more complex. More staff meant more requirements for housing, transport, administrative support, and office space. US government regulations governed residential security (stringent and expensive), work locations (even more stringent and expensive), procurement, and much more. A restriction that plagued the CDC was lack of authority to undertake construction overseas, despite ability to "renovate." Generous interpretation of this phrase was still often insufficient to rapidly provide working space necessary for progress. Adding staff needed approval from the embassy through a complex authorizing process that had to go back to the State Department in Washington, DC.

I benefited from good relations with different US ambassadors in Nairobi who were strongly supportive of the CDC's work and expansion. Johnnie Carson was one of the doyens of American diplomacy, charged with rebuilding the embassy in Kenya after its bombing in 1998, as well as later helping ease President Moi out of power. Carson was one of the first diplomats to speak out loudly on HIV/AIDS and rang the alarm at highest levels of the US government about the pandemic's implications for Africa.

Carson and his administrative staff required the CDC to be better coordinated, demanding in an official cable not to have "CDC splinter groups." What this referred to were uncoordinated, frequent visits by disease-specific experts, some of whom occasionally got into trouble or required embassy assistance, with nobody in-country apparently in oversight mode. I saw the importance of avoiding siloed approaches in the field, even if that was how technical groups at headquarters in Atlanta were funded and organized.

I forced groups in the field to work in a more coordinated way and operate as "one CDC." Although this seemed obviously necessary, it met with some resistance from technical specialists who deemed their autonomy restricted or expertise sidelined. Later, CDC Director Tom Frieden furthered this vision with his creation of the CDC's Center for Global Health, of which I was the founding director. Nevertheless, this necessity to operate as one global agency for maximal public health impact is not universally understood, and the risk of splinter groups and their negative impact on other CDC work remains. It is sometimes accentuated by groups with narrow technical focus allowing elitism to creep into attitudes toward others working in broader programs such as for HIV or malaria.

Over the following years, we were able to graft on additional infectious disease work, and, importantly, to initiate the Kenya Field Epidemiology Training Program, the international version of CDC's EIS program. We had attempted in earlier years to broaden training through RETRO-CI in West Africa, but now we were operating at a much higher, better funded and better coordinated level. CDC Kenya, as our expanded country office became known, helped advance thinking of how the agency should conduct its global operations in an expanding number of countries.

As we labored to implement nascent programmatic interventions for HIV, we also edged into HIV research. An initial activity was to measure the severity of HIV and associated risk factors in the area of the DSS. Pauli Amornkul oversaw the field work. The overall prevalence of HIV in people 13 to 34 years old in 2003–2004 was 15%, but in women aged 25–29 years and men aged 30–34 years, it was 37% and 41%, respectively.[34] Risk factors for HIV were age, number of sex partners, being widowed, and herpes simplex virus infection. These baseline data were useful for comparison with later studies assessing the impact of interventions, including male circumcision, prevention of HIV transmission by breastfeeding ("the Kisumu Breastfeeding Study"),[35] and ART scale-up.

The CDC's investments in KEMRI infrastructure, including in laboratory strengthening, allowed wider collaboration including with NIH research networks. Years later, in 2021, I was saddened to learn that the CDC was cutting its research support and, henceforth, the Kenya HIV work would consist exclusively of prevention and treatment implementation under PEPFAR. Research on HIV became increasingly interventional, required multicenter studies and large study populations, and were best conducted by universities and academic investigators.

ART implementation resulted in an almost halving the death rate among persons with HIV, and a reduction of more than one-fourth in the overall death rate of the general population.[36] These observations stress the astonishing demographic impact that AIDS was having in this African population, as well as the powerful public health effect of HIV treatment. Separate analyses led by Martien Borgdorff, senior Dutch epidemiologist and subsequent director of CDC Western Kenya, showed that the rate of new HIV infections also fell by nearly one-half.[37] The DSS showed its value by facilitating direct measurement of HIV incidence, prevalence, and mortality, rather than relying on mathematical modeling to estimate trends.

Relations between malaria and HIV workers were cordial, but early on there was fear on the part of CDC malaria staff that HIV, with its considerably greater resources and attention, would push malaria work aside. HIV was still a taboo subject in the communities around Lake Victoria in the early 2000s, despite the astonishingly high rates of HIV infection. Lack of resources earlier for HIV work, as well as this ingrained reluctance to face the subject, meant that malaria work had continued in isolation, as if the raging AIDS epidemic was not relevant.

In 2001, we organized a meeting in Atlanta to discuss research priorities for the Kisumu field station, with participation of key

Kenyan scientists, including the late John Vulule, KEMRI's local director and a senior malaria researcher. Robert ("Bob") Bailey, an established HIV researcher from Chicago, had approached me to ask if the CDC would partner in a randomized clinical trial evaluating the HIV preventive efficacy of male circumcision. Vulule and others felt the topic was too controversial and could have a negative impact on malaria research. Bailey successfully completed his trial, one of three such studies that rank among the most important HIV prevention studies of all time.[38-40] I realize wistfully that the CDC missed out.

Experience with program scale-up under PEPFAR is described in other works.[2,32] With expansion in diverse areas of CDC work, our staff increased to more than thirty direct-hire Americans and close to one hundred and fifty Kenyan nationals. Our first recruits for PEPFAR work were the husband-and-wife team of Lawrence ("Larry") and Elizabeth Marum who previously had been working in Uganda. Along with Barbara ("Barb") Marston (coincidentally also Larry Slutsker's wife), the Marums were instrumental in the success of the CDC's early PEPFAR work in Kenya.

Marston drove treatment scale-up, Elizabeth Marum spearheaded policies and practice on HIV testing and counseling, and Larry Marum headed our work in blood transfusion and surveillance. Close ties with the Ministry of Health, including embedding Larry Marum in the surveillance unit, were critical for trust and impact. Larry Marum's early surveillance work strengthened capacity for subsequent national surveys assessing the country's HIV epidemic, studies to which the CDC gave strong technical support.[41-49]

The stigma of HIV/AIDS remained deep. People recognized the problem but did not think or accept it could be relevant to them. Several of our Kenyan staff fell ill with undiagnosed HIV disease, sometimes life-threatening, despite their own daily work in HIV testing and prevention. A member of our team working on HIV with the Kenya military, the partner of the director of a non-governmental organization devoted to AIDS policy, died shortly after his delayed diagnosis of cryptococcal meningitis, to her shock and disbelief. The wife of one of our drivers died of AIDS, the staff member clearly unwell himself. I was called to a private hospital because a laboratory colleague, who spent his days instructing others on HIV testing, was ill with *Pneumocystis* pneumonia. With time, attitudes changed. The driver who lost his wife accessed treatment, regained his health, rebuilt his life, and obtained a more senior position at the embassy. Such individual stories illustrate the impact of PEPFAR.

It's Never All Technical

Increased funding and greater visibility are inevitably accompanied by calls for greater accountability. The systems and flexibility "to get the job done" that supported early CDC field work were steadily replaced by requirements for more rigorous administrative organization. For the first two decades of the malaria research in Kenya, funds were transferred to the US embassy in Nairobi by cable, and CDC staff would disburse funds to KEMRI and others as required. A British man who had set up a small nongovernmental operation assisted with fiscal administration and oversaw a bank account supporting operations, referred to as "The Jeremy Account." Work got done, field staff were paid, procurements were made, and all went swimmingly, outside of US government systems, until it didn't.

A few months into my tenure in Kenya in 2000, I received a call from the US embassy's financial management officer, refusing my request to transfer money to KEMRI. He emphasized that he was personally responsible for any funds used outside of regulations.

Henceforth, he would not sign off on CDC requests. My appeal that this meant he was effectively shutting down our operations met with no sympathy. To their credit, CDC supervisors in Atlanta sprang into action. The head of the CDC's overall financial management office, a patrician southerner, made an emergency visit to Kenya and negotiated establishment of a cooperative agreement with KEMRI.

Cooperative agreements are funding tools whose nature is captured in their title—they are binding agreements, and they define cooperation. The CDC transfers the money to the recipient for an agreed body of work on which the two parties will cooperate over a specified period. Cooperative agreements, administratively distinct from grants (equivalent to gifts) or contracts ("I will pay you to do what I ask"), are the principal way the CDC funds its partners. The Kenya cooperative agreement was the first of its kind for the CDC's international work, and this tool became standard for PEPFAR and other work.

Cooperating is different from directing. Once transferred, the funds belong to the recipient, who is supposed to lead the work and provide regular financial and technical reports, all with support, but not direction, from the CDC. Kayla Laserson followed Slutsker as director of CDC activities in western Kenya. She invested heavily in the DSS and other scientific work, as well as reinforcing bonds with KEMRI. Outstanding technical work was done, infrastructure was strengthened, and administrative requirements appeared met. Sometimes, unfortunately, things did not go well.

Around 2006–2007, coincidentally or not within a year of Kenya's upcoming presidential election, almost a quarter of a million dollars went missing from the accounts. Even more funds disappeared from KEMRI's own coffers, the institute's pension fund having been cleaned out. These monies appeared to have been diverted by the then KEMRI director, Davy Koech, who was eventually removed, prosecuted, and, much later, imprisoned but released after 1 year*.[50]

In 2015, the cooperative agreement ran out of money 6 months ahead of schedule. Investigations showed that, this time, almost $3 million could not be accounted for, and an audit showed numerous financial system weaknesses. By now, KEMRI was receiving large amounts of funding from diverse international partners and donors, but tracking these funds going into similar activities and infrastructure was difficult. Elizabeth ("Beth") Barr, a later director of the CDC's western Kenya activities, analyzed funding flows from the CDC and other partners. Her diagram resembled a complex rail network or freeway spaghetti junction. KEMRI received substantial funding from diverse international partners, but overall money streams were almost impossible to disentangle.

I negotiated with different ministers of health concerning the missing CDC funds which, to Kenya's honor, have been repaid. I was amused that on a visit by KEMRI leadership to Atlanta to discuss all this around 2017, their deputy director was able to claw back $1 million from the debt owed, because the CDC itself had miscalculated the debt owed.

Another challenge has been the issue of security. Ambassador Carson was prescient in his post–9/11 comments, predicting that Somalia would become a hub of extremism and terrorism after the expulsion of Al-Qaeda from Afghanistan. In 2002, an attack on a hotel at the coast killed thirteen people and injured many more, and two missiles were fired at an Israeli jetliner leaving from Mombasa, without damage. Carson looked weary as I encountered him in a corridor one day, and he shared how worried he was about Kenya's security situation.

---

* Davy Koech died in September 2024.

On September 21, 2013, terrorists attacked Westgate mall in Nairobi, an up-market shopping venue widely frequented by expatriates and staff of international agencies. The Islamic terrorist organization Al-Shabaab claimed the attack was retribution for Kenyan military involvement in Somalia. The standoff and siege lasted more than two days and left sixty-seven dead. In 2019, an attack on a hotel and commercial complex in Nairobi resulted in twenty-two deaths, the security forces performing in a more effective and coordinated way than was the case in the Westgate debacle.[51] In summaries I have seen of security incidents in Kenya, dozens of attacks occurred over the years, something unknown to many; because most did not involve internationals, they received little attention.

Although our staff were fortunately not directly affected by terrorism, anxiety increased. Security of US government personnel became an ever-higher priority, especially after the events in Benghazi, Libya, in 2012 when Ambassador J. Christopher Stevens was killed. Stevens had practiced hands-on diplomacy, emphasizing the importance of deep and personal interaction with the local population. Diplomatic security began to trump the needs of day-to-day field work and interactions, unquestionably reducing the ability of the CDC to do its global work.

Insecurity from crime has also been a problem. In 2005, the young son of an American visiting researcher was shot in Kisumu in an attempted robbery. Fortunately, his injuries were not life-threatening. Less fortunate were two Kenyan physicians working on tuberculosis under our PEPFAR program, who died violent deaths in 2012. One colleague died in a car crash that some deemed suspicious, and the other was shot in Kisumu in a possible robbery. That both were working in the same program and died within a few months of each other raised speculation that these were not random events, although we had no evidence their deaths were related. These incidents emphasized that the Kenyan environment could be unpredictable and insecure, despite its simultaneous hospitality and generosity.

Conclusions

What do I take away from these nontechnical experiences? First, that medical epidemiologists and researchers are not well placed to design, correct, or oversee administrative and financial systems. Internationally, CDC administrative systems do not match the sophistication of the agency's technical work. Some KEMRI officials understandably felt left in the lurch when they alone were held responsible for money difficulties, while the CDC emphasized that scientific achievements were jointly owned.

Power imbalances affect these international relationships and are influencing the very notion of global health and associated research. Navigating these waters shows the need for global health diplomacy. Regrettably, I have seen examples of clumsy behaviors, including in the world of PEPFAR, where withholding of funding was sometimes used as a blunt tool to correct faulty management but sometimes to impose programmatic or technical decisions, such as restrictions on HIV testing.[52]

Equally, mismanagement of funds or corruption should not be tolerated. There is now increasing emphasis on country ownership and listening to country voice, giving partners in the Global South greater independence in priority setting and decision-making. This inevitably will come up against calls for greater control and scrutiny when financial or administrative mismanagement occurs, as it does in high- as well as lower-income settings.

My time in Kenya for the CDC left me with broad conclusions about how the agency should best function internationally, but also about how global health was changing. If the CDC remains fragmented and balkanized across its technical divisions, it will not have maximal impact. Repeatedly, the CDC's effectiveness in Kenya was shown to be enhanced by collaboration between the agency's technical groups.[53]

That was perhaps my main philosophy as I took up the directorship of the CDC's newly created Center for Global Health in 2010, emphasizing three broad conclusions: that the CDC had to operate as one agency overseas ("One CDC"); that global health action was in the field, not in Atlanta ("global health is global"); and that the CDC had to engage in a coordinated way at the highest political levels in individual countries and globally ("take a seat at the high table"). It is not all technical, I came to realize, and there is much that does not get into the materials and methods of a paper. Sometimes that omitted material and the associated stories are even more important than the study results.

CHAPTER 13

Health Bureaucracy

Careers are judged on appointments and achievements summarized in résumés, but these ignore an important fundamental: the passage of time. The Peter Principle, that in a hierarchy employees rise to their level of incompetence, contains truth as well as cynicism. At the CDC, there was a jibe that there were three ways to deal with troublesome or awkward employees: promote them to a position of nonsupervisory, ill-defined responsibility; put them in charge of a long-term working group; or send them away on long-term training. Ensuring organizational efficiency and impact can be challenged by the daily needs of just getting by.

Individual excellence is vital, but we overlook the cohort effect that propels us into positions of increasing authority as older colleagues age still further, vacating positions that then need filling. With seniority come administrative burdens, responsibility for others, and distancing from the front line. Suddenly, ruefully, you find that you have become a bureaucrat. You miss field work, research, or the direct impact of treating sick patients. Introspection can offer insight but too easily leads to self-doubt and the melancholia that afflicts many in mid- to late career. "Is this all there is, is this what it was all for?" you ask. The gloom can border on despair, threaten marriages and partnerships, and lead to impulsive and unwise decisions.

Yet, taking on the mantle of seniority is as important as obtaining degrees and experience in earlier life, is essential to drive change in the world, and merits its own preparation. The world needs capable and inspirational health bureaucrats.

On Leadership and Administration

Organizations, large or small, need structure that defines who is who and who does what. Organizational structure may not be important in small groups where everybody is reasonable, all get along, and everyone works toward a common cause. More commonly, not everyone sees eye to eye, opinions and temperaments differ, and tensions lie close below the surface. In such instances, ambiguity about roles and responsibilities, lines of authority, and channels of communication can derail the most talented of groups. It was practical experience of such challenges that made me aware of the importance of leadership, management, and organizational structure. Leadership and management are different. Both are essential. Neither was taught at my medical school or during subsequent training.

Multiple definitions exist for these concepts. The simplest are the most useful because they convey essence, if not comprehensiveness. You recognize good leadership and administration when you see them. Leadership is the ability to get others to do what needs to be done. It is different from hierarchy, which simply describes authority. Getting others to do what needs to be done means that leadership should take account of lines of authority, but it reminds one that being in authority does not guarantee leadership. As is said in politics, you can be in office but not in power.

Leadership can also be exerted horizontally without formal authority over others, upstream to those who have authority over us, and to actors outside the organization. Good leadership is required to decide what needs to be done, strong administration is needed to see that it gets done. Organizational structure is an administrative tool to facilitate actions and activities aimed at doing what needs to get done, and its absence or defects can handicap or scupper the overriding essential—getting everyone to do what needs to be done.

It is useful to distinguish among leadership, authority, power, and influence. Ideally, formal authority would be aligned with good leadership, but this is not always the case. Leadership, by contrast, can be exerted without formal authority. Power is usually associated with authority, and in public health or other areas, especially the work of governments, this generally goes along with funding. In global health, for example, donor and philanthropic agencies may seem more powerful than the CDC because of their flexibility and scope for allocation of targeted funding. Influence, however, is not guaranteed by money or sheer power, and impactful innovations and change can derive from incisive leadership without formal authority, power, or great resources.

An example is the influence WHO exerts over global health through its convening authority and technical guidelines. The CDC mostly influences the world of health through specific technical work and its reputation, not through power. Leaders must think strategically of their position in the ecosystem, the tools and attributes at their disposal, how they can influence what needs to be done, and how they can best work toward getting it done.

Why Are You Here?

A useful question in early adulthood is "what man or woman do you want to be?" Clinical medicine provided me with daily routines and the structure of clinics, ward rounds, teaching, and research that allowed avoidance of the question "why am I here?"

Moving to the CDC and into public health took away that security and instilled anxiety about the need to constantly define purpose. I recalled earlier instances of decisive action clinically or in field work that changed events, which I might later have considered examples of leadership, but I never benefited from education in the subject.

As a clinician and then EIS officer, I did not lead groups or have substantial authority. I did not think much about leadership but saw individual examples of excellence in mentors whom I admired and then thought to emulate. My first substantial position of authority was in Cote d'Ivoire, where we established the CDC's Projet RETRO-CI that grew from a staff of two—our laboratory director Anne Porter and myself—to more than fifty.[1] We achieved a lot, but not without hiccups or anguish along the way that were lessons for the administratively uneducated such as I.

An early observation concerned the need to distinguish between friendship and business. The work was so intense, the group so small, and interactions with the early staff so close that overall functioning was informal. Dividing lines between work and friendship were blurred. Yet, we worked within the regulatory framework of the US government and embassy, more rigid than highly educated, itinerant, individualistic internationals sometimes understood. Although regulations can be maladaptive—for example, CDC's domestically oriented regulatory framework sometimes handicaps international work—they usually exist for a reason and have been hammered out based on experience.

I learned that trying to adapt regulations or rules to accommodate individuals usually exacerbated problems rather than solving them. I saw the importance of being sympathetic and supportive as a supervisor but applying rules consistently. Trying to adjust to individual circumstances beyond the ordinary often leads to further problems down the road.

Alan Greenberg succeeded me as Projet RETRO-CI director after my 5-year tenure. He undertook a strategic review and reorganization of the project, most importantly reorienting the mission from one of descriptive and analytic epidemiology to evaluation of interventions and strengthening laboratory science. This example of strategic thinking was eye opening to me, as was Greenberg's self-identified course after RETRO-CI. He persuaded the CDC to support him for 2 years of further education at Harvard, obtaining a master's degree in public health as well as attending courses at the John F. Kennedy School of Government, the university's public policy school. I envied him this further education that contributed to his widely lauded skill in strategic thinking and organization, which I later called on several times.

My entry into real bureaucracy at the CDC began in 1997, when Helene Gayle appointed me as director of the Division of HIV/AIDS Prevention–Surveillance and Epidemiology. This division had about two hundred employees and an annual budget of approximately $100 million. I selected Greenberg as chief of the Epidemiology Branch, where he immediately applied his analytic thinking. The branch had contributed substantially to understanding HIV epidemiology and transmission but had not questioned its mission for some time. We found that a substantial proportion of the budget was devoted to mother-to-child transmission of HIV, although only a small fraction of the tens of thousands of new infections annually in the United States were in infants, and interventions were succeeding in reducing this number still further.

This epidemiology budget simply did not reflect the trends or burden of HIV infection and disease in the United States at the time. Budgets are boring but represent political and policy choices. Budgets are administrative statements, but they also are the skeleton on which the flesh and blood of activities and interventions hang. The epidemiology budget we incisively revised illustrated lack of previous regular review of purpose and impact.

"If you keep doing what you've always done, you'll get what you always got" was a statement the CDC's tuberculosis leader at the time, Dixie Snider, said about approaches to that disease. Organizations need to review their identity and *raison d'être* every few years. Leaders need to prioritize, decide on budget proposals, and balance current with evolving challenges. "Skate to where the puck is going to be, not where it was," they say in ice hockey, a maxim that is relevant to making organizational choices.

On Vision, Mission, and Structure

Mention consultants and many think of expensive firms and slick PowerPoint presentations. Yet, outside views can be critically important for organizations, which, like individuals, can be paralyzed by daily routines and responsibilities that obscure the need for new directions. Stability offers comfort but not necessarily the adaptability needed to face an unpredictable environment. When I was appointed director of the Department of HIV/AIDS at WHO's headquarters in Geneva, I invited Greenberg to assist us in strategic planning. He took me through the process of defining vision, mission, and strategic objectives and action steps.

To persuade and motivate staff and other stakeholders, it is more important for leaders and their organizations to communicate why they do something rather than what they do.[2] A vision statement concerns the *why* of an organization, its fundamental reason for existing. It is difficult to make a difference if you do not know *why* you are doing something. Mission then concerns *how* the organization's vision might be attained, and strategic objectives and action steps the *what*, the specifics of the collective work.

Defining these essentials is not simply a theoretical exercise. If you don't define where you want to go, you could end up anywhere. And if the organization has not communicated its aspirations and intent, it is difficult to evaluate whether it is up or down, succeeding or failing. An editorial in *The Economist* years ago used breakfast cereal as an analogy for life: crunchy or soggy.[3] With crunchy cereal, you know what you are eating, even if it sometimes makes the teeth hurt. Soggy breakfast fare may not need teeth at all. Sogginess allows institutions to drift; crunchiness is oriented toward results. By contrast, crunchiness can be uncomfortable. If an organization is not adequately crunchy, cannot explain succinctly why it exists or measure whether it is succeeding or failing, it will be difficult to garner financial or political support. These insights were helpful in my progression through seniority, offering structure and purpose for what otherwise might have been diffuse areas of work conducted simply because that is what we always did.

Vision, mission, objectives, and activities cannot be implemented without a sound organizational structure. In that regard, avoiding duplication and overlap of function is important, unless redundancy is a specific intent. My tenure as director of the newly established CDC Division of HIV/AIDS Prevention–Surveillance and Epidemiology was tested by the existence of another division with a rather similar name that was responsible for prevention programs and led by a colleague of equal rank. This inevitably led to competitive ambiguity about who had authority to speak on HIV.

The multitude of agencies in the United Nations system with HIV activities leads to predictable overlap and conflict. In defining strategy and structure, it is important to scan the environment for competitors. The most challenging competitors will be those who most resemble you, an observation attributed to the management guru Bruce Henderson. Organizations derive their advantage by the extent to which they offer something unique or, in other words, how different they are from competitors.

A useful approach at the CDC, highlighted by former director Bill Foege, has been the pairing of epidemiologists, usually the supervisors, with public health advisors responsible for administration, finance, and implementation.[4] If leadership is not the same as administration, bad administration can certainly sink good leadership. In larger groups or organizations, the leader may benefit from choosing a deputy who focuses predominantly on the internal workings of the organization, leaving the director to deal with higher-level and external responsibilities. A director and deputy function best when they commit to complete trust and information sharing, allowing the deputy to act for the director as necessary.

One of the greatest challenges to directors or leaders is to let others do what they need to do without interference. A senior leader, and my supervisor, once said to me that he attributed his success to micromanagement. Peripatetic activity can allay individual anxiety and give the impression of making a difference. This is rarely strategic, however, especially for leaders and directors whose most precious commodity is time. Directors should think strategically about their use of time, devoting it principally to what only they can do and delegating what can be done equally well by others. The human tendency will always be to revert to that with which one is most comfortable, not necessarily that which is most important or strategic.

The World Health Organization

The WHO must be the most misunderstood organization in global health, and the extreme disparity between what the world expects and the resources it provides to the agency is not widely recognized. I described some of my personal experiences at WHO earlier in this book. Despite the challenges, my time at the helm of the agency's global HIV work, two decades after Jon Mann ini-

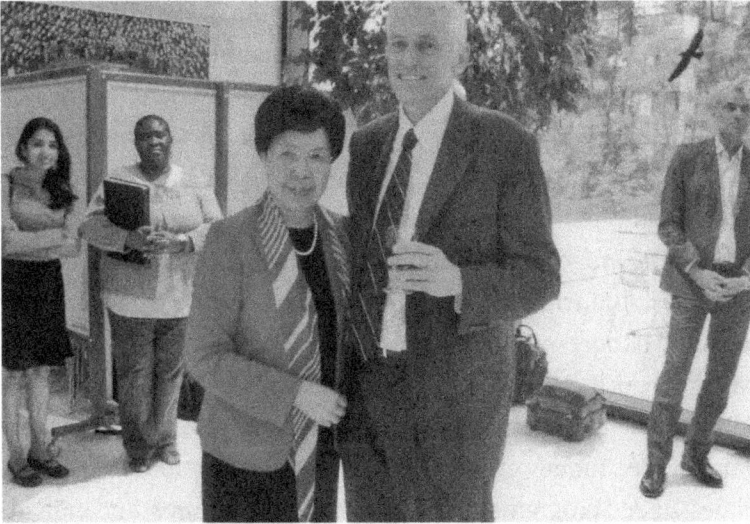

Figure 13.1   Leaving WHO, June 2009. (*left to right, front*) Margaret Chan, director general; Kevin De Cock, director, Department of HIV/AIDS. (Kevin De Cock, personal collection)

tiated the agency's focus on this pandemic, was uniquely meaningful to me (Figure 13.1).

If the organization is often perceived as slow and bureaucratic, it is useful to dissect out causes in relation to leadership, management, funding, rules and regulations, organizational structure, and geopolitics. Blowing it up will not help, but innovative thinking of how to improve and make it fit for purpose for the twenty-first century would be useful. Unfortunately, member states protect vested interests associated with the status quo, as is seen throughout UN organizations, including the Security Council. WHO's weaknesses are unlikely to be solved by cautious, incremental fiddling.

The CDC's 1-year budget request for 2024 was for $11.6 billion.[5] The Bill and Melinda Gates Foundation spent approximately $6 billion on all its global programs in 2022, and is an important donor to WHO.[6,7] By contrast, WHO's 2-year aspirational budget is just over $6 billion for its work across the globe.[8] In line with the emphasis the George W. Bush administration placed on supporting faith-based organizations in global health work, we joked when I was at WHO that the agency itself was one because we had faith that money would come sooner or later.

In addition to limited funding, there is the complication that an increasing proportion of funds are provided as "voluntary contributions," financial support that may have strings attached. The biennial budget must be approved by WHO's governing body, the World Health Assembly, but this does not guarantee that member states will deliver the approved sums. The result is that the real budget (i.e., money available) resembles a Christmas tree of partially funded programs, administrative expenditures, and individual earmarks.

WHO is hierarchical in a way difficult to imagine in a modern university or business, structurally as well as in relations between staff. Its constitution defines WHO's cumbersome global structure with Geneva-based headquarters, six regional offices, and some one hundred fifty country offices. WHO is more of a confederation than a single organization with a unified purpose.

Every year in May, ministers of health and their delegations from WHO's 194 member states converge on Geneva for the World Health Assembly, the senior decision-making body in global health. The week-long meeting is a mixture of technical prioritization, bureaucracy, diplomacy, and raw politics around controversial issues such as sexual and reproductive health and universal health coverage. The august Palais des Nations, built in the 1930s and overlooking Lake Geneva and the Swiss Alps, is a building from another era that somehow matches the feel of the organization itself.

There have been calls from member states for "WHO reform," but what this truly means is unclear and the fate of the organization really rests with the member states themselves. Not only are public health agencies like the CDC or the European Centre for Disease Prevention and Control (the European CDC) more active internationally, but the activities and influence of nongovernmental organizations like the Bill and Melinda Gates Foundation and Médecins Sans Frontières also have increased. WHO does not have sole pride of place as it did decades ago.

Most WHO staff I worked with were deeply committed and hard working. Bureaucratic requirements nonetheless affected personnel and human resources. Although appointments were said to be made on merit, there was constant need to ensure representativeness and national diversity, avoiding dominance of any geographic block. This resulted in some less-than-ideal appointments, technical capability sometimes not being the prime consideration.

Financial shortages meant many staff were hired on repeated short-term contracts, depriving them of long-term benefits. Staff on fixed-term appointments were afraid about the long-term viability of their positions in the face of often shifting priorities and financial and political turbulence. For younger colleagues, WHO was an exciting place for a brief period but not a substitute for practical field experience. Sometimes very senior people arrived in Geneva—deans, professors, or former ministers of health from low- or middle-income countries—who then found themselves unsupported and isolated, both professionally and socially, in a rigid organization that left some feeling diminished.

Not everyone at WHO would necessarily be able to regain a position in their home country, and the anxiety of staff who might face termination of their contracts was intense. How well specific programs were funded was not solely under WHO's control and did not reflect the global burden of disease. Individual and programmatic insecurity understandably limited opportunity for challenging and open debate or for mutual support across the organization.

Comments shared with me by a senior health official from an African country conveyed aspirations from this essential organization: to help deal with numerous external partners and their divergent requirements; to provide the necessary guidance for the health sector response to HIV/AIDS and other major health challenges; to ensure the country was "doing things the right way"; and to be "the country's conscience."

The debate should be about the WHO we need and how to attain it, not just about deficiencies of an irreplaceable organization we do not adequately support. And to better define what we need from WHO, we might start with analyses of its leadership at different levels; its organizational structure based on its mission; its administration and budget; and its communications. It needs to be crunchy.

Surviving as a Health Bureaucrat

The rewards of field research or clinical medicine are immediate. In positions of seniority, removed from the direct fray, it is natural to question whether one is making a difference. Delving into activities younger colleagues should be carrying out, engaging in technical work previously excelled in but that is now another's responsibility, focusing on more easily controlled minutiae—these exemplify the natural tendency to retreat into areas of reassuring familiarity. The extent to which these temptations are resisted is one of the tests for leaders of their inner strength and self-awareness. At the same time, fear of losing expertise should be a concern for a technical person rising through the ranks of an organization. Maintaining broad technical knowledge contributes to credibility as one increases in seniority.

I found it useful to think of big goals as well as small ones. If your only criterion for success is the organization's vision—a world without malaria, for example-you are likely to end up disappointed. William Blake wrote of the importance of "Minute Particulars," dismissing "General Good" as the domain of "the scoundrel, hypocrite and flatterer." Combine measurable, discrete elements of a big agenda into chains of plausibility toward progress, and it is easier to see that that forward motion has, indeed, occurred. Find time for smaller and separate aspirations still relevant to one's role—teaching, editing a journal, chairing important workgroups—and satisfaction can emerge from a list of specific achievements additional to the higher-level vision. Ultimately, the competition is with oneself.

Change such as a more senior position or retirement lead people to ask "What will I do?" Even more important is the question "Who will I be?" Two extremes in leadership styles are a disruptive approach on the one hand, and a confirmatory one on the other. Jonathan Mann was disruptive in his leadership setting up WHO's Global Programme on AIDS.[1] His work had long-lasting impact, still felt today in how the world addresses the HIV pandemic. He challenged the status quo, forcing the world to adapt to his radically new vision. Such an approach leaves little room for compromise or second chances—you cannot leap in two stages, and if you try to kill the king, you have to succeed the first time.

When my CDC colleague Rob Newman took over WHO's Global Malaria Programme in 2009, I recommended he read biographies of two long-term United Nations insiders, Sérgio Vieira de Mello[9] and Kofi Annan.[10] Vieira de Mello, the UN high commissioner for Human Rights, died in a bomb attack on his hotel in Baghdad in 2003, and former Secretary General Annan from natural causes in 2018. Their two lives illustrated the fundamental purpose and importance of the United Nations, why the organization matters, but also different leadership and management trajectories. Vieira de Mello's was more action-packed and abrasive, Annan's smoother and more traditionally administrative.

Disruptive leaders can change the world but can also leave chaos behind them, and their own ends are frequently dire. By contrast, confirmatory leaders' quest for stability can amount to what is best called reckless caution, impeding sorely needed change. Such hesitancy can stymie an organization or agenda, condemning them to just more of the same.

Few have the skill with which Mann, Vieira de Mello, or Annan acted on the global stage. For most, what is achievable is a middle ground between risk aversion that paralyzes groups and audacity that compromises an organization's functioning. Recognizing opportunities and seizing the right ones are tests of judgment essential for success. "When you come to a fork in the road, take it," Yogi Berra wisely said, but first you must recognize the fork.

Autocrats may have impact by wielding their power, but they are rarely good leaders. An essential quality is humility, an attribute autocrats lack, and without which one fails to learn from mistakes or to listen rather than always talk. Perhaps it was my experience as a clinician that led me to recognize that if you listen, people will tell you, and often more than they should. Authority, like rights, often must be taken, but excessively autocratic or manipulative approaches are rarely the answer. My former CDC colleague Anna Likos said, "You get what you give, but you can't give to get, because people see through that."

Respect for senior leaders and managers stems from their personal charisma and quality, but authority derives from the desk behind which they sit. That authority can be corrupting, lead to failure to listen, and blind one to the need for change. It is lack of insight and humility that causes people—academics, politicians, others in leadership—to hold on to outmoded ideas, agendas, or their own positions for too long. Knowing when to quit or abandon a particular course of action is important, and not just to poker players.[11] Quit when you are ahead, not when it is too late.

My father's words "tall trees catch the wind" have stayed with me, especially as I took on more senior positions. At WHO, where it is difficult to remove someone who has flouted regulations or not performed, a staff member with his own agenda tried different routes to evict me from my position. Years later, an anonymous letter to the CDC director and the *Lancet* resulted in questioning of my competence as lead for global health at the CDC.[12] It is difficult not to be defensive about these and other experiences. Yet, they come with the territory, and I have found the best approach in moments of controversy is to focus on the mission and resist self-pity.

In complex environments or large institutions, tensions and conflicts between people and groups are frequent. Comments I made once while at WHO about lack of generalized HIV spread outside of Africa were taken out of context in the international press.[1] Sister agencies made hay, and there were calls for my resignation. I learned that it is almost never enough just to be right. WHO's deputy director general at the time, Asamoa-Baah, likened the interagency space to a jungle where tigers and leopards pounce, never changing their stripes or spots. His point was not to be surprised by such events, nor to take them personally.

The term resilience best captures the attribute required to weather difficult situations that are an inescapable accompaniment to leadership. In 2012, when our CDC group in Kenya was fearful after the violent deaths of two colleagues, I invited the State Department's regional psychiatrist to meet with staff. She chose to speak on resilience, citing an investigation of what factors protected the mental health of prisoners of war compared with peers who fared badly.[13] Like leadership, resilience may come naturally to some but also can be taught and purposefully developed.

Much help and advice go toward younger colleagues starting their careers, but little to seniors on the meaningful closure of official working lives. When the great transplant surgeon Thomas ("Tom") Starzl died in 2017, his obituary in the *Lancet* cited six attributes contributing to his success: intelligence, creativity, ambition, curiosity, hard work, and ability to get along with people.[14] I agreed with this tribute but thought it incomplete. Others who had achieved much shared additional characteristics including experience, having been there and borne witness; communication, the ability to persuade and inspire; character and integrity, being able to overcome inner fears and stay true; and judgment, a necessary quality for decision-making in clinical medicine and public health that investigations and data alone cannot replace.

Health bureaucrats might find it useful to reflect on these life tests and qualities, assess how well they meet them, and how they could strengthen them. And they should avoid taking themselves too seriously, mindful of the words of the French philosopher François de La Rochefoucauld: "*Qui vit sans folie n'est pas si sage qu'il croit*" ("he who lives without folly is not as wise as he thinks").

Epilogue

Health is a human story, and the ultimate equalizer. Anguish in childhood or fears of mortality in old age feel similar to the prince as to the pauper. Politics and conflicts will have their short-term impacts, but the quest for better health is for the ages. For these and other reasons, I remain an optimist.

Health is inherently political, because it requires decisions on policy and funding. This book is not political. Good medicine and public heath need open-mindedness and clear thinking. I have attempted to draw meaning from journeys and experiences as objectively as possible.

2025—Contradictions

The global health community has been stunned by the extent and rapidity of organizational and programmatic change in the United States over the first months of 2025. Intermittent review of activities and funding is appropriate, but the speed and breadth of the cuts, elimination of programs, and firings of staff for domestic and global health have raised concerns and communicated uncertainty.[1] Reductions in health programs abroad have seemed arbitrary and have cost lives.

Programmatic, financial, and staffing cuts at the CDC run counter to aspirations for a healthier nation. Increased focus on noncommunicable diseases, the leading cause of death in the United States and the world as a whole, is welcome. Principal remediable risk factors include salt, sugar, tobacco, alcohol and other drugs, processed and other unhealthy foods, and air pollution. Whether political will exists to take on the commercial interests benefiting from such hazards remains to be seen.

Controversial support for reinvigorating coal mining contrasts with the initial elimination of the CDC's program to monitor and address black lung disease, the leading occupational health risk for coal workers.[2,3] President Trump's acclaimed initiative in 2019 to end the domestic HIV epidemic in the United States aimed to reduce new HIV infections by 90% by 2030.[4] On April 1, 2025, approximately one-quarter of the CDC's HIV prevention staff were terminated. Such contradictions hamper attainment of public health goals.

Advice and commentaries from critics of the CDC on how the agency should be reorganized have been diverse. Project 2025 advised splitting the agency into an epidemiology section and a public health part, totally separated.[5] Others have opined that the CDC should concentrate on infectious diseases, its traditional focus.[6] There has been talk of reducing the agency further and moving some of its programs elsewhere. Criticism abounds, but no cohesive view has been presented on how the infectious and noninfectious challenges of the era will be comprehensively addressed. There must be concern that the cuts and changes envisaged will irrevocably handicap the reach and impact of the CDC, long considered the leading public health agency in the world.

As repeatedly emphasized, one of the CDC's prime functions is disease surveillance. In this area of work, which no other agency is equipped to conduct, diversity cannot be a forbidden word. Disease must be tracked in all communities and locations where it occurs—unvaccinated religious minorities with measles, for example, or immigrant communities with tuberculosis. The HIV epidemic is concentrated in key populations such as sexual minorities and people who inject drugs. Eliminating focus on vulnerable groups, either by cutting surveillance or denying such groups' self-identity, obscures but does not solve public health problems. Invisibility allows challenges to fester until they erupt into the mainstream.

There has been criticism of globalization for its negative economic and social effects on some regions and populations. Irrespective of moves to counter adverse consequences, what is irreversible is the globalization of public health risk. Global health is influenced by the spread of accurate information and misinformation, cultural practices, drugs and other unsafe products, infectious diseases, and more. Today's world is too interconnected for isolationism to protect any country against infectious and noninfectious health risks. In global health, no country can go it alone.

Reflections to a Younger Self

Former CDC Director Bill Foege advised public health students not to make a life plan, because events are too random and scientific advances too rapid for any plan to hold. In the face of predictable unpredictability, he urged investment in a life ethos, a philosophy for the ages. For students or younger colleagues, "What man or woman do I want to be?" is a more pertinent question than simply "What should I do?"

It is important to have the right training and education, but after a certain point learning must come from doing. The Pareto Principle, or 80/20 rule, states that 80% of outcomes come from 20% of causes. Think health, where poverty or exclusion drive a large proportion of ill health. Extending the principle, basic technical skills allow one to address most health challenges. I always felt I needed more training but now recognize field experience was the best teacher. At some time, you have to hold your nose and jump, and you cannot do it in two leaps.

I have tried in this book to convey the excitement of work in global health. Like any career, it has had its rewards and disappointments, but it has rarely been dull. Some opportunities I had would not be available today, but, equally, some aspects of today's world were unimaginable when I was young. Diagnostic imaging; molecular biology for development of vaccines, drugs, and diagnostics; immunotherapy; and antiviral medications count among the more obvious advances. That information is instantly retrievable with a stroke on a keyboard or mobile phone, and almost anywhere in the world, is a distant reality from what I faced scouring archived journals for my doctoral thesis.

Many comment that careers today are more challenging than they were in earlier times, but are they really? Or are they just different? Environments and their problems differ across the world, but people are the same. Disruptive innovations have driven social change across the ages. Moore's law—that the number of transistors on a chip will double every 2 years, increasing computing power exponentially—may apply to science but not to human nature.

Certain realities remain constant. People are people, wherever they live. They aspire to a better life and a better future for their children. Talent exists everywhere, but opportunity does not. Never mistake lack of education for lack of intelligence. Biology is stronger than culture; the cultural environment changes rapidly, human nature stays the same.

"Vices are sometimes only virtues carried to excess" is a saying attributed to Charles Dickens. Humility is good, but its extension to low self-esteem is not. Pride in one's work is positive but can morph into arrogance. Being right is important but never enough to assure what is right gets done. And self-righteousness is insufferable. The rules and methods of science are universally applicable, but resources for implementation differ widely by geographic region or topic. No matter where you have worked, always ensure you can get a job in your own country.

The turbulence of 2025 will pose inevitable questions for career opportunities and choices. What it will not affect is the nature of health disparities in the world, a world that will keep on turning. Global health will still require bright minds and trained, committed people. Foege's teaching still applies.

Global Health, 2025—Contradictions and Uncertainties

"The past is a foreign country; they do things differently there." (L. P. Hartley, 1953)[7]

Diverse forces are bearing down on global health, a discipline that in many ways is in crisis. The debates and uncertainty have implications for the traditional learning institutes as well as for research funding and development agencies—in fact, for all involved in today's global health. Recent reductions in development assistance for health have made the uncertainties more acute.

A seminal article in the *Lancet* by a former CDC director, Jeff Koplan, and colleagues in 2009 attempted to define global health, the subject that emerged from earlier visions of international health and tropical medicine and their political contexts.[8] Tropical medicine was emblematic of the colonial era, and international health was largely concerned with donor-supported health activities in the early postcolonial years.

The European schools of tropical medicine have considered changing their names now that their curricula extend far beyond colonial medicine. They have refrained from doing so largely because their brands are so famous, but they recognize that history has moved on. Colleagues and I wrote an opinion piece some decades ago saying that tropical medicine would best be absorbed into infectious diseases, which should incorporate parasitic diseases, travel medicine, and sexually transmitted infections.[9]

Koplan and colleagues discussed whether global health encompasses national and cross-border issues (yes); whether it concerned more than infectious diseases (yes); the importance of globalization (important); and its multidisciplinary nature. Insofar as the quest for equity is core to public health, they considered this relevant also. Health equity, similar health outcomes irrespective of the inputs required, offers the parameter by which we can assess progress. Optimistically, the discipline of global health heralded a different relationship between countries, away from the "us" and "them" of earlier North-South relationships. It is, in part, this incompletely realized vision that lies at the root of today's controversies about global health.

From the CDC, colleagues and I discussed global health through the prism of development, health security, and public health.[10] Development was an unspoken aim of traditional international health activities in nutrition and maternal and child health, while health security took account of trends in emerging and epidemic-prone infectious diseases. The recent epidemics of Ebola and the COVID-19 pandemic demonstrated how health security must be an integral part of global health. A simple definition might be that global health is concerned with the response to globalized public health risk, what we do as a global community to assure the world is healthy.[11]

The nature and identity of global health face some inherent contradictions. Recognized global health experts are mostly practitioners from the Global North who study problems in the Global South. Professionals in the South rarely describe themselves as global health specialists, and they certainly do not focus exclusively on the health priorities of the other side of the world. Global health practice and research have been heavily influenced by funding from the Global North, funding that does not match the actual burden of disease but reflects northern choices. Monies allocated affect perceptions of what global health is more than do analyses of the health of the world. Global health, in sum, is not global.

Development assistance for health has been heavily skewed toward maternal and child health, HIV, tuberculosis, and malaria, which have accounted for about two-thirds of funding.[12] Research support in the Global South has been mainly oriented to infectious diseases, although these are no longer the leading causes of death in the world.

When I left Europe in 1979 for my university appointment in Nairobi, there were more than twelve million annual deaths in children younger than 5 years. This number has more than halved since then. Maternal mortality has declined, and women are having fewer children. More children are becoming healthy adults and aging, increasing life expectancy. Development assistance for health has achieved impressive results and is faced with the choice between addressing changing patterns of disease or simply adhering to its original aims.

As childhood and infectious causes of death declined, new health challenges have come to the fore. Intentional and unintentional injuries are important causes of morbidity and mortality in people of working age. Mental health, long neglected, is more prominent. Noncommunicable diseases have emerged as leading causes of death, even in poor countries. In some, a dual burden exists, with old problems such as tuberculosis and HIV but also high and rising rates of obesity and diabetes presenting new challenges. To date, little funding has gone toward these newer priorities. An attitude exists that "lifestyle" diseases such as obesity and diabetes are personal responsibilities, ignoring the relevance of social determinants or of the commercialization of foods and beverages.

Although improving health trends are widespread, they are staggered in time across countries, and progress is unequal. Close to one-fifth of the world's countries are in disarray from natural or man-made disasters, conflict, or mismanagement, and the optimistic assessments just cited may not apply to all. There is still extensive need for humanitarian assistance in our world, as well as support for the unfinished traditional priorities such as HIV and child survival.

The world population is expected to grow from around 8 billion people currently and stabilize late this century at around 10.4 billion.[13] More than half of population growth before 2050 will be in Africa; Africa will account for more than one-fourth of the world population by 2050 and almost 40% by 2100. Fertility is declining in sub-Saharan Africa but from a higher level—4.6 children on average per woman—than elsewhere. The great majority of future youth in the world will be African, and they will need education and jobs. Radicalization or recruitment into gangs are often driven more by financial need than ideology. Not least because of these population trends, Africa will feature more prominently in world affairs, including in health, than it has to date.

The more than one hundred million displaced people in the world have been driven from their homes by conflict, persecution, and a host of other challenges that render them incapable of supporting themselves or their families.[14] A disproportionate number of the displaced from Africa, the Middle East, and Asia have been taken in by other low- and middle-income countries, but media attention is principally focused on the borders of the United States and Europe. Tens of thousands of migrants have died crossing hostile territory such as the Sahara or have drowned at sea, but migrant health has lagged as a global health concern.

Much speculation, and gradually increasing evidence, concerns the impact on health of climate change.[15] The most direct and measurable effects are short term, such as deaths among the elderly during heat waves. There are already examples of vectors of arboviruses and parasitic infections extending their geographic range. The effects on agriculture and the environment may affect the ability of whole communities to sustain themselves, including nutritionally. Rising sea levels will make some environments uninhabitable.

These major forces affect health directly but also interact: Environments rendered inhospitable or no longer arable because of climate change may lead to conflict. Conflict and displacement drive migration, as do conditions of diminishing opportunity. Migrants are susceptible to a variety of infectious diseases for which recipient countries need to assure services as well as vigilance. Problems feed on problems, and the short-term response of increased walls and barriers in the Global North will not provide meaningful resolution.

Governance and control have become increasingly controversial, as seen by the emergence of a movement to "decolonize global health" and global health education.[16,17] Technologic innovations such as distance-based learning are allowing northern educational institutions to collaborate with partners in the Global South more cost-effectively. By contrast, as discussed earlier, the concepts of equity, inclusiveness, and diversity have become political lightning rods. Global health discussions are becoming fraught.

Inevitably, the balance of power in global health leadership, decision-making, funding, and knowledge ownership will have to shift away from the previously colonizing North to the more populous, low- and middle-income South. Good governance and accountability, frequent sources of tension everywhere, will have to be assured whatever model is used for funding. Northern politicians question endless development assistance for health in the face of diverse disparities and challenges at home. The debate about global health must include consideration of respective responsibilities of the Global North and South, and how long-term funding of HIV and other programs will be assured.

Hartley's quote conveys that analysis of earlier events through the attitudes of today can be misleading or incomplete. The process of change in global health and its research and funding may be frustrating if too slow but damaging to the health of populations if too abrupt. Judgment will be required to manage shifts in global health if the vulnerable are not to be abandoned to their own lot.

Conclusions

The Millennium Development Goals take the world up to the year 2030. Now is the time to frame the debate about the nature and future of global health, its funding, how it is managed and led, and what its priorities are for coming decades. Politics, development, climate, conflict, migration, demography, the epidemiologic transition, health trends, and equity—all are relevant to a broadened discipline.

Amid the new uncertainties are opportunities for current and future health professionals to forge their own paths in search of meaningful careers and a safer, healthier world. There is still need for nurses, doctors, and other health cadres to aid vulnerable, marginalized, or poor individuals and populations. There will be continued dependence on civil society and faith-based organizations, working with governments, to deliver services. There is still need for health research and response for neglected topics, underserved geographic areas, and health emergencies.

Opportunities are not fewer in global health today; they are just different from when I first stepped onto a plane bound for Africa. Whatever the direction taken, field experience is essential for authority, integrity, and respect. Field work taught me more than I was able to contribute.

ACKNOWLEDGMENTS

One does not get through training and a career in medicine and public health without extensive assistance and support. Listing individuals is risky because some will inevitably be omitted, potentially causing hurt and offense. I have elected, therefore, to cite the institutions that I passed through on three continents and in that way express gratitude to the many to whom I owe thanks.

The University of Bristol, United Kingdom, provided my entry into medicine. My medical school class recently celebrated at a splendid reunion its fiftieth anniversary since graduation. Certain teachers were especially encouraging or supportive, even without knowing the influence they had on young students or doctors. Deep friendships were made in those early years that have endured.

Experience in hospitals in Bristol and Torquay, along with supportive supervision, prepared me for my first international responsibilities practicing and teaching internal medicine at the University of Nairobi. My early contacts with the Liverpool School of Tropical Medicine and the London School of Hygiene and Tropical Medicine had long-lasting influence. Later, in the 1990s, I returned to teach at the London School and to work as a senior clinician on the AIDS unit at the Middlesex Hospital, then part of University College London. I am deeply grateful to the academic and clinical colleagues at these institutions.

My work on the Liver Unit at the University of Southern California (USC) in Los Angeles in the early 1980s led me to the CDC.

Strong friendships were made in a busy clinical environment where several seniors served as role models in dedication and integrity. USC's medical community and the CDC were exceptionally welcoming and open to outsiders like me. Work at the CDC, including the 2-year EIS program, gave entry to a global network and exposure to diverse and important health events. I have commented on several supervisors and mentors in this book and thank them for their guidance.

While this book focuses most on international work, I spent some years in supervisory positions in Atlanta, heading HIV epidemiology and surveillance, and later the newly established Center for Global Health. It was a privilege to serve in those positions and to work with such capable and dedicated staff. I am grateful to the CDC leaders who selected me for diverse appointments. I am pained by recent government decisions reducing CDC funding and staffing. Reducing CDC capacity and influence is detrimental not only to the United States, but to the world as a whole.

Heading WHO's global work on HIV/AIDS in the 2000s gave unique insight into the crucial role of this organization. Once again I found competent, committed professionals and colleagues who provided guidance, friendship, and support. I fear for our world if it does not attempt to strengthen the UN and its agencies rather than denigrate or evade them.

What molded me the most and I consider most important was field work in different countries in Africa, especially in Cote d'Ivoire and Kenya. I owe thanks to the legion of students and colleagues internationally who accepted me and worked with me. I am grateful to the CDC for the opportunities and support provided in diverse locations, and again marvel at the quality of colleagues with whom I collaborated. Many became friends. Host country officials and professional counterparts were supportive and essential for any successes.

As a government agency, the CDC operates in the field under the aegis of the local US embassy. The assistance provided by embassy staff in different countries, from ambassadors to more junior ranks, needs highlighting. Seeing how an embassy works and the wide roles it plays has been an interesting aspect of my field experience. I was fortunate in being exposed to the practice of diplomacy in real time, increasing my respect for the discipline.

I have a few regrets looking back, and most were my own fault. I regret that I did not recognize earlier in my career that spoon feeding cannot be provided and that developing expertise, with or without degrees—in technical epidemiology and biostatistics, for example—is one's own responsibility. I think of specific individuals who helped or guided me over the years, or simply showed kindness, whom I did not thank, and I wish I could apologize.

I am grateful for the planned and unexpected paths that my career took, ever thankful for the identity of a doctor. That identity has been more meaningful than I can express. And finally, I express deep thanks to Sopiato and my family for love, tolerance, and support in an itinerant career and its challenges.

Kevin M. De Cock, MD
Nairobi, April 2025

NOTES

Prologue

1. Rosling H. *Factfulness: Ten Reasons We're Wrong About The World—And Why Things Are Better Than You Think*. Flatiron Books; 2018.
2. Carlisle C. *Philosopher of the Heart: The Restless Life of Søren Kierkegaard*. Penguin Random House; 2019.
3. Frame JD, Baldwin JM J, Gocke DJ, Troup JM. Lassa fever, a new virus disease of man from West Africa: I. Clinical description and pathological findings. Am J Trop Med Hyg 1970;19:670-676.
4. CDC. Marburg hemorrhagic fever (Marburg HF). https://www.cdc.gov/vhf/marburg/resources/outbreak-table.html
5. Report of an International Commission. Ebola haemorrhagic fever in Zaire, 1976. Bull World Health Organ. 1978;56:271-293.
6. De Cock KM, Jaffe HW, Curran JW. *Dispatches from the AIDS Pandemic: A Public Health Story*. Oxford University Press; 2023.
7. De Cock KM, Jaffe HW, Curran JW. Reflections on 40 years of AIDS. Emerg Infect Dis. 2021; 27:1553-1560.
8. WHO. Antimicrobial resistance. https://www.who.int/news-room/fact-sheets/detail/antimicrobial-resistance
9. Der Arzt by Ivo Saliger. Dimensions:73 cm × 53.4 cm https://artsci.case.edu/dittrick/collections/images/prints/
10. Frieden TR, Koplan JP. Stronger national public health institutes for global health. Lancet. 2010;376:1721-1722.
11. Etheridge EW. *Sentinel for Health. A History of the Centers for Disease Control*. University of California Press; 1991.
12. Pendergrast M. *Inside the Outbreaks: The Elite Medical Detectives of the Epidemic Intelligence Service*. Houghton Mifflin Harcourt; 2010.
13. Koplan JP, Bond TC, Merson MH, et al. Towards a common definition of global health. Lancet 2009;373:1993-1995.
14. Affun-Adegbulu C, Cosaert T, Meudec M, et al. Decolonisation initiatives at the Institute of Tropical Medicine, Antwerp, Belgium: ready for change? BMJ Global Health 2023;7:e011748. doi:10.1136/bmjgh-2023-01174

15. Callaway E. "It is chaos": US funding freezes are endangering global health. Nature 2025. Accessed April 14, 2025. https://www.nature.com /articles/d41586-025-00385-9

16. De Cock KM, Mbori-Ngacha D, Marum E. Shadow on the continent: public health and HIV/AIDS in Africa in the 21st century. Lancet 2002;360:67-72.

17. The Heritage Foundation. *Mandate for Leadership: The Conservative Promise.* Project 2025, Presidential Transition Project. Accessed April 14, 2025. https://static.project2025.org/2025_MandateForLeader ship_FULL.pdf

Chapter 1. Why Medicine, Not Politics?

1. White Fathers. Wikipedia. Updated February 19, 2025. Accessed February 21, 2025. https://en.wikipedia.org/wiki/White_Fathers

2. Hergé. *Tintin au Congo.* Casterman; 2005.

3. Lee L. *As I Walked Out One Midsummer Morning.* Penguin Books; 1971.

4. Lourdes sanctuaire. Sanctuaire Notre-Dame de Lourdes. Accessed February 21, 2025. https://www.lourdes-france.org/en/

5. Hochschild A. *King Leopold's Ghost.* Mariner Books; 1998.

6. Ladycross School. Wikipedia. Updated February 28, 2024. Accessed February 21, 2025. https://en.wikipedia.org/wiki/Ladycross_School

7. Greene G. *A Sort of Life.* Simon and Schuster; 1971.

8. Brel J. "Le plat pays." YouTube. 2016. https://www.youtube.com /watch?v=rzeZcdW4Pbo

9. Griffin J. *Black Like Me.* Houghton Mifflin; 1961.

10. Stonyhurst College. Wikipedia. Updated February 15, 2025. Accessed February 28, 2025. https://en.wikipedia.org/wiki/Stonyhurst_College

11. Ross A. The UK boarding school identity crisis. *FT Weekend.* October 25, 2019;2.

12. Renton A. *Stiff Upper Lip: Secrets, Crimes and the Schooling of a Ruling Class.* Weidenfeld and Nicolson; 2017.

13. Beard R. *Sad Little Men: Private Schools and the Ruin of England.* Harvill Secker; 2021.

14. Turner D. *The Old Boys: The Decline and Rise of the Public School.* Yale University Press; 2015.

15. Spencer C. *A Very Private School: A Memoir.* William Collins; 2024.

16. Stonyhurst hit by abuse charges. *Catholic Herald* archive. April 30, 1999. Accessed February 28, 2025. https://archive.catholicherald.co.uk /article/30th-april-1999/2/stonyhurst-hit-by-abuse-charges

17. Monastier M, Brügger A. *Paix, Pelle et Pioche. Histoire du Service civil international de 1919 à 1965.* Service civil international; 1965.

18. Gillette A. *One Million Volunteers: The Story of Volunteer Youth Service.* Penguin Books; 1968.

Chapter 2. Medicine

1. Epstein MA, Achong BG, Barr YM. Virus particles in cultured lympho-blasts from Burkitt's lymphoma. Lancet. 1964;1:702–703.
2. Burkitt D. A sarcoma involving the jaws in African children. Br J Surg. 1958;46:218–223.
3. Henle G, Henle W, Diehl V. Relation of Burkitt's tumor-associated herpes-type virus to infectious mononucleosis. Proc Natl Acad Sci U S A. 1968;59:94–101.
4. Damania B, Kenney SC, Raab-Traub N. Epstein-Barr virus: biology and clinical disease. Cell. 2022;185:3652–3670.
5. Crawford DH, Rickinson A, Johannessen I. *Cancer Virus: The Story of Epstein-Barr Virus.* Oxford University Press; 2014.
6. Obituaries. Bert Geoffrey Achong. BMJ. 1997;314:150.
7. De Cock KM, Rees JR. Staphylococcal aortic valve endocarditis with aortic root to right atrial fistula. Postgrad Med J. 1978;54:413.
8. DeCock KM, Thorne MS. The treatment of pyoderma gangrenosum with sodium cromoglycate. Brit J Derm. 1980;102:231–233.
9. De Cock KM, Wakley EJ, Rees JR. Propranolol in thyroid storm with simultaneous Addisonian crisis. East Afr Med J. 1981;58:364–367.
10. Gottlieb MS, Schanker HM, Fan PT, et al. *Pneumocystis* pneumonia—Los Angeles. MMWR Morb Mortal Wkly Rep. 1981;30:250–252.
11. Marshall AJ, Baddeley H, Barritt DW, et al. Practolol peritonitis. A study of 16 cases and a survey of small bowel function in patients taking beta adrenergic blockers. Q J Med. 1977;46:135–149.

Chapter 3. Tropical Medicine

1. International Conference on Primary Health Care. Declaration of Alma-Ata. 1978. Accessed March 9, 2025. https://cdn.who.int/media /docs/default-source/documents/almaata-declaration-en.pdf?sfvrsn =7b3c2167_2
2. De Cock KM. Personal view. BMJ. 1983;287:1139.
3. Bahemuka M. Benign brain stem strokes of unknown cause in young people. East Afr Med J. 1982;59:133–144.
4. Bahemuka M. Cerebrovascular accidents in 207 Kenyans; general peculiarities and prognosis of stroke in an urban medical centre. East Afr Med J. 1985;62:315–322.
5. Bahemuka M. Malignant hypertension: a review of the neurological features in 34 consecutive patients. East Afr Med J. 1985;62: 560–565.

6. Poulter N, Khaw KT, Hopwood BE, Mugambi M, Peart WS, Sever PS. Salt and blood pressure in various populations. J Cardiovasc Pharmacol. 1984;6:S197-S203.

7. Poulter N, Khaw KT, Hopwood BE, et al. Blood pressure and associated factors in a rural Kenyan community. Hypertension. 1984; 6:810-813.

8. Poulter NR, Khaw K, Hopwood BE, Mugambi M, Peart WS, Sever PS. Determinants of blood pressure changes due to urbanization: a longitudinal study. J Hypertens Suppl. 1985;3:S375-S377.

9. Poulter NR, Khaw KT, Mugambi M, Peart WS, Rose G, Sever P. Blood pressure patterns in relation to age, weight and urinary electrolytes in three Kenyan communities. Trans R Soc Trop Med Hyg. 1985;79:389-392.

10. Poulter NR, Khaw KT, Mugambi M, Peart WS, Sever PS. Migration-induced changes in blood pressure: a controlled longitudinal study. Clin Exp Pharmacol Physiol. 1985;12:211-216.

11. Poulter NR, Khaw KT, Hopwood BE, et al. The Kenyan Luo migration study: observations on the initiation of a rise in blood pressure. BMJ. 1990;300:967-972.

12. Dzudie A, Rayner B, Ojji D, et al. Roadmap to achieve 25% hypertension control in Africa by 2025. Glob Heart. 2018;13:45-59.

13. Watkins DA, Johnson CO, Colquhoun SM, et al. Global, regional, and national burden of rheumatic heart disease, 1990-2015. N Engl J Med. 2017;377:713-722.

14. McLarty DG, Pollitt C, Swai AB. Diabetes in Africa. Diabet Med. 1990;7:670-684.

15. Calder JF, De Cock KM, Stass B. Diagnostic ultrasound in abdominal disease - first experience in Kenya. East Afr Med J. 1980;57:607-614.

16. De Cock KM, Calder JF. Ultrasonic diagnosis of abdominal disease in Kenya. Trans Roy Soc Trop Med Hyg. 1981;75:632-636.

17. De Cock KM, Gatei DF, Shah MV. Aspiration cytology in the diagnosis of liver cancer. East Afr Med J. 1981;58:636-640.

18. Mwaungulu GS, Wankya BM, Thomas SE, De Cock KM, Shah MV. Clinical value of fibreoptic endoscopy in the diagnosis of gastric malignancy at Kenyatta National Hospital. East Afr Med J. 1983; 60:328-331.

19. Thomas SE, Mwaungulu GS, Wankya BM, De Cock KM. Acute upper gastrointestinal haemorrhage at Kenyatta National Hospital, Kenya: a prospective endoscopic study. East Afr Med J. 1983;60:428-431.

20. Thomas SE, De Cock KM, Raja RS. Comparison of barium swallow and fibreoptic oesophagoscopy for diagnosis of oesophageal varices in Nairobi, Kenya. Trop Doct. 1984;14:76-77.

21. Raja RS, Talwar VK, De Cock KM. Percutaneous transhepatic cholangiography with a fine gauge (Chiba) needle - initial experience in Nairobi. East Afr Med J. 1982;59:11–19.
22. De Cock KM, Raja RS, Talwar VK. A review of cholestatic jaundice and its diagnosis. East Afr Med J. 1982;59:20–28.
23. De Cock KM, Bhatt KM, Bhatt SM, et al. Management of liver abscesses. Lancet. 1982;1:743.
24. De Cock KM, Gikonyo DK, Lucas SB, Were JBO. Metastatic tumour of right atrium mimicking constrictive pericarditis and tricuspid stenosis. BMJ. 1982; 285:1314.
25. De Cock KM, Kasili EG. Hairy cell leukemia (leukemic reticuloendotheliosis) at Kenyata National Hospital. East Afr Med J. 1983; 60:113–118.
26. De Cock KM, Kasili EG, Lucas SB, Radia K, Gichuyia NR, Wankya BM. Kaposi's sarcoma associated with hairy cell leukemia. Postgrad Med J. 1983;59:32–33.
27. De Cock KM, Govindarajan S, Bertrand J, et al. Infection with the delta agent in Nairobi, Kenya. Trans Roy Soc Trop Med Hyg. 1985;79:734.
28. El Sayed NM, Gomatos PJ, Beck-Sagué CM, et al. Epidemic transmission of human immunodeficiency virus in renal dialysis centers in Egypt. J Infect Dis. 2000;181:91–97.
29. De Cock KM, Armitage J, Markey AC, Draper CC. A possible case of RIII chloroquine-resistant malaria from East Africa. Lancet. 1983;1:773–774.
30. Center for Global Health (US), Office of the Director for Global Health. Centers for Disease Control and Prevention—Kenya: Annual Report 2018. Accessed March 9, 2025. https://archive.cdc.gov/www_cdc_gov /globalhealth/countries/kenya/reports/2018/index.html
31. Herman-Roloff A, Aman R, Samandari T, Kasera K, et al. Adapting longstanding public health collaborations between Government of Kenya and CDC Kenya in response to the COVID-19 pandemic, 2020–2021. Emerg Infect Dis. 2022;28:S159–S167.
32. De Cock KM. Hepatosplenic schistosomiasis: a clinical review. Gut. 1986;27:734–745.
33. De Cock KM, Rees PH, Klauss V, Kasili EG, Kager PA, Schattenkerk JK. Retinal hemorrhages in kala-azar. Am J Trop Med Hyg. 1982;31:927–930.
34. World Health Organization. Neglected tropical diseases. January 8, 2025. Accessed March 9, 2025. https://www.who.int/news-room /questions-and-answers/item/neglected-tropical-diseases
35. Molyneux DH, Asamoa-Bah A, Fenwick A, Savioli L, Hotez P. History of the neglected tropical disease movement. Trans R Soc Trop Med Hyg. 2021;115:169–175.

36. Lutumba P, Robays J, Miaka mia Bilenge C, et al. Trypanosomiasis control, Democratic Republic of Congo, 1993-2003. Emerg Infect Dis. 2005;11:1382-1388.

37. World Health Organization. Podoconiosis: endemic non-filarial elephantiasis. n.d. Accessed March 9, 2025. https://www.who.int /teams/control-of-neglected-tropical-diseases/lymphatic-filariasis /podoconiosis-endemic-non-filarial-elephantiasis

38. Rees P, Gatei DG, De Cock KM, Toswill J. Some preliminary observations of the investigation of splenomegaly in Kenya. East Afr Med J. 1982;59:658-664.

39. De Cock KM, Hodgen AN, Jupp RA, Slavin B, Arap Siongok TK, Rees PH. Chronic splenomegaly in Nairobi, Kenya: I Epidemiology, malarial antibody and immunoglobulin levels. Trans Roy Soc Trop Med Hyg. 1987;81:100-106.

40. De Cock KM, Hodgen AN, Jupp RA, et al. Immunoglobulin M and malarial antibody levels in hyper-reactive malarial splenomegaly. J Hyg Trop Med. 1986;89:119-121.

41. De Cock KM, Hodgen AN, Jupp RA, Slavin B, Arap Siongok TK, Rees PH. A comparison of immunoglobulin and malarial antibody levels in rural Kenyans. BMJ. 1984;289:1422-1423.

42. Bryceson A, Fakunle YM, Fleming AF, et al. Malaria and splenomegaly. Trans Roy Soc Trop Med Hyg. 1983;77:879.

43. De Cock KM, Hodgen AN, Lillywhite JE, Arap Siongok TK, Lucas SB, Rees PH. Hepatosplenic schistosomiasis in Nairobi, Kenya: an assessment of the enzyme-linked immunosorbent assay (ELISA). Trop Geogr Med. 1986;35:285-290.

44. De Cock KM, Hodgen AN, Channon J, Arap Siongok TK, Rees PH, Lucas SB. Enzyme-linked immunosorbent assay (ELISA) for the diagnosis of visceral leishmaniasis in Kenya. J Infect Dis. 1985;151:750-752.

45. De Cock KM, Awadh S, Raja RS, Wankya BM, Lucas, SB. Oesophageal varices in Nairobi, Kenya - a study of 68 cases. Am J Trop Med Hyg. 1982;31:579-588.

46. De Cock KM, Awadh S, Raja RS, et al. Portal hypertension in Nairobi, Kenya. Bull Soc Pathol Exot Filiales. 1983;76:567-570.

47. De Cock KM, Awadh S, Raja RS, et al. Chronic splenomegaly in Nairobi, Kenya: II Portal hypertension. Trans Roy Soc Trop Med Hyg. 1987;81:107-110.

48. De Cock KM, Lucas SB, Rees PH, Hodgen AN, Jupp RA, Slavin B. Obscure splenomegaly in the tropics that is not the tropical splenomegaly syndrome. BMJ. 1983;287:1347-1348.

49. De Cock KM. *Splenomegaly and Portal Hypertension in Nairobi, Kenya. A Study in Geographical Medicine*. MD thesis. University of Bristol; 1984.

Chapter 4. Hepatitis and HIV in the City of Angels

1. Centers for Disease Control and Prevention. Pneumocystis pneumonia—Los Angeles. MMWR Morb Mortal Wkly Rep. 1981;30:1–3.
2. Terrence Higgins Trust. Website homepage. Accessed March 14, 2025. https://www.tht.org.uk/
3. Starzl TE. *The Puzzle People: Memoirs of a Transplant Surgeon*. University of Pittsburgh Press; 1992.
4. Boyer TD. Obituary. Telfer B. Reynolds, M.D. (1921–2004). Hepatology 2004;40:512–513.
5. Fong T-L, Hoofnagle JH. Obituary. Allan G. Redeker, M.D. (1924–2021). Hepatology 2021;73:2621–2623.
6. McIntyre N. An obituary. Sheila. Professor Dame Sheila Sherlock (1918–2001). Hepatology 2002;35:507–509.
7. Kuo G, Choo QL, Alter HJ, et al. An assay for circulating antibodies to a major etiologic virus of human non-A, non-B hepatitis. Science. 1989;244:362–364.
8. Krugman S. The Willowbrook hepatitis studies revisited: ethical aspects. Rev Infect Dis. 1986;8:157–162.
9. Akriviadis EA, Redeker AG. Fulminant hepatitis A in intravenous drug users with chronic liver disease. Ann Intern Med. 1989;110:838–839.
10. Most H. Manhattan: "a tropic isle"? Am J Trop Med Hyg. 1968;17:333–354.
11. Centers for Disease Control and Prevention. Hepatitis A among drug abusers. MMWR Morb Mortal Wkly Rep. 1988;37;297–300,305.
12. Spitters C, Moran J, Kruse D, et al. Wound botulism among black tar heroin users - Washington, 2003. MMWR Morb Mortal Wkly Rep. 2003;52;885–886.
13. De Cock KM, Bradley DW, Sandford NG, Govindarajan S, Maynard J, Redeker AG. Epidemic non-A, non-B hepatitis in patients from Pakistan. Ann Int Med. 1987;106:227–230.
14. World Health Organization. Hepatitis. 2025. Accessed March 14, 2025. https://www.who.int/health-topics/hepatitis#tab=tab_1
15. Rizzetto M, Canese MG, Arico S, et al. Immunofluorescence detection of a new antigen-antibody system (delta/anti-delta) associated with hepatitis B virus in liver and in serum of HBsAg carriers. Gut. 1977;18:997–1003.
16. De Cock KM, Govindarajan S, Chin KP, Redeker AG. Delta hepatitis in the Los Angeles area: a study of 126 cases. Ann Int Med. 1986; 105:108–114.
17. De Cock KM, Govindarajan S, Redeker AG. HDV infection in the Los Angeles area. In: Rizzetto M, Gerin JL, Purcell RH, eds. *The Hepatitis Delta Virus and Its Infection*. Progress in Clinical and Biological Research. Alan R Liss; 1987: 234:167–179.

18. De Cock KM, Jones B, Govindarajan S, Redeker AG. Prevalence of hepatitis delta virus infection: a seroepidemiologic study in the Los Angeles County-University of Southern California Medical Center. West J Med. 1988;148:307–309.

19. Govindarajan S, De Cock KM, Redeker AG. Natural course of delta superinfection in chronic hepatitis B virus infected patients - histopathologic study with multiple liver biopsies. Hepatology. 1986;6:640–644.

20. Craig JR, Govindarajan S, De Cock KM. Delta viral hepatitis. Histopathology and course. Pathol Annu. 1986;21(pt. 2):1–21.

21. De Cock KM, Govindarajan S, Redeker AG. Fulminant delta hepatitis in chronic hepatitis B infection. JAMA. 1984;252:2746–2748.

22. Govindarajan S, Kanel GC, De Cock KM, Redeker AG, Falzarano JS. Delta agent superinfection: rapidly progressive liver disease in a hepatitis B carrier. Arch Path Lab Med. 1985;109:395–397.

23. Govindarajan S, De Cock KM, Peters RL. Morphology and immunohistochemistry of fulminant delta hepatitis with follow-up studies. Human Pathol. 1985;16:262–267.

24. De Cock KM. Govindarajan S, Redeker AG. Acute delta hepatitis without circulating HBsAg. Gut. 1985;26:212–214.

25. Govindarajan S, Smedile A, De Cock KM, Valinluck B, Redeker AG, Gerin JL. Study of reactivation of chronic hepatitis delta virus infection. J Hepatol. 1989;9:204–208.

26. Ponzetto A, Hoofnagle JH, Seeff LB. Antibody to the hepatitis B virus-associated delta-agent in immune serum globulins. Gastroenterology. 1984;87(6):1213–1216.

27. De Cock KM, Govindarajan S, Redeker AG. Non-percutaneous spread of delta infection. J Infect Dis. 1985;152:845.

28. Fong TL, De Cock KM, Govindarajan S, Ashcavai M, Yamada S, Redeker AG. Clustering of delta hepatitis in a family from Lebanon. J Infect Dis. 1986;154:912–913.

29. Beasley RP, Hwang LY, Lin CC, Chien CS. Hepatocellular carcinoma and hepatitis B virus. A prospective study of 22 707 men in Taiwan. Lancet. 1981;2:1129–1133.

30. World Health Organization. Hepatitis B. Accessed March 14, 2025. https://www.who.int/teams/health-product-policy-and-standards /norms-and-standards /vaccine-standardization/hep-b

31. Rees PH. HIV/AIDS: the first 25 years—a view from Nairobi. East Afr Med J. 2008;85:292–300.

32. Cooper DA, Gold J, Maclean P, Donovan B, et al. Acute AIDS retrovirus infection. Definition of a clinical illness associated with seroconversion. Lancet. 1985;1:537–540.

33. Buitrago B, Hadler SC, Popper H, et al. Epidemiologic aspects of Santa Marta hepatitis over a 40-year period. Hepatology. 1986;6:1292–1296.
34. Bensabath G, Hadler SC, Soares MC, et al. Hepatitis delta virus infection and Labrea hepatitis. Prevalence and role in fulminant hepatitis in the Amazon Basin. JAMA. 1987;258:479–483.
35. Hahn BH, Shaw GM, De Cock KM, Sharp PM. AIDS as a zoonosis: scientific and public health implications. Science. 2000;287:607–614.
36. De Cock KM, Niland JC, Lu HP, et al. Experience with human immunodeficiency virus infection in patients with hepatitis B virus and hepatitis delta virus infection in Los Angeles, 1977–1985. Am J Epidemiol. 1988,127:1250–1260.

Chapter 5. Chance and the Prepared Mind

1. Etheridge EW. *Sentinel for Health. A History of the Centers for Disease Control.* University of California Press; 1991.
2. Pendergrast M. *Inside the Outbreaks. The Elite Medical Detectives of the Epidemic Intelligence Service.* Houghton Mifflin Harcourt Publishing Company; 2010.
3. De Cock KM, Jaffe HW, Curran JW. *Dispatches from the AIDS Pandemic. A Public Health Story.* Oxford University Press; 2023.
4. Smith GCS, Pell JP. Parachute use to prevent death and major trauma related to gravitational challenge: systematic review of randomised controlled trials. BMJ 2003;327:1459–1461
5. Centers for Disease Control and Prevention. *Pneumocystis* pneumonia—Los Angeles. 1981. MMWR Morb Mortal Wkly Rep. 1996;45:729–733.
6. De Cock KM, Niland JC, Lu HP, et al. Experience with human immunodeficiency virus infection in patients with hepatitis B virus and hepatitis delta virus infections in Los Angeles, 1977–1985. Am J Epidemiol. 1988;127:1250–1260.
7. Report of an International Commission. Ebola haemorrhagic fever in Zaire, 1976. Bull World Health Organ. 1978;56:271–293.
8. Piot P. *No Time to Lose. A Life in Pursuit of Deadly Viruses.* W.W. Norton and Co; 2012.
9. McCormick JB, Fisher-Hoch S. *Level 4: Virus Hunters of the CDC.* Turner Publishing, Inc.; 1996.
10. Piot P, Quinn TC, Taelman H, et al. Acquired immunodeficiency syndrome in a heterosexual population in Zaire. Lancet 1984;2:65–69.
11. Nzilambi N, De Cock KM, Forthal DN, et al. The prevalence of infection with human immunodeficiency virus over a 10-year period in rural Zaire. N Engl J Med. 1988;318:276–279.

12. Henderson RH, Sundaresan T. Cluster sampling to assess immunization coverage: a review of experience with a simplified sampling method. Bull World Health Organ. 1982;60:253–260.
13. Greenberg AE, Nguyen-Dinh P, Mann JM, et al. The association between malaria, blood transfusions, and HIV seropositivity in a pediatric population in Kinshasa, Zaire. JAMA 1988;259:545–549.
14. Greenberg AE, Ntumbanzondo M, Ntula N, Mawa L, Howell J, Davachi F. Hospital-based surveillance of malaria-related paediatric morbidity and mortality in Kinshasa, Zaire. Bull World Health Organ. 1989;67:189–196.

Chapter 6. An Unknown Disease in Nigeria

1. Cain K, Postlewait H, Thomson A. *Emergency Sex (and Other Desperate Measures)*. Ebury Press; 2006.
2. Warah R. *Lords of Impunity. How the United Nations Failed the World and What Can Be Done to Transform It*. Lens&Pens Publishing; 2022.
3. Gregg MB. *Field Epidemiology*. 3rd ed. Oxford University Press; 2008.
4. Centers for Disease Control and Prevention. Yellow fever. Accessed March 15, 2025. https://www.cdc.gov/yellowfever/index.html
5. Monath TP. Yellow fever: an update. Lancet Infect Dis. 2001;1:11–20.
6. Centers for Disease Control and Prevention. Guinea worm. Updated March 14, 2024. Accessed March 15, 2025. https://www.cdc.gov/guinea-worm/about/?CDC_AAref_Val=https://www.cdc.gov/parasites/guinea worm/
7. Global Polio Eradication Initiative. Homepage. Accessed March 15, 2025. https://polioeradication.org/
8. Monath TP. Yellow fever: a medically neglected disease. Report on a seminar. Rev Infect Dis. 1987;9:165–75.
9. Mohammed I, Nasidi A, Chikwem JO, et al. HIV infection in Nigeria. AIDS, 1988;2:61–62.
10. De Cock KM, Monath TP, Nasidi A, et al. Epidemic yellow fever in eastern Nigeria, 1986. Lancet. 1988;1:630–632.
11. De Cock KM, Barrere B, Lafontaine M-F, et al. Mortality trends in Abidjan, (Cote d'Ivoire), 1983–1988. AIDS. 1991;4:393–398.
12. Monath TP, Nasidi A. Should yellow fever vaccine be included in the expanded program of immunization in Africa? A cost-effectiveness analysis for Nigeria. Am J Trop Med Hyg. 1993;48:274–299.
13. Nasidi A, Monath TP, DeCock K, et al. Urban yellow fever epidemic in western Nigeria, 1987. Trans R Soc Trop Med Hyg. 1989;83:401–406.
14. Lindsey NP, Horton J, Barrett ADT, et al. Yellow fever resurgence: an avoidable crisis? NPJ Vaccines. 2022;7(1):137.

15. De Cock KM, Jaffe HW, Curran JW. Reflections on 40 years of AIDS. Emerg Infect Dis. 2021;27:1553–1560.

Chapter 7. Outbreaks in Kenya

1. Gregg MB, ed. *Field Epidemiology*. Oxford University Press; 1996.
2. De Cock KM, Jaffe HW, Curran JW. *Dispatches from the AIDS Pandemic. A Public Health Story*. Oxford University Press; 2023.
3. Centers for Disease Control and Prevention. History of anthrax. https://www.cdc.gov/anthrax/basics/anthrax-history.html
4. Jernigan DB, Raghunathan PL, Bell BP, et al. Investigation of bioterrorism-related anthrax, United States, 2001: epidemiologic findings. Emerg Infect Dis. 2002;8:1019–1028.
5. Cole LA. *The Anthrax Letters. A Medical Detective Story*. Joseph Henry Press; 2003.
6. Theme Issue. Bioterrorism-related anthrax. October 2002. Accessed March 15, 2025. https://wwwnc.cdc.gov/eid/articles/issue/8/10/table-of-contents
7. Muturi M, Gachohi J, Mwatondo A, et al. Recurrent anthrax outbreaks in humans, livestock, and wildlife in the same locality, Kenya, 2014–2017. Am J Trop Med Hyg. 2018;99:833–839.
8. Vugia DJ, Kiehlbauch JA, Yeboue K, et al. Pathogens and predictors of fatal septicemia associated with human immunodeficiency virus infection in Ivory Coast, West Africa. J Infect Dis. 1993;168:564–570.
9. Polyak CS, Macy JT, De La Cruz MI, et al. Bioterrorism-related anthrax: International response by the Centers for Disease Control and Prevention. Emerg Infect Dis. 2002;8:1056–1059.
10. Peers FG, Linsell CA. Dietary aflatoxins and liver cancer—a population based study in Kenya. Br J Cancer. 1973;27:473–84.
11. De Cock KM. *Splenomegaly and Portal Hypertension in Nairobi, Kenya: A Study in Geographical Medicine*. MD dissertation, Bristol University; 1983.
12. Linsell CA. Cancer incidence in Kenya 1957–63. Br J Cancer. 1967; 21:465–473.
13. Ngindu A, Johnson BK, Kenya PR, et al. Outbreak of acute hepatitis caused by aflatoxin poisoning in Kenya. Lancet. 1982;1:1346–1348.
14. Rose G. *Rose's Strategy of Preventive Medicine*. Oxford University Press; 2008.
15. Lewis L, Onsongo M, Njapau H, et al. Aflatoxin contamination of commercial maize products during an outbreak of acute aflatoxicosis in Eastern and Central Kenya. Environ Health Perspect. 2005;113:1763–1767.
16. Azziz-Baumgartner E, Lindblade K, Gieseker K, et al. Case-control study of an acute aflatoxicosis outbreak—Kenya-2004. Environ Health Perspect. 2005;113:1779–1783.

17. Centers for Disease Control and Prevention. Outbreak of aflatoxin poisoning—eastern and central provinces, Kenya, January–July 2004. MMWR Morb Mortal Wkly Rep. 2004;53:790–793.

18. Probst C, Njapau H, Cotty PJ. Outbreak of an acute aflatoxicosis in Kenya in 2004: identification of the causal agent. Appl Environ Microbiol. 2007;73:2762–2764.

19. Strosnider H, Azziz-Baumgartner E, Banziger M, et al. Workgroup Report: public health strategies for reducing aflatoxin exposure in developing countries. Environ Health Perspect. 2006;114:1898–1903.

20. Daniel JH, Lewis LW, Redwood YA, et al. Comprehensive assessment of maize aflatoxin levels in Eastern Kenya, 2005–2007. Environ Health Perspect. 2011;119:1794–1799.

21. Yard EE, Daniel JH, Lewis LS, et al. Human aflatoxin exposure in Kenya, 2007: a cross-sectional study. Food Addit Contam Part A Chem Anal Control Expo Risk Assess. 2013;30:1322–1331.

22. Schleicher RL, McCoy LF, Powers CD, Sternberg MR, Pfeiffer CM. Serum concentrations of an aflatoxin-albumin adduct in the National Health and Nutrition Examination Survey (NHANES) 1999–2000. Clin Chim Acta. 2013;423:46–50.

23. Azziz-Baumgartner E. When your food glows blue. In: Dworkin MS, ed. *Cases in Field Epidemiology: A Global Perspective*. Jones & Bartlett Learning; 2011: Chapter 24.

Chapter 8. From Exotic Infection to Global Health Priority

1. Fukuyama F. *The End of History and the Last Man*. Free Press; 1992.

2. Report of an International Commission. Ebola haemorrhagic fever in Zaire, 1976. Bull World Health Organ. 1978;56:271–93.

3. World Health Organization. Ebola haemorrhagic fever in Sudan, 1976. Report of a WHO/International Study Team. Bull World Health Organ. 1978;56:247–270.

4. Centers for Disease Control and Prevention. History of Ebola disease outbreaks. https://www.cdc.gov/vhf/ebola/history/chronology.html

5. Swanepoel R, Leman PA, Burt FJ, et al. Experimental inoculation of plants and animals with Ebola virus. Emerg Infect Dis. 1996;2:321–5.

6. Spengler JR, Ervin ED, Towner JS, Rollin PE, Nichol ST. Perspectives on West Africa Ebola Virus Disease Outbreak, 2013–2016. Emerg Infect Dis. 2016 22:956–63.

7. Centers for Disease Control and Prevention. Ebola disease. April 23, 2024. Accessed March 18, 2025. https://www.cdc.gov/vhf/ebola/index .html

8. Lo TQ, Marston BJ, Dahl BA, De Cock KM. Ebola: anatomy of an epidemic. Annu Rev Med. 2017;68:359–370.

9. CDC Ebola Response Oral History Project. Joel Montgomery. *The Global Health Chronicles*. May 10, 2016. Accessed March 18, 2025. https://globalhealthchronicles.org/items/show/7804

10. Centers for Disease Control and Prevention. CDC Emergency Operations Center (EOC). https://www.cdc.gov/orr/eoc/eoc.htm

11. CDC Ebola Response Oral History Project. Tom Frieden. *The Global Health Chronicles*. January 6, 2016. Accessed March 18, 2025. https://www.globalhealthchronicles.org/items/show/8132

12. CDC Ebola Response Oral History Project. Inger K. Damon. *The Global Health Chronicles*. May 17, 2016. Accessed March 18, 2025. https://globalhealthchronicles.org/items/show/7849

13. CDC Ebola Response Oral History Project. Pierre Rollin. *The Global Health Chronicles*. May 23, 2016, and June 27, 2016. Accessed March 18, 2025. https://globalhealthchronicles.org/items/show/7858

14. CDC Ebola Response Oral History Project. Deborah R. Malac. *The Global Health Chronicles*. February 15, 2017. Accessed March 18, 2025. https://globalhealthchronicles.org/items/show/7902

15. Kanagasabai U, Ballah JB. A historical review of Liberia's public health evolution-past, present & future. Hygiene 2022;2:251-266.

16. van den Ende MC, Brotman B, Prince AM. An open air holding system for chimpanzees in medical experiments. Dev Biol Stand. 1980; 45:95-98.

17. CDC Ebola Response Oral History Project. Satish K. Pillai. *The Global Health Chronicles*. September 19, 2016. Accessed March 18, 2025. https://globalhealthchronicles.org/items/show/7913

18. CDC Ebola Response Oral History Project. Tai-Ho Chen. *The Global Health Chronicles*. August 24, 2018. Accessed March 18, 2025. https://globalhealthchronicles.org/items/show/7846

19. CDC Ebola Response Oral History Project. Edward Rouse. *The Global Health Chronicles*. September 30, 2016. Accessed March 18, 2025. https://globalhealthchronicles.org/items/show/7745

20. Shuaib F, Gunnala R, Musa EO, et al. Ebola virus disease outbreak - Nigeria, July–September 2014. MMWR Morb Mortal Wkly Rep. 2014;63:867-872.

21. Cohen J. Ebola survivor II, Nancy Writebol: 'We just don't even have a clue what happened.' ScienceInsider. October 2, 2014. Accessed March 18, 2025. https://www.science.org/content/article/ebola-survivor-ii-nancy-writebol-we-just-dont-even-have-clue-what-happened#:~:text=I%20never%20crossed%20those%20lines,what%20would%20I%20do%20differently.

22. Forrester JD, Hunter JC, Pillai SK, et al. Cluster of Ebola cases among Liberian and U.S. health care workers in an Ebola treatment unit and

adjacent hospital—Liberia, 2014. MMWR Morb Mortal Wkly Rep. 2014;63:925–929.

23. Ebola patients discharged from Emory University Hospital. https:// video.samaritanspurse.org/ken-isaacs-cspan/

24. Frayer L. Excalibur, the dog exposed to Ebola, is euthanized. Goats and Soda, National Public Radio. October 8, 2014. Accessed March 18, 2025. https://www.npr.org/sections/goatsandsoda/2014/10/08 /354568673/excalibur-the-dog-exposed-to-ebola-awaits-his-fate #:~:text=Excalibur%2C%20a%20sandy-colored%20mixed-breed%20 mutt%2C%20belonged%20to%20a,for%20treatment%20but%20 died%20in%20August%20and%20September

25. Qiu X, Wong G, Audet J, et al. Reversion of advanced Ebola virus disease in nonhuman primates with ZMapp. Nature. 2014; 514:47–53

26. Matanock E, Arwady A, Ayscue P, et al. Ebola virus disease cases among health care workers not working in Ebola treatment Units—Liberia, June–August, 2014. MMWR Morb Mortal Wkly Rep. 2014;63:1077–1081.

27. Pillai SK, Nyenswah T, Rouse E, et al. Developing an incident management system to support Ebola response—Liberia, July–August 2014. MMWR Morb Mortal Wkly Rep. 2014;63:930–933.

28. Forrester JD, Pillai SK, Beer KD, et al. Assessment of Ebola virus disease, health care infrastructure, and preparedness—four counties, southeastern Liberia, August 2014. MMWR Morb Mortal Wkly Rep. 2014;63:891–893.

29. Médecins Sans Frontières. Pushed to the limit and beyond. A year into the largest ever Ebola outbreak. 2015. Accessed March 18, 2025. http://www.msf.org/sites/msf.org/files/msf1yearebolareport_en _230315.pdf

30. Arwady MA, Bawo L, Hunter J, et al. Evolution of Ebola virus disease from exotic infection to global health priority, Liberia, mid-2014. Emerg Infect Dis. 2015;21:578–584.

31. Agence France-Presse. Ebola quarantine in Liberia's capital sparks violence in slum. The Guardian. August 21, 2014. Accessed March 18, 2025. https://www.theguardian.com/society/2014/aug/21/ebola -quarantine-violence-west-point-monrovia-liberia

32. Hudson D. A major increase in our response to the Ebola outbreak. September 16, 2014. Accessed March 18, 2025. https://obamawhitehouse .archives.gov/blog/2014/09/16/major-increase-our-response-ebola -outbreak

33. Sifferlin A, Worland J. Here's who's blaming who for Ebola. Time. October 16, 2014. Accessed March 18, 2025. https://time.com/3513274 /ebola-cdc-obama-blame/

34. Fauci AS. *On Call: A Doctor's Journey in Public Service.* Viking; 2024.
35. McNeil DG Jr. Ebola response in Liberia is hampered by infighting. *New York Times.* November 19, 2014. Accessed March 18, 2025. https://www.nytimes.com/subscription/all-access?campaignId=8QWWY
36. Frieden TR, Damon IK. Ebola in West Africa—CDC's Role in epidemic detection, control, and prevention. Emerg Infect Dis. 2015 21:1897–1905.
37. CDC Ebola Response Oral History Project. Tolbert G. Nyenswah. *The Global Health Chronicles.* March 10, 2017. Accessed March 18, 2025. https://globalhealthchronicles.org/items/show/7941
38. Nyenswah T. Collapse and Resiliency: *The Inside Story of Liberia's Unprecedented Ebola Response.* Johns Hopkins University Press, 2023.
39. CDC Ebola Response Oral History Project. Alex Gasasira. *The Global Health Chronicles.* March 8, 2017. Accessed March 18, 2025. https://globalhealthchronicles.org/items/show/7826
40. United Nations. UN Mission for Ebola Emergency Response (UNMEER). Accessed March 18, 2025. https://ebolaresponse.un.org/un-mission-ebola-emergency-response-unmeer
41. Schafer IJ, Knudsen E, McNamara LA, Agnihotri S, Rollin PE, Islam A. The Epi Info Viral Hemorrhagic Fever (VHF) application: A resource for outbreak data management and contact tracing in the 2014–2016 West Africa Ebola epidemic. J Infect Dis. 2016;214(suppl 3):S122–S136.
42. Rosling H. *Factfulness: Ten Reasons We're Wrong About the World—and Why Things Are Better Than You Think.* Flatiron Books, 2018.
43. Berglof AM. At home: statistician Hans Rosling. *Financial Times.* April 6, 2013. Accessed March 18, 2025. https://www.ft.com/content/31eb93be-a80e-11e2-8e5d-00144feabdc0
44. Meltzer MI, Atkins CY, Santibanez S, et al. Estimating the future number of cases in the Ebola epidemic—Liberia and Sierra Leone, 2014–2015. MMWR Suppl. 2014;63:1–14.
45. CDC Ebola Response Oral History Project. Martin I. Meltzer. *The Global Health Chronicles.* February 23, 2016. Accessed March 18, 2025. https://globalhealthchronicles.org/items/show/7790
46. *PBS Newshour.* What's the worst-case scenario if Ebola can't be slowed? September 22, 2014. Accessed March 18, 2025. https://www.pbs.org/newshour/show/ebola-cdc
47. Nyenswah T, Fahnbulleh M, Massaquoi M, et al. Ebola epidemic—Liberia, March–October 2014 [published correction appears in MMWR Morb Mortal Wkly Rep 2014;63:1094]. MMWR Morb Mortal Wkly Rep 2014;63:1082–1086.
48. CDC Ebola Response Oral History Project. Kimberly A. Lindblade. *The Global Health Chronicles.* June 8, 2016. Accessed March 18, 2025. https://globalhealthchronicles.org/items/show/7918

49. Kateh F, Nagbe T, Kieta A, et al. Rapid response to Ebola outbreaks in remote areas—Liberia, August–December 2014, MMWR Morb Mortal Wkly Rep. 2015; 64:188–192.

50. Lindblade KA, Kateh F, Nagbe T, et al. Decreased Ebola transmission after rapid response to outbreaks in remote areas, Liberia, 2014. Emerg Infect Dis 2015;21:1800–1807.

51. Baker A. Liberia burns its bodies as Ebola fears run rampant. *Time*. October 7, 2014. Accessed March 18, 2025. https://time.com/3478238 /ebola-liberia-burials-cremation-burned/

52. CDC Ebola Response Oral History Project. Mosoka P. Fallah. *The Global Health Chronicles*. March 8, 2017. Accessed March 18, 2025. https://www.globalhealthchronicles.org/items/show/7908

53. CDC Ebola Response Oral History Project. Barbara Marston. *The Global Health Chronicles*. August 1, 2018. Accessed March 18, 2025. https://globalhealthchronicles.org/items/show/8127

54. CDC Ebola Response Oral History Project. John Hoover. *The Global Health Chronicles*. March 23, 2017. Accessed March 18, 2025. https:// globalhealthchronicles.org/items/show/7915

55. Lindblade KA, Nyenswah T, Keita S, et al. Secondary infections with Ebola virus in rural communities, Liberia and Guinea, 2014–2015. Emerg Infect Dis 2016;22:1653–1655.

56. Nyenswah T, Fallah M, Sieh S, et al. Controlling the last known cluster of Ebola virus disease - Liberia, January–February 2015 [published corrections appear in MMWR Morb Mortal Wkly Rep. 2015;64:806 and 2015;64:1180]. MMWR Morb Mortal Wkly Rep. 2015;64:500–504.

57. Vedantam S. A gang killed a guy with Ebola. Will they agree to be quarantined? December 15, 2016. Accessed March 18, 2025. https:// www.npr.org/sections/goatsandsoda/2016/12/15/505658504/a-gang -killed-a-guy-with-ebola-will-they-agree-to-be-quarantined

58. CDC Ebola Response Oral History Project. Desmond Williams. *The Global Health Chronicles*. April 1, 2016, and June 9, 2016. Accessed March 18, 2025. https://globalhealthchronicles.org/items/show /7889

59. Rodriguez LL, De Roo A, Guimard Y, et al. Persistence and genetic stability of Ebola virus during the outbreak in Kikwit, Democratic Republic of the Congo, 1995. J Infect Dis. 1999;179(Suppl 1):S170–S176.

60. Christie A, Davies-Wayne GJ, Cordier-Lasalle T, et al. Possible sexual transmission of Ebola virus more than three months after recovery, Liberia 2015. MMWR Morb Mortal Wkly Rep. 2015;64;479–481

61. Mate S, Kugelman J, Nyenswah T, et al. Molecular evidence for sexual transmission of Ebola virus. New Engl J Med. 2015;373:2448–2454.

62. Den Boon S, Marston BJ, Nyenswah TG, et al. Ebola virus infection associated with transmission from survivors. Emerg Infect Dis. 2019; 25:249–255.

63. Deen GF, Broutet N, Xu W, et al. Ebola RNA persistence in semen of Ebola virus disease survivors - final report. N Engl J Med. 2017; 377:1428–1437.

64. Purpura LJ, Rogers E, Baller A. Ebola virus RNA in semen from an HIV-positive survivor of Ebola. Emerg Infect Dis. 2017;23:714–715.

65. Keita AK, Koundouno FR, Faye M, et al. Resurgence of Ebola virus in 2021 in Guinea suggests a new paradigm for outbreaks. Nature. 2021; 597:539–543.

66. PREVAIL III Study Group; Sneller MC, Reilly C, Badio M, et al. A longitudinal study of Ebola sequelae in Liberia. N Engl J Med. 2019; 380:924–934.

67. Varkey JB, Shantha JG, Crozier I, et al. Persistence of Ebola virus in ocular fluid during convalescence. N Engl J Med. 2015;372:2423–2427.

68. Jacobs M, Rodger A, Bell DJ, et al. Late Ebola relapse causing meningo-encephalitis: a case report. Lancet. 2016; 388:498–503.

69. CDC Ebola Response Oral History Project. Dr. Kevin M. De Cock, Dr. H. Clifford Lane, Dr. Frank J. Mahoney, and Dr. Oliver W. Morgan. *The Global Health Chronicles.* July 14, 2016. Accessed March 18, 2025. https://globalhealthchronicles.org/items/show/7946

70. Fallah MP, Lane HC, Higgs ES, et al. Clinical research as a critical component of epidemic response: the case of PREVAIL in Liberia. Lancet Glob Health. 2023;11:e321–e323.

71. Henao-Restrepo AM, Camacho A, Longini IM, et al. Efficacy and effectiveness of an rVSV-vectored vaccine in preventing Ebola virus disease: final results from the Guinea ring vaccination, open-label, cluster-randomised trial (Ebola Ça Suffit!) [published correction appears in Lancet. 2017;389:504]. Lancet. 2017;389:505–518.

72. van Griensven J, Edwards T, de Lamballerie X, et al. Evaluation of convalescent plasma for Ebola virus disease in Guinea. N Engl J Med. 2016;374:33–42.

73. Kerber R, Lorenz E, Duraffour S, et al. Laboratory findings, compassionate use of favipiravir, and outcome in patients with Ebola virus disease, Guinea, 2015 - a retrospective observational study. J Infect Dis. 2019;220:195–202.

74. World Health Organization. Situation Report. Ebola virus disease. 10 June, 2016. Accessed March 18, 2025. https://apps.who.int/iris/bitstream/handle/10665/208883/ebolasitrep_10Jun2016_eng.pdf;jsessionid=EBF CAB99AB8CB3D77CB236B397E376BD?sequence=1

75. von Drehle D, Baker A. Person of the Year: The Ebola Fighters. *Time*. December 10, 2014. Accessed March 18, 2025. https://time.com/time -person-of-the-year-ebola-fighters/

76. Moon S, Sridhar D, Pate MA, et al. Will Ebola change the game? Ten essential reforms before the next pandemic. The report of the Harvard-LSHTM Independent Panel on the Global Response to Ebola. Lancet. 2015;386:2204–2221.

77. Committee on Microbial Threats to Health, Institute of Medicine. Emerging Infections: Microbial Threats to Health in the United States. National Academies Press; 1992.

78. Garrett L. *The Coming Plague. Newly Emerging Diseases in a World Out of Balance*. Farrar, Straus and Giroux; 1994.

79. Centers for Disease Control and Prevention. Global Health Security. December 12, 2024. Accessed March 18, 2025. https://www.cdc.gov /globalhealth/security/what-is-ghsa.htm

80. Marston BJ, Dokubo EK, van Steelandt A, et al. Response impact on public health programs, West Africa, 2014–2017. Emerg Infect Dis. 2017;23:S25–S32.

81. Glynn JR, Bower H, Johnson S, et al. Asymptomatic infection and unrecognised Ebola virus disease in Ebola-affected households in Sierra Leone: a cross-sectional study using a new non-invasive assay for antibodies to Ebola virus. Lancet Infect Dis. 2017;17:645–653.

82. Bloland P, Simone P, Burkholder B, Slutsker L, De Cock KM. The role of public health institutions in global health system strengthening efforts: the US CDC's perspective. PLoS Med. 2012;9:e1001199.

83. Green A. Remembering health workers who died from Ebola in 2014. Lancet. 2014;384:2201–2206.

84. David J. Sencer CDC Museum. Monrovia Medical Unit. Accessed March 18, 2025. https://cdcmuseum.org/exhibits/show/ebola/public -health/isolation-treatment/mmu#:~:text=The%20United%20 States%20Government%20opened%20the%20Monrovia%20 Medical,was%20staffed%20by%20U.S.%20Public%20Health%20 Service%20clinicians.

85. CDC Ebola Response Oral History Project. Patricia M. Simone. The *Global Health Chronicles*. July 14, 2017. Accessed March 18, 2025. https://globalhealthchronicles.org/items/show/7886

86. CDC Ebola Response Oral History Project. Kevin M. De Cock. *The Global Health Chronicles*. June 8, 2016. Accessed March 18, 2025. https://globalhealthchronicles.org/items/show/7899

87. CDC Ebola Response Oral History Project. Ebola. *The Global Health Chronicles*. Accessed March 18, 2025. https://globalhealthchronicles .org/ebola

Chapter 9. Ebola in the Democratic Republic of the Congo

1. Centers for Disease Control and Prevention. Global Health Security Agenda. Accessed April 7, 2025. https://www.hhs.gov/about/agencies /oga/global-health-security/agenda/index.html.

2. Report of an International Commission. Ebola haemorrhagic fever in Zaire, 1976. Bull World Health Organ. 1978;56:271–293.

3. Centers for Disease Control and Prevention. History of Ebola disease outbreaks. https://www.cdc.gov/vhf/ebola/history /chronology.html

4. World Health Organization. Cluster of presumptive Ebola cases in North Kivu in the Democratic Republic of the Congo. August 2018. Accessed March 21, 2025. https://www.who.int/news-room/detail/01 -08-2018-cluster-of-presumptive-ebola-cases-in-north-kivu-in-the -democratic-republic-of-the-congo

5. World Health Organization. Ebola outbreak in the Democratic Republic of the Congo declared a Public Health Emergency of International Concern. July 2019. Accessed March 21, 2025. https:// www.who.int/news/item/17-07-2019-ebola-outbreak-in-the-democratic -republic-of-the-congo-declared-a-public-health-emergency-of-inter national-concern

6. Naipaul VS. *A Bend in the River.* Alfred Knopf; 1979.

7. Stearns J. *Dancing in the Glory of Monsters: The Collapse of the Congo and the Great War of Africa.* Public Affairs; 2012.

8. Wrong M. *Do Not Disturb: The Story of a Political Murder and an African Regime Gone Bad.* Harper Collins; 2021.

9. Maxmen A. "The world has never seen anything like this": WHO chief on battling Ebola in a war zone. Nature. May 2, 2019. Accessed March 21, 2025. https://www.nature.com/articles/d41586-019-01432-y

10. Global Ebola Response. UN Mission for Ebola Emergency Response (UNMEER). Accessed March 21, 2025. https://ebolaresponse.un.org /un-mission-ebola-emergency-response-unmeer

11. World Health Organization. Ebola: Équateur, Democratic Republic of the Congo, May–July 2018. Accessed March 21, 2025. https://www.who .int/emergencies/situations/Ebola-2018-drc

12. United Nations Secretary General. Mr. David Gressly of the United States of America - United Nations Emergency Ebola Response Coordinator (EERC). June 2019. Accessed March 21, 2025. https:// www.un.org/sg/en/content/sg/personnel-appointments/2019-06-27 /mr-david-gressly-of-the-united-states-of-america-united-nations -emergency-ebola-response-coordinator-%28eerc%29

13. Ministère de la Santé. Strategic Response Plan for the Ebola virus disease outbreak in the provinces of North Kivu and Ituri, Democratic

Republic of the Congo, July–December 2019. https://www.who.int
/docs/default-source/documents/drc-srp4-9august2019.pdf

14. Burke J, Giuffrida A. Italian ambassador to DR Congo dies in attack on
UN convoy. February 22, 2021. Accessed March 21, 2025. https://www
.theguardian.com/world/2021/feb/22/italian-ambassador-to-dr
-congo-dies-in-attack-un-convoy-luca-attanasio

15. Park S-J, Brown H, Wema KM, et al. 'Ebola is a business': an analysis of
the atmosphere of mistrust in the tenth Ebola epidemic in the DRC.
Crit Public Health. 2023;33:297-307.

16. Adebamowo C, Bah-Sow O, Binka F, et al. Randomised controlled trials
for Ebola: practical and ethical issues. Lancet. 2014;384:1423-1424.

17. van Griensven J, Edwards T, de Lamballerie X, et al. Evaluation of
convalescent plasma for Ebola virus disease in Guinea. N Engl J Med.
2016;374:33-42.

18. PREVAIL II Writing Group; Multi-National PREVAIL II Study Team;
Davey RT Jr, Dodd L, Proschan MA, Neaton J. A randomized, controlled trial of ZMapp for Ebola virus infection. N Engl J Med.
2016;375:1448-1456.

19. Mulangu S, Dodd LE, Davey RT Jr, et al. A randomized, controlled trial
of Ebola virus disease therapeutics. N Engl J Med. 2019;381:2293-2303.

20. Di Paola N, Sanchez-Lockhart M, Zeng X, et al. Viral genomics in
Ebola virus research. Nat Rev Microbiol. 2020;18:365-378.

21. Henao-Restrepo AM, Camacho A, Longini IM, et al. Efficacy and
effectiveness of an rVSV-vectored vaccine in preventing Ebola virus
disease: Final results from the Guinea ring vaccination, open-label,
cluster-randomised trial (Ebola Ça Suffit!) [published correction
appears in Lancet. 2017;389:504]. Lancet. 2017;389:505-518.

22. Ishola D, Manno D, Afolabi MO, et al. Safety and long-term immuno-
genicity of the two-dose heterologous Ad26.ZEBOV and MVA-BN-Filo
Ebola vaccine regimen in adults in Sierra Leone: A combined open-
label, non-randomised stage 1, and a randomised, double-blind,
controlled stage 2 trial. Lancet Infect Dis. 2022;22:97-109.

23. Jerving S, Ravelo JL. Suspected Ebola in Tanzania highlights importance of transparency. September 24, 2019. Accessed March 21, 2025.
https://www.devex.com/news/suspected-ebola-in-tanzania
-highlights-importance-of-transparency-95674

24. Branswell H. WHO signals alarm over possible unreported Ebola cases
in Tanzania. September 21, 2019. Accessed March 21, 2025. https://
www.statnews.com/2019/09/21/who-signals-alarm-over-possible
-unreported-ebola-cases-in-tanzania/

25. Branswell H. U.S. and U.K. alert travelers to Tanzania about possible
unreported Ebola cases. September 27, 2019. Accessed March 21, 2025.

https://www.statnews.com/2019/09/27/ebola-tanzania-travelers
-alerted-to-possible-unreported-cases/

26. World Health Organization. Tanzanian authorities inform WHO they
have no cases of Ebola. September 18, 2019. Accessed March 21, 2025.
https://www.afro.who.int/news/tanzanian-authorities-inform-who
-they-have-no-cases-ebola

27. Dahir AL, John Magufuli, Tanzania leader who played down Covid,
dies at 61. *New York Times*. March 17, 2021. Updated March 19, 2021.
https://www.nytimes.com/2021/03/17/world/africa/tanzania-president
-magufuli-dead.html

28. Rollin PE. Ebola in eastern DRC. Lancet Infect Dis.
2019;19:1049–1050.

29. Daniel Levine-Spound. Backlash in Beni: Understanding anger against
the UN Peacekeeping Mission in the DRC. December 18, 2021. Center
for Civilians in Conflict. December 18, 2019. Accessed March 21, 2025.
https://civiliansinconflict.org/blog/backlash-in-beni/#:~:text
=On%20November%2025%2C%202019%2C%20angry%20protest-
ers%20in%20the,Stabilization%20Mission%20in%20the%20
DRC%2C%20known%20as%20MONUSCO

30. UN News. Armed groups kill Ebola health workers in eastern DR
Congo. November 28, 2019. Accessed March 21, 2025. https://news.un
.org/en/story/2019/11/1052421

31. Associated Press. Ebola response workers are killed in Congo. *New
York Times*. November 29, 2019. Accessed March 21, 2025. https://www
.nytimes.com/2019/11/28/world/africa/ebola-congo.html

32. World Health Organization. 10th Ebola outbreak in the Democratic
Republic of the Congo declared over; vigilance against flare-ups and
support for survivors must continue. June 25, 2020. Accessed March 21,
2025. https://www.who.int/news/item/25-06-2020-10th-ebola
-outbreak-in-the-democratic-republic-of-the-congo-declared-over
-vigilance-against-flare-ups-and-support-for-survivors-must-continue

33. Cheap Asian motorcycles are transforming African cities. *The Economist*. August 15, 2024; 36. Accessed March 21, 2025. https://www
.economist.com/middle-east-and-africa/2024/08/15/cheap-asian
-motorcycles-are-transforming-african-cities

Chapter 10. The Pandemic

1. World Health Organization. Archived: WHO Timeline - COVID-19.
April 27, 2020. Accessed March 22, 2025. https://www.who.int/news
/item/27-04-2020-who-timeline---covid-19

2. Wu JT, Leung K, Leung GM. Nowcasting and forecasting the potential
domestic and international spread of the 2019-nCoV outbreak

originating in Wuhan, China: a modelling study. Lancet. 2020;395: 689–697.

3. Gostin LO, Gronvall GK. The origins of Covid-19 - why it matters (and why it doesn't). N Engl J Med. 2023;388:2305–2308.

4. Centers for Disease Control and Prevention. SARS basics fact sheet. Last reviewed December 6, 2017. Accessed March 22, 2025. https:// www.cdc.gov/sars/about/fs-sars.html

5. World Health Organization. Listings of WHO's response to COVID-19. June 29, 2020. Accessed March 22, 2025. https://www.who.int/news /item/29-06-2020-covidtimeline

6. BBC. Welcome to Fever: The hunt for COVID's origin. May 23, 2023. Accessed March 22, 2025. https://www.bbc.co.uk/sounds/brand /m001mdfw

7. Chan A, Ridley M. *Viral: The Search for the Origin of COVID-19*. Harper; 2021.

8. Quammen D. The ongoing mystery of COVID's origin. *New York Times Magazine*. July 25, 2023; revised August 18, 2023. Accessed March 22, 2025. https://www.nytimes.com/2023/07/25/magazine/covid-start .html?searchResultPosition=2

9. Birx D. *Silent Invasion: The Untold Story of the Trump Administration, Covid-19, and Preventing the Next Pandemic Before It's Too Late*. Harper; 2022.

10. Fauci AS. *On Call: A Doctor's Journey in Public Service*. Viking, 2024.

11. Gilbert S, Green C. Vaxxers: *The Inside Story of the Oxford AstraZeneca Vaccine and the Race Against the Virus*. Hodden and Stroughton; 2021.

12. Calvert J, Arbuthnott G. *Failures of State: The Inside Story of Britain's Battle With Coronavirus*. Mudlark; 2021.

13. World Health Organization. Statement on the first meeting of the International Health Regulations (2005) Emergency Committee regarding the outbreak of novel coronavirus (2019-CoV). January 23, 2020. Accessed March 22, 2025. https://www.who.int/news/item/23 -01-2020-statement-on-the-meeting-of-the-international-health -regulations-(2005)-emergency-committee-regarding-the-outbreak-of -novel-coronavirus-(2019-ncov)

14. World Health Organization. WHO Director-General's statement on the advice of the IHR Emergency Committee on Novel Coronavirus. January 23, 2020. Accessed March 22, 2025. https://www.who.int /director-general/speeches/detail/who-director-general-s-statement -on-the-advice-of-the-ihr-emergency-committee-on-novel-coronavirus

15. World Health Organization. Coronavirus disease (COVID-19): herd immunity, lockdowns and COVID-19. December 31, 2020. Accessed

March 22, 2025. https://www.who.int/news-room/questions-and
-answers/item/herd-immunity-lockdowns-and-covid-19

16. Reuters Staff. Wuhan lockdown 'unprecedented', shows commitment
to contain virus: WHO representative in China. January 23, 2020.
Accessed March 22, 2025. https://www.reuters.com/article/us-china
-health-who-idUSKBN1ZM1G9

17. Reuters Staff. China building 1,000-bed hospital over the weekend to
treat coronavirus. January 24, 2020. Accessed March 22, 2025. https://
www.reuters.com/article/us-china-health-hospital-idUSKBN1ZN07U

18. Jones JM, Saad L. Americans sour on IRS, rate CDC and FBI most
positively. May 23, 2013. Accessed March 22, 2025. https://news.gallup
.com/poll/162764/americans-views-irs-sharply-negative-2009.aspx

19. Jones JM. Government agency ratings: CIA, FBI up; Federal Reserve
down. October 5, 2022. Accessed March 22, 2025. https://news.gallup
.com/poll/402464/government-agency-ratings-cia-fbi-federal-reserve
-down.aspx

20. Centers for Disease Control and Prevention. First travel-related case of
2019 novel coronavirus detected in United States. January 21, 2020.
Accessed March 22, 2025. https://www.cdc.gov/media/releases/2020
/p0121-novel-coronavirus-travel-case.html

21. Holshue ML, DeBolt C, Lindquist S, et al. First case of 2019 novel
coronavirus in the United States. N Engl J Med. 2020;382:929–936.

22. Vetter P, Vu DL, L'Huillier, SG, Schibler M, Kaiser L, Jacquerioz F.
Clinical features of covid-19. BMJ. 2020;369:m1470. Accessed March 22,
2025. https://www.bmj.com/content/bmj/369/bmj.m1470.full.pdf

23. Cohen J. The United States badly bungled coronavirus testing—but
things may soon improve. Science. February 28, 2020. Accessed
March 22, 2025. https://www.science.org/content/article/united
-states-badly-bungled-coronavirus-testing-things-may-soon-improve

24. US Senate Committee on Homeland Security and Governmental Affairs.
Historically unprepared. Examination of the Federal Government's
pandemic preparedness and initial COVID-19 response. Accessed
March 22, 2025. https://www.hsgac.senate.gov/wpcontent/uploads/imo
/media/doc/221208_HSGACMajorityReport_Covid-19.pdf

25. Johansson MA, Quandelacy TM, Kada S, et al. SARS-CoV-2 transmission from people without COVID-19 symptoms. JAMA Netw Open.
2021;4:e2035057.

26. Foege WH. The Fears of the Rich, the Needs of the Poor: My Years at
the CDC. Johns Hopkins University Press; 2018.

27. Frieden TR, Koplan JP. Stronger national public health institutes for
global health. Lancet. 2010;376:1721–1722.

28. Frieden T. What's a national public health institute to do? Health Affairs. December 7, 2022. Accessed March 22, 2025. https://www.healthaffairs .org/content/forefront/s-national-public-health-institute-do

29. Centers for Disease Control and Prevention. Crisis & Emergency Risk Communication (CERC). Accessed March 22, 2025. https://emergency .cdc.gov/cerc/index.asp

30. HHS. Public Health Emergencies and Major Disaster Declarations. Public Health Emergency Determination. Accessed July 7, 2025. https://hhs.com/assets/docs/Disaster%20Primer.pdf

31. Mandavilli A. A C.D.C. official who early on warned that the coronavirus would upend American lives resigns. May 7, 2021. Accessed March 22, 2025. https://www.nytimes.com/2021/05/07/world/messonier -virus-cdc-resign.html

32. The White House. Vice President Pence announces Ambassador Debbie Birx to serve as the White House Coronavirus Response Coordinator. February 27, 2020. Accessed March 22, 2025. https:// trumpwhitehouse.archives.gov/briefings-statements/vice-president -pence-announces-ambassador-debbie-birx-serve-white-house -coronavirus-response-coordinator/

33. HHS Secretary Azar to name Robert R. Redfield, M.D., Director of the Centers for Disease Control and Prevention. March 21, 2018. Accessed March 22, 2025. https://www.einpresswire.com/article/438090258 /hhs-secretary-azar-to-name-robert-r-redfield-m-d-director-of-the -centers-for-disease-control-and-prevention

34. Piller C. How CDC foundered: the agency's missteps were multiplied by political interference. Science. 2020;370:396. Accessed March 22, 2025 https://www.science.org/doi/full/10.1126/science.370.6515.396 ?adobe_mc=MCMID%3D2817298552916626681147207380464842571 0%7CMCORGID%3D242B6472541199F70A4C98A6%2540AdobeOr g%7CTS%3D1689315506

35. Gostin LO, Koh HH, Williams M, et al. US withdrawal from WHO is unlawful and threatens global and US health and security. Lancet. 2020;396:293–295.

36. Murphy B, Stein L. 'It is a slaughter': public health champion asks CDC director to expose White House, orchestrate his own firing. USA Today. October 6, 2020. Accessed March 22, 2025. https://www.usatoday.com /story/news/investigations/2020/10/06/expert-cdcs-redfield-should -expose-trump-covid-failures-leave-post/5899724002/

37. Foege B. Letter from Bill Foege, past CDC director, to Robert Redfield, current CDC director. Epimonitor. Accessed March 22, 2025. https:// www.epimonitor.net/Foege-Letter-to-CDC-Director.htm#:~:text =Letter%20from%20Bill%20Foege%2C%20Past%20CDC%20

Director%2C%20to,first%20thing%20would%20be%20to%20
face%20the%20truth

38. Bass E. *To End a Plague*. Public Affairs; 2021.

39. Rupar A. Deborah Birx praised Trump as attentive to scientific literature and details. Nope. March 27, 2020. Accessed March 22, 2025. https://www.vox.com/2020/3/27/21197074/deborah-birx-praised -trump-scientific-literature-coronavirus

40. President Trump claims injecting people with disinfectant could treat coronavirus. YouTube. Accessed March 22, 2025. https://www.bing .com/videos/search?q=trump+inject+bleach&view=detail&mid=2B6 6C7923B8ADD72ACD02B66C7923B8ADD72ACD0&FORM=VIRE

41. McGraw M, Stein S. It's been exactly one year since Trump suggested injecting bleach. We've never been the same. Politico. April 23, 2021. Accessed March 22, 2025. https://www.politico.com/news/2021/04/23 /trump-bleach-one-year-484399

42. Owermohle S. 'You don't want to go to war with a president'. Politico. March 3, 2020. Accessed March 22, 2025. https://www.politico.com /news/2020/03/03/anthony-fauci-trump-coronavirus-crisis-118961

43. Piller C. Undermining CDC. October 14, 2020. Accessed March 22, 2025. https://www.science.org/content/article/inside-story-how -trumps-covid-19-coordinator-undermined-cdc

44. Banco E. CDC chief tries to rebuild her agency's reputation—and morale. Politico. March 5, 2021. Accessed March 22, 2025. https://www .politico.com/news/2021/03/05/rochelle-walensky-cdc-rebuild-473841

45. Ghebreyesus, TA; World Health Organization. WHO Director-General's opening remarks at the media briefing on COVID-19 - 11 March 2020. Accessed March 22, 2025. https://www.who.int/director -general/speeches/detail/who-director-general-s-opening-remarks-at -the-media-briefing-on-covid-19---11-march-2020

46. Office of the Historian, Department of State. 20 STATE 28418. Accessed March 22, 2025. https://history.state.gov/departmenthistory /timeline/2020-2029

47. Herman-Roloff A, Aman R, Samandari T, et al. Adapting longstanding public health collaborations between Government of Kenya and CDC Kenya in response to the COVID-19 pandemic, 2020–2021. Emerg Infect Dis. 2022;28:S159–S167.

48. Nyagwange J, Ndwiga L, Muteru K et al. Epidemiology of COVID-19 infections on routine polymerase chain reaction (PCR) and serology testing in Coastal Kenya. Wellcome Open Res. 2022;7:69.

49. Adetifa IMO, Uyoga S, Gitonga JN, et al. Temporal trends of SARS-CoV-2 seroprevalence during the first wave of the COVID-19 epidemic in Kenya. Nat Commun. 2021;12:3966.

50. Havers FP, Reed C, Lim T, et al. Seroprevalence of antibodies to SARS-CoV-2 in 10 sites in the United States, March 23–May 12, 2020. JAMA Intern Med. 2020;180:1576–1586.

51. Johns Hopkins Coronavirus Resource Center. COVID-19 dashboard. Accessed March 22, 2025. https://coronavirus.jhu.edu/map.html

52. Institute for Health Metrics and Evaluation. COVID-19 projections. Accessed March 22, 2025. https://covid19.healthdata.org/global?view =cumulative-deaths&tab=trend

53. Our World in Data. Coronavirus pandemic (COVID-19). 2020. Accessed March 22, 2025. https://ourworldindata.org/coronavirus

54. World Health Organization. COVID-19 cases, world. Accessed March 22, 2025. https://covid19.who.int/

55. *The Economist.* The pandemic's true death toll. October 25, 2022. Accessed March 22, 2025. https://www.economist.com/graphic-detail /coronavirus-excess-deaths-estimates

56. Feuer A, Rashbaum WK. 'We ran out of space': bodies pile up as N.Y. struggles to bury its dead. *New York Times.* April 30, 2020; updated November 18, 2020. Accessed March 22, 2025. https://www.nytimes .com/2020/04/30/nyregion/coronavirus-nyc-funeral-home-morgue -bodies.html

57. Odone A, Delmonte D, Scognamiglio T, Signorelli C. COVID-19 deaths in Lombardy, Italy: data in context [published correction published in Lancet Public Health. 2020;5:e315]. Lancet Public Health. 2020;5:e310.

58. Anderson RM, Heesterbeek H, Klinkenberg D, Hollingsworth TD. How will country-based mitigation measures influence the course of the COVID-19 epidemic? Lancet. 2020;395:931–934.

59. Anderson RM, Vegvari C, Truscott J, Collyer BS. Challenges in creating herd immunity to SARS-CoV-2 infection by mass vaccination. Lancet. 2020;396:1614–1616.

60. Brand SPC, Ojal J, Aziza R, et al. COVID-19 transmission dynamics underlying epidemic waves in Kenya. Science. 2021;374:989–994.

61. Mwananyanda L, Gill C J, MacLeod W, et al. Covid-19 deaths in Africa: prospective systematic postmortem surveillance study. BMJ. 2021;372:n334.

62. Wadman M. An advocate for Africa. Science. October 6, 2022. Accessed March 22, 2025. https://www.science.org/content/article /covid-19-sleuth-making-friends-and-foes-advocating-african-science

63. Larson HJ, Gakidou E, Murray CJL. The vaccine-hesitant moment. N Engl J Med. 2022;387:58–65.

64. Centers for Disease Control and Prevention. CDC Museum COVID-19 timeline. July 8, 2024. https://www.cdc.gov/museum/timeline /covid19.html

65. Slaoui M, Hepburn M. Developing safe and effective Covid vaccines—Operation Warp Speed's strategy and approach. N Engl J Med. 2020;383:1701–1703.

66. Baker S, Koons C. Inside Operation Warp Speed's $18 billion sprint for a vaccine. Bloomberg. October 29, 2020. Accessed March 22, 2025. https://www.bloomberg.com/news/features/2020-10-29/inside -operation-warp-speed-s-18-billion-sprint-for-a-vaccine

67. Centers for Disease Control and Prevention. National Center for Health Statistics. COVID-19 mortality by state. Accessed March 22, 2025. https://www.cdc.gov/nchs/pressroom/sosmap/covid19 _mortality_final/COVID19.htm

68. Kamarck E. COVID-19 is crushing red states. Why isn't Trump turning his rallies into mass vaccination sites? Brookings. July 29, 2021. Accessed March 22, 2025. https://www.brookings.edu/articles/covid -19-is-crushing-red-states-why-isnt-trump-turning-his-rallies-into -mass-vaccination-sites/

69. Walensky R. A call to action for new investigators: opportunities in research and public health. February 19, 2023. Accessed March 22, 2025. https://www.croiwebcasts.org/portal/

70. Centers for Disease Control and Prevention. CDC launches new Center for Forecasting and Outbreak Analytics. April 19, 2022. Accessed March 22, 2025. https://www.cdc.gov/media/releases/2022 /p0419-forecasting-center.html

71. Miller BJ, Gowda N, Ranasinghe P, Phan P, Cullen TA, Lushniak BD. A vision for supporting and reforming the CDC. Health Affairs. June 10, 2022. Accessed March 22, 2025. https://www.healthaffairs.org/content /forefront/vision-supporting-and-reforming-cdc

72. Frieden T. Three solutions for public health—and one dangerous idea. *The Atlantic.* August 31, 2022. Accessed March 22, 2025. https://www .theatlantic.com/ideas/archive/2022/08/cdc-reform-covid/671296/

73. Foege W, Roper W, Koplan J, Gerberding J, Frieden T, Fitzgerald B, Redfield R, Walensky R. Eight former CDC directors: hollowing out the CDC is a prescription for disaster. STAT. September 5, 2024. Accessed April 8, 2025. https://www.statnews.com/2024/09/05/cdc -directors-funding-core-mission/#:~:text=William%20Foege%20 (1977%2D1983),Walensky%20(2021%2D2023)

74. World Health Organization. WHO Director-General's opening remarks at the media briefing—5 May 2023. Accessed March 22, 2025. https://www.who.int/news-room/speeches/item/who-director -general-s-opening-remarks-at-the-media-briefing---5-may-2023

75. WHO Director-General's report to Member States at the 76th World Health Assembly—22 May 2023. Accessed March 22, 2025. https://

www.who.int/director-general/speeches/detail/who-director-general
-s-report-to-member-states-at-the-76th-world-health-assembly---22
-may-2023

76. Centers for Disease Control and Prevention. End of the Federal
COVID-19 Public Health Emergency (PHE) Declaration. Updated
September 12, 2023. Accessed March 22, 2025. https://www.cdc.gov
/coronavirus/2019-ncov/your-health/end-of-phe.html

77. World Health Organization. Weekly epidemiological update on
COVID-19 - 25 May 2023. Accessed March 22, 2025. https://www.who
.int/publications/m/item/weekly-epidemiological-update-on-covid
-19---25-may-2023

78. Centers for Disease Control and Prevention. Accessed March 22, 2025.
https://covid.cdc.gov/covid-data-tracker/#trends_weeklydeaths
_select_00

79. Mandavilli A, Weiland N. Walensky resigns as C.D.C. director. *New
York Times*. May 5, 2023. Accessed March 22, 2025. https://www
.nytimes.com/2023/05/05/health/walensky-cdc-resignation.html

80. LaFraniere S, Weiland N. Walensky, citing botched pandemic response, calls for C.D.C. reorganization. *New York Times*. Accessed
March 22, 2025. https://www.nytimes.com/2022/08/17/us/politics
/cdc-rochelle-walensky-covid.html

81. De Cock KM, Jaffe HW, Curran JW. *Dispatches from the AIDS Pandemic: A Public Health Story*. Oxford University Press; 2023:282–303).

82. Roper WL. Bill Roper: You cannot remove politics from public health.
April 11, 2022. Accessed March 22, 2025. https://www.youtube.com
/watch?v=MBtfRx6OwkY

83. David Sencer interview. CDC Connects. August 20, 2010.

Section III. Bureaucrat

1. De Cock KM, Jaffe HW, Curran JW. *Dispatches from the AIDS Pandemic: A Public Health Story*. Oxford University Press; 2023.

Chapter 11. More than Just a Disease: Tuberculosis

1. Ali M, Nelson AR, Lopez AL, Sack DA. Updated global burden of
cholera in endemic countries. PLoS Negl Trop Dis. 2015;9:e0003832.

2. Korenromp EL, Rowley J, Alonso M, et al. Global burden of maternal
and congenital syphilis and associated adverse birth outcomes-
estimates for 2016 and progress since 2012 [published correction appears
in PLoS One. 2019;14(7):e0219613]. PLoS One. 2019;14:e0211720.

3. World Health Organization. Global Tuberculosis Report 2022. World
Health Organization; 2022.

4. De Cock KM, Jaffe HW, Curran JW. *Dispatches from the AIDS Pandemic: A Public Health Story.* Oxford University Press; 2023.

5. Dubos R, Dubos J. *The White Plague.* Little, Brown, and Company; 1952.

6. Snider DE. Tuberculosis: the world situation. History of the disease and efforts to combat it. In: Porter JDH, McAdam KPWJ, eds. *Tuberculosis: Back to the Future.* John Wiley and Sons; 1994:13-33.

7. Daniel TH, Bates JH, Downes KA. History of tuberculosis. In: Bloom BR, ed. *Tuberculosis: Pathogenesis, Protection, and Control.* ASM Press; 1994:13-24.

8. Ryan F. *Tuberculosis: The Greatest Story Never Told.* Swift Publishers; 1992.

9. Keats J. Ode to a nightingale.

10. Toman K. *Tuberculosis Case-Finding and Chemotherapy: Questions and Answers.* World Health Organization; 1979.

11. Iseman D. *A Clinician's Guide to Tuberculosis.* Lippincott, Williams, and Wilkins; 2000.

12. Murray JF. A century of tuberculosis. Am J Respir Crit Care Med. 2004;169:1181-1186.

13. Mann T. *The Magic Mountain.* 1924.

14. Frieden TR, Lerner BH, Rutherford BR. Lessons from the 1800s: tuberculosis control in the new millennium. Lancet. 2000;355: 1088-1092.

15. International Union Against Tuberculosis and Lung Disease. Homepage. Accessed March 22, 2025. https://theunion.org/

16. AMFAR. Making AIDS history. Accessed March 22, 2025. https://www.amfar.org/

17. Elizabeth Glaser Pediatric AIDS Foundation. Accessed March 22, 2025. https://www.pedaids.org/

18. Evans DK, Goldstein M, Popova A. Health-care worker mortality and the legacy of the Ebola epidemic. Lancet Global Health. 2015;3: e439-e440.

19. World Health Organization. Health and care worker deaths during COVID-19. October 20, 2021. Accessed March 22, 2025. https://www.who.int/news/item/20-10-2021-health-and-care-worker-deaths-during-covid-19

20. Galgalo T, Dalal S, Cain KP, et al. Tuberculosis risk among staff of a large public hospital in Kenya. Int J Tuberc Lung Dis. 2008 12:949-54.

21. Centers for Disease Control and Prevention. TB infection control in health care settings. Accessed March 22, 2025. https://www.cdc.gov/tb/topic/infectioncontrol/TBhealthCareSettings.htm

22. De Cock KM. Impact of interaction with HIV. In: Porter JDH, McAdam KPWJ, eds. *Tuberculosis: Back to the Future*. John Wiley and Sons; 1994: 36–49.

23. Jones JL, Hanson DL, Dworkin MS, DeCock KM; Adult/Adolescent Spectrum of HIV Disease Group. HIV-associated tuberculosis in the era of highly active antiretroviral therapy. The Adult/Adolescent Spectrum of HIV Disease Group. Int J Tuberc Lung Dis. 2000;4:1026–1031.

24. Lucas SB, Hounnou A, Peacock C, et al. The mortality and pathology of HIV infection in a West African city. AIDS. 1993;7:1569–1579.

25. Mann JM, Snider DE, Francis H, et al. Association between HTLV-III/LAV infection and tuberculosis in Zaire. JAMA. 1986;256:346.

26. De Cock KM, Gnaore E, Adjorlolo G, et al. Increased risk for tuberculosis in persons with HIV-1 and HIV-2 infections in Abidjan, Cote d'Ivoire. BMJ. 1991;302:496–499.

27. Corbett EL, Watt CJ, Walker N, et al. The growing burden of tuberculosis: global trends and interactions with the HIV epidemic. Arch Intern Med. 2003;163:1009–1021.

28. Selwyn PA, Hartel D, Lewis VA, et al. A prospective study of the risk of tuberculosis among intravenous drug users with human immunodeficiency virus infection. N Engl J Med. 1989;320:545–550.

29. Mallory KF, Churchyard GJ, Kleinschmidt I, De Cock KM, Corbett EL. The impact of HIV infection on recurrence of tuberculosis in South African gold miners. Int J Tuberc Lung Dis. 2000;4:455–462.

30. Suthar AB, Lawn SD, del Amo J, Antiretroviral therapy for prevention of tuberculosis in adults with HIV: a systematic review and meta-analysis. PLoS Med. 2012;9(7):e1001270.

31. De Cock KM, Marston B. The sound of one hand clapping: tuberculosis and antiretroviral therapy in Africa. Am J Respir Crit Care Med. 2005;172:3–4.

32. De Cock KM, Soro B, Coulibaly IM, Lucas SB. Tuberculosis and HIV infection in sub-Saharan Africa. JAMA. 1992;268:1581–1587.

33. Marston B, Miller B. Tuberculosis: the elephant in the AIDS clinic? AIDS. 2006;20:1323–1325.

34. WHO Global Tuberculosis Programme. *TB: A Global Emergency, WHO Report on the TB Epidemic*. World Health Organization. 1994. Accessed March 22, 2025. https://apps.who.int/iris/handle/10665/58749

35. Rieder HL. *Epidemiologic Basis of Tuberculosis Control*. 1st ed. International Union Against Tuberculosis and Lung Disease; 1999.

36. Rieder HL. *Interventions for Tuberculosis Control and Elimination*. International Union Against Tuberculosis and Lung Disease; 2002.

37. World Health Organization. *What is DOTS? A Guide to Understanding the WHO-Recommended TB Control Strategy Known as DOTS*. Word

Health Organization; 1999. Accessed March 22, 2025. https://apps.who
.int/iris/bitstream/handle/10665/65979/WHO_CDS_CPC_TB_99
.270.pdf;jsessio

38. Nunn P, Kibuga D, Gathua S, et al. Cutaneous hypersensitivity
reactions due to thiacetazone in HIV-1 seropositive patients treated for
tuberculosis. Lancet. 1991;337:627–630.

39. De Cock KM, Wilkinson D. Tuberculosis control in resource poor
countries: novel approaches in the era of HIV. Lancet.
1995;346:675–677.

40. Wilkinson D, De Cock KM. Tuberculosis control in South Africa: time
for a new paradigm? S Afr Med J. 1996;86:33–35.

41. De Cock KM. Tuberculosis control in resource-poor settings with high
rates of HIV infection. Am J Public Health. 1996;86:1071–1073.

42. Kenyon TA, Mwasekaga MJ, Huebner R, Rumisha D, Binkin N,
Maganu E. Low levels of drug resistance amidst rapidly increasing
tuberculosis and human immunodeficiency virus co-epidemics in
Botswana. Int J Tuberc Lung Dis. 1999;3:4–11.

43. De Cock KM, Chaisson RE. Will DOTS do it? A reappraisal of tuberculosis control in countries with high rates of HIV infection. Int J Tuberc
Lung Dis. 1999;3:457–465.

44. Frieden TR, Fujiwara PI, Washko RM, Hamburg MA. Tuberculosis in
New York City—turning the tide. N Engl J Med. 1995;333:229–233.

45. De Cock KM. Plus ça change . . . antiretroviral therapy, HIV prevention and the HIV treatment cascade. Clin Infect Dis.
2014;58:1012–1014.

46. Kassim S, Sassan-Morokro M, Ackah A, et al. Two-year follow-up of
persons with HIV-1- and HIV-2-associated pulmonary tuberculosis
treated with short course chemotherapy in West Africa. AIDS.
1995;9:1185–1191.

47. Richards SB, St Louis M, Nieburg P, et al. Impact of the HIV epidemic
on tuberculosis in Abidjan, Cote d'Ivoire. Tuber Lung Dis.
1995;76:11–16.

48. Yuen CM, Weyenga HO, Kim AA, et al. Comparison of trends in
tuberculosis incidence among adults living with HIV and adults
without HIV—Kenya, 1998-2012. PLoS One. 2014;9:e99880.

49. Surie D, Borgdorff MW, Cain KP, Click ES, De Cock KM, Yuen CM.
Assessing the impact of antiretroviral therapy on tuberculosis notifica-
tion rates among people with HIV: a descriptive analysis of 23 countries
in sub-Saharan Africa, 2010-2015. BMC Infect Dis. 2018;18:481.

50. Williams BG, Granich R, De Cock K, Glaziou P, Sharma A, Dye C.
Anti-retroviral therapy for tuberculosis control in in nine African
countries. Proc Natl Acad Sci U S A. 2010;107:19485–19489.

51. Suthar AB, Lawn SD, del Amo J, et al. Antiretroviral therapy for prevention of tuberculosis in adults with HIV: a systematic review and meta-analysis. PLoS Med. 2012;9:e1001270.

52. Centers for Disease Control and Prevention. National action plan to combat multidrug-resistant tuberculosis. MMWR Recomm Rep. 1992;41;5-48.

53. Dheda K, Gumbo T, Maartens G, et al. The epidemiology, pathogenesis, transmission, diagnosis, and management of multidrug-resistant, extensively drug-resistant, and incurable tuberculosis. Lancet Respir Med. 2017:S2213-2600(17)30079-6.

54. Global Programme on Tuberculosis and Lung Health, Guidelines Review Committee. *WHO Consolidated Guidelines on Tuberculosis. Module 4: Treatment - Drug-Resistant Tuberculosis Treatment, 2022 Update*. World Health Organization; 2022.

55. Yong Kim J, Shakow A, Mate K, Vanderwarker C, Gupta R, Farmer P. Limited good and limited vision: multidrug-resistant tuberculosis and global health policy. Soc Sci Med. 2005;61:847-859.

56. Friedland G, Harries A, Coetzee D. Implementation issues in tuberculosis/HIV program collaboration and integration: 3 case studies. J Infect Dis. 2007;196:S114-123.

57. Vegter I. Welkom to a world where mining dies. Institute of Race Relations March 26, 2019. Accessed March 22, 2025. https://irr.org.za/media/welkom-to-a-world-where-mining-dies-the-star

58. Corbett EL. *Mycobacterial Disease in South African Gold Miners: Associations With HIV Infection and Occupational Lung Disease*. PhD Thesis. London School of Hygiene and Tropical Medicine; 2002.

59. De Greef K. The dystopian underworld of South Africa's illegal gold mines. *The New Yorker*. February 20, 2023. Accessed March 22, 2025. https://www.newyorker.com/magazine/2023/02/27/the-dystopian-underworld-of-south-africas-illegal-gold-mines

60. Crush J, James W, eds. *Crossing Boundaries: Mine Migrancy in a Democratic South Africa*. Institute for Democracy in South Africa and the International Development Research Center; 1995.

61. Masekela H. "Stimela (The Coal Train)." 1974. Accessed March 22, 2025. https://genius.com/Hugh-Masekela-stimela-the-coal-train-lyrics

62. Corbett EL, Churchyard GJ, Charalambos S, et al. Morbidity and mortality in South African gold miners: impact of untreated disease due to human immunodeficiency virus. Clin Infect Dis. 2002;34:1251-1258.

63. Coovadia HM, Benatar SR, eds. *A Century of Tuberculosis: South African Perspectives*. Oxford University Press, 1991.

64. Del Amo J, Petruckevitch A, Phillips A, et al. Spectrum of disease in Africans with AIDS in London. AIDS. 1996;10:1563-1569.

65. Del Amo J, Petruckevitch A, Phillips A, et al. Disease progression and survival in HIV-1-infected Africans in London. AIDS. 1998;12:1203-1209.

66. Petruckevitch A, Del Amo J, Phillips A, et al. Disease progression and survival following specific AIDS-defining conditions: a retrospective cohort study of 2048 HIV-infected persons in London. AIDS. 1998;12:1007-1013.

67. Grant AD, Djomand G, Smets P, et al. Profound immunosuppression across the spectrum of opportunistic disease among hospitalized HIV-infected adults in Abidjan, Cote d'Ivoire. AIDS. 1997;11:1357-1364.

68. Grant AD, Djomand G, De Cock KM. Natural history and spectrum of disease in adults with HIV/AIDS in Africa. AIDS. 1997;11:S43-S54.

69. Grant AD, Kassim S, Domoua K, et al. Spectrum of disease among HIV-infected adults hospitalised in a respiratory medicine unit in Abidjan, Cote d'Ivoire. Int J Tuberc Lung Dis. 1998;2:926-934.

70. The Aurum Institute. Homepage. Accessed March 22, 2025. https://auruminstitute.org/

71. Churchyard GL, Kleinschmidt I, Corbett L, Mulder D, De Cock KM. Mycobacterial disease in South African gold miners in the era of HIV infection. Int J Tuberc Lung Dis. 1999;3:791-798.

72. Churchyard GJ, Kleinschmidt I, Corbett EL, Mulder D, De Cock KM. Drug resistant tuberculosis in South African gold miners: incidence and associated factors. Int J Tuberc Lung Dis. 2000;4:433-440.

73. Corbett EL, Hay M, Churchyard GJ, et al. *Mycobacterium kansasii* and *M. scrofulaceum* isolates from HIV-negative South African gold miners: incidence, clinical significance and radiology. Int J Tuberc Lung Dis. 1999;3:501-507.

74. Corbett EL, Churchyard GJ, Hay M, et al. The impact of HIV infection on *Mycobacterium kansasii* disease in South African gold miners. Am J Resp Crit Care Med. 1999;160:10-14.

75. Corbett EL, Blumberg L, Churchyard GJ, et al. Nontuberculous mycobacteria: defining disease in a prospective cohort of South African miners. Am J Respir Crit Care Med. 1999;160:15-21.

76. Corbett EL, Murray J, Churchyard GJ, et al. Use of mini-radiographs to detect silicosis: comparison of radiological with autopsy findings. Am J Respir Dis Crit Care Med. 1999;160:2012-2017.

77. Corbett EL, Churchyard GJ, Clayton T, et al. Risk factors for pulmonary mycobacterial disease in South African gold miners: a case-control study. Am J Respir Crit Care Med. 1999;159:94-99.

78. Charlambous S, Churchyard GJ, Murray J, De Cock KM, Corbett EL. Persistent radiological changes following miliary tuberculosis in miners exposed to silica dust. Int J Tuberc Lung Dis. 2001;5:1044-1050.

79. Corbett EL, Charlbambous S, Moloi VM, et al. Human immunodeficiency virus and the prevalence of undiagnosed tuberculosis in African goldminers. Am J Respir Dis Crit Care Med. 2004;170: 673–679.

80. Churchyard GJ, Fielding K, Roux S, et al. Twelve-monthly versus six-monthly radiological screening for active case-finding of tuberculosis: a randomized controlled trial. Thorax. 2011;66:134–139.

81. Mallory KF, Churchyard GJ, Kleinschmidt I, De Cock KM, Corbett EL. Impact of HIV infection on rates of recurrence after treatment for tuberculosis in South African gold miners. Int J Tuberc Lung Dis. 2000;4:455–462.

82. Charlambous S, Grant AD, Moloi V, et al. Contribution of reinfection to recurrent tuberculosis in South African gold miners. Int J Tuberc Lung Dis. 2008;12:942–948.

83. Churchyard GJ, Corbett EL, Kleinschmidt I, Murray J, Smit J, De Cock KM. Factors associated with an increased case-fatality rate in HIV-infected and non-infected South African gold miners. Int J Tuberc Lung Dis. 2000;4:705–712.

84. Corbett EL, Churchyard GJ, Clayton TC, et al. HIV infection and silicosis: the impact of two potent risk factors on the incidence of mycobacterial disease in South African miners. AIDS. 2000;14:2759–2768.

85. Charlambous S, Day JH, Fielding K, De Cock KM, Churchyard GJ, Corbett EL. HIV infection and chronic chest disease as risk factors for bacterial pneumonia: a case control study in South African gold miners. AIDS. 2003;17:1531–1537.

86. Corbett EL, Mozzato-Chamay N, Butterworth AE, et al. Polymorphisms in the tumor necrosis factor α gene promoter may predispose to severe silicosis in black South African miners. Am J Respir Crit Care Med. 2002;165:690–3.

87. Corbett EL, Charlambous S, Fielding K, et al. Stable tuberculosis incidence rates among HIV-negative South African gold miners during a decade of epidemic HIV-associated tuberculosis. J Infect Dis. 2003;188:1156–1163.

88. Churchyard GJ, Fielding K, Charlambous S, et al. Efficacy of secondary isoniazid preventive therapy among HIV-infected Southern Africans: time to change policy? AIDS. 2003;17:2063–2070.

89. Grant AD, Charalambous S, Fielding KL, et al. Effect of routine isoniazid preventive therapy on tuberculosis among HIV-infected men in South Africa: a novel randomized incremental recruitment study. JAMA. 2005;293:2719–2725.

90. Murray J, Davies T, Rees D. Occupational lung disease in the south African mining industry: research and policy implementation. J Public Health Policy. 2011;32:S65-79.

91. Kistnasamy B, Yassi A, Yu J, et al. Tackling injustices of occupational lung disease acquired in South African mines: recent developments and ongoing challenges [published correction appears in Global Health. 2018;14:78]. Global Health. 2018;14:60.

92. van Halsema CL, Fielding KL, Chihota VN, Lewis JJ, Churchyard GJ, Grant AD. Trends in drug-resistant tuberculosis in a gold-mining workforce in South Africa, 2002–2008. Int J Tuberc Lung Dis. 2012; 16:967-973.

93. Churchyard GJ, Fielding KL, Lewis JJ, et al. A trial of mass isoniazid preventive therapy for tuberculosis control. N Engl J Med. 2014;370:301-310.

94. Fitzpatrick S, Jakens F, Kuehne J. *Tuberculosis in South Africa's Gold Mines: A United Call to Action.* 2013. Accessed March 22, 2025. http://www.catalogue.safaids.net/sites/default/files/publications/Tuberculosis%20in%20South%20Africa.pdf

95. Chang ST, Chihota VN, Fielding KL, et al. Small contribution of gold mines to the ongoing tuberculosis epidemic in South Africa: a modeling-based study [published correction appears in BMC Med. 2018;16:242]. BMC Med. 2018;16:52.

96. Lurie MN, Williams BG, Zuma K, et al. Who infects whom? HIV-1 concordance and discordance among migrant and non-migrant couples in South Africa. AIDS. 2003;17:2245-2252.

97. Webb A. Gold production over the past and next 25 years. March 2021. Accessed March 22, 2025. https://www.lbma.org.uk/alchemist/issue -100/gold-production-over-the-past-and-next-25-years

98. Lurie MN, Williams BG. Migration and health in southern Africa: 100 years and still circulating. Health Psychol Behav Med. 2014;2:34-40.

99. Marmot M, Wilkinson RG. *Social Determinants of Health.* 2nd ed. Oxford University Press; 2005.

100. Dooyema CA, Neri A, Lo YC, et al. Outbreak of fatal childhood lead poisoning related to artisanal gold mining in northwestern Nigeria, 2010. Environ Health Perspect. 2012;120:601-607.

101. Corbett EL, De Cock KM. The clinical significance of interactions between HIV and TB: more questions than answers. Int J Tuberc Lung Dis. 2001;5:205-207.

102. Corbett EL, Marston B, Churchyard GJ, De Cock KM. Tuberculosis in sub-Saharan Africa: opportunities, challenges, and change in the era of antiretroviral therapy. Lancet. 2006;367:926-937.

103. De Cock KM. HIV infection, tuberculosis and World AIDS Day, 2006. Int J Tuberc Lung Dis. 2006;10:1305.

104. De Cock KM. HIV/AIDS 2007: an end-of-year commentary. Int J Tuberc Lung Dis. 2007;11:1267–1269.

105. Nunn P, Reid A, De Cock KM. Tuberculosis and HIV infection: the global setting. J Infect Dis. 2007;196:S5–14.

106. Nunn P, De Cock K. Measuring progress towards integrated TB-HIV treatment and care services: are countries doing what needs to be done? Int J Tuberc Lung Dis. 2008;12:1

107. Odhiambo J, Kizito W, Njoroge A, et al. Provider-initiated HIV testing and counseling for TB patients and suspects in Nairobi, Kenya. Int J Tuberc Lung Dis. 2008;12:S63–S68.

108. De Cock KM. HIV/AIDS and global health in 2010: from the old to the old and the new. Int J Tuberc Lung Dis. 2010;14:1500–1503.

109. Harries AD, Zacharias R, Corbett EL, et al. The HIV-associated tuberculosis epidemic—when will we act? Lancet. 2010;375: 1906–1919.

110. Lawn SD, Wood R, De Cock KM, Churchyard GJ. Antiretrovirals and isoniazid preventive therapy in the prevention of HIV-associated tuberculosis in settings with limited health-care resources. Lancet Infect Dis. 2010;10:489–498.

111. Lawn SD, Harries AD, Williams BG, et al. Antiretroviral therapy and the control of HIV-associated tuberculosis. Will ART do it? Int J Tuberc Lung Dis. 2011;15;571–581.

112. Marston BJ, De Cock KM. How can this be? Preventing death in patients with HIV-associated tuberculosis. Int J Tuberc Lung Dis. 2012;16:569–570.

113. Borgdorff MW, Cain KP, De Cock KM. The molecular epidemiology of tuberculosis in settings with a high HIV prevalence: implications for control. J Infect Dis. 2014;11:8–9.

114. Cain K, Marano N, Kamene M, et al. The movement of multidrug-resistant tuberculosis across borders in East Africa needs a regional solution. PLoS Med. 2015;12:e1001791.

115. Van't Hoog A, Laserson KF, Githui WA, et al. High prevalence of tuberculosis and inadequate case finding in rural Western Kenya. Am J Respir Crit Care Med. 2011;183:1245–1253.

116. Fox GJ, Nhung NV, Sy DN, et al. Household-contact investigation for detection of tuberculosis in Vietnam. N Engl J Med. 2018;378: 221–229.

117. Marks GB, Nguyen NV, Nguyen PTB, et al. Community-wide screening for tuberculosis in a high-prevalence setting. N Engl J Med. 2019;381:1347–1357.

118. Wood R, Lawn SD, Johnstone-Robertson S, Bekker LG. Tuberculosis control has failed in South Africa—time to reappraise strategy. S Afr Med J. 2011;101:111–114.

119. Dye C, Williams BG. The population dynamics and control of tuberculosis. Science. 2010;328:856–861.

120. Houben RMGJ, Dodd PJ. The global burden of latent tuberculosis infection: a re-estimation using mathematical modelling. PLoS Med. 2016;13:e1002152.

121. UNAIDS. *The Path That Ends AIDS: UNAIDS Global AIDS Update 2023*. Joint United Programme on HIV/AIDS; 2023.

Chapter 12. Health Diplomacy

1. Kickbusch I, Liu A. Global health diplomacy—reconstructing power and governance. Lancet. 2022;399:2156–2166.

2. De Cock KM, Jaffe HW, Curran JW. *Dispatches From the AIDS Pandemic: A Public Health Story*. Oxford University Press; 2023.

3. De Cock KM. AIDS: an old disease from Africa? Br Med J. 1984;289: 306–308.

4. De Cock KM, Low N. HIV and AIDS, other sexually transmitted diseases, and tuberculosis in ethnic minorities in United Kingdom: is surveillance serving its purpose? BMJ. 1997;314:1747–1751.

5. Daskalakis D, McClung RP, Mena L, Mermin J; Centers for Disease Control and Prevention's Monkeypox Response Team. Monkeypox: avoiding the mistakes of past infectious disease epidemics. Ann Intern Med. 2022;175:1177–1178.

6. Odehouri K, De Cock KM, Krebs JW, et al. HIV-1 and HIV-2 infection associated with AIDS in Abidjan, Côte d'Ivoire. AIDS. 1989;3:509–512.

7. Greenberg, Alan. The Global Health Chronicles. July 26, 2017. Accessed March 23, 2025. https://globalhealthchronicles.org/items /show/7907

8. De Cock, Kevin. The Global Health Chronicles. June 13, 2016. Accessed March 23, 2025. https://globalhealthchronicles.org/items/ show/6481

9. Sassan-Morokro M, Greenberg AE, Coulibaly IM, et al. High rates of sexual contact with female sex workers, sexually transmitted diseases, and condom neglect among HIV-infected and uninfected men with tuberculosis in Abidjan, Côte d'Ivoire. J Acquir Immune Defic Syndr Hum Retrovirol. 1996;11:183–187.

10. Lucas SB, Hounnou A, Peacock C, et al. The mortality and pathology of HIV infection in a west African city. AIDS. 1993;7:1569–1579.

11. De Cock KM, Soro B, Coulibaly IM, Lucas SB. Tuberculosis and HIV infection in sub-Saharan Africa. JAMA. 1992;268:1581–1587.

12. De Cock KM, Adjorlolo G, Ekpini E, et al. Epidemiology and transmission of HIV-2. Why there is no HIV-2 pandemic. JAMA. 1993;270: 2083–2086.

13. Gottlieb GS, Raugi DN, Smith RA. 90-90-90 for HIV-2? Ending the HIV-2 epidemic by enhancing care and clinical management of patients infected with HIV-2. Lancet HIV. 2018;5:e390–e399.

14. Mulder DW, Nunn AJ, Wagner HU, Kamali A, Kengeya-Kayondo JF. HIV-1 incidence and HIV-1-associated mortality in a rural Ugandan population cohort. AIDS. 1994;8:87–92.

15. Shilts R. And the Band Played On. St. Martin's Press; 1987.

16. De Cock KM, Johnson AM. From exceptionalism to normalisation: a reappraisal of attitudes and practice around HIV testing. BMJ. 1998;316:290–293.

17. Janssen RS, Holtgrave DR, Valdiserri RO, Shepherd M, Gayle HD, De Cock KM. The serostatus approach to fighting the HIV epidemic: prevention strategies for HIV-infected individuals. Am J Public Health. 2001;91:1019–1024.

18. De Cock KM, Mbori-Ngacha D, Marum E. Shadow on the continent - public health and HIV/AIDS in Africa in the 21st century. Lancet. 2002;360:67–72.

19. De Cock KM, Marum EL, Mbori-Ngacha D. A serostatus-based approach to HIV/AIDS prevention in Africa. Lancet. 2003;362:1847–1849.

20. De Cock KM, Bunell R, Mermin J. Unfinished business—expanding HIV testing in developing countries. New Engl J Med. 2006;354:440–442.

21. World Health Organization, UNAIDS. Guidance on Provider-Initiated HIV Testing and Counseling in Health Facilities. World Health Organization; 2007.

22. Cohen MS, Chen YQ, McCauley M, et al. Prevention of HIV-1 infection with early antiretroviral therapy. N Engl J Med. 2011;365:493–505.

23. Eisinger RW, Dieffenbach CW, Fauci AS. HIV viral load and transmissibility of HIV infection: undetectable equals untransmittable. JAMA. 2019;321:451–452.

24. Fleming PL, Ward JW, Janssen RS, et al. Guidelines for human immunodeficiency virus case surveillance, including monitoring for human immunodeficiency virus infection and acquired immunodeficiency syndrome. MMWR Recomm Rep. 1999;48:1–27.

25. Benkimoun P. How Lee Jong-wook changed WHO. Lancet. 2006;367:1806–1808.

26. The western Kenya insecticide-treated bed net trial. Am J Trop Med Hyg. 2003;68:1–173.

27. Adazu K, Lindblade KA, Rosen DH, et al. Health and demographic surveillance in rural western Kenya: a platform for evaluating inter-

ventions to reduce morbidity and mortality from infectious diseases. Am J Trop Med Hyg. 2005;73:1151-1158.

28. Phillips-Howard PA, Odhiambo FO, Hamel M, et al. Mortality trends from 2003 to 2009 among adolescents and young adults in rural western Kenya using a health and demographic surveillance system. PLoS One. 2012;7:e47017.

29. Odhiambo F, Lasersson KF, Sewe M, et al. Profile: the KEMRI/CDC health and demographic surveillance system—Western Kenya. Int J Epidemiol. 2012;41:977-987.

30. Odhiambo FO, Beynon CM, Ogwang S, et al. Trauma-related mortality among adults in rural western Kenya: analysis of data from a health and demographic surveillance system. PLoS One. 2013;8: e79840.

31. Phillips-Howard PA, Laserson KF, Amek N, et al. Deaths ascribed to non-communicable diseases are proportionately increasing: evidence from a health and demographic surveillance system, 2003-2010. PLoS One. 2014:9:e114010.

32. Bass E. *To End a Plague: America's Bold Quest to Defeat AIDS in Africa*. PublicAffairs; 2021.

33. Centers for Disease Control and Prevention. *CDC Kenya Annual Report 2018*. Reviewed September 2019. Accessed March 23, 2025. https://archive.cdc.gov/#/details?url=https://www.cdc.gov /globalhealth/countries/kenya/reports/index.html

34. Amornkul P, Vandenhoudt H, Nasokho P, et al. HIV prevalence and associated risk factors among individuals aged 13-34 years in rural western Kenya. PLoS One. 2009;4:e6470.

35. Thomas TK, Masaba R, Borkowf CB, et al. Triple-antiretroviral prophylaxis to prevent mother-to-child HIV transmission through breastfeeding - the Kisumu Breastfeeding Study, Kenya: a clinical trial. PLoS Med. 2011;8:e1001015.

36. Otieno GO, Whiteside YO, Achia T, et al. Decreased HIV-associated mortality rates during the scale-up of antiretroviral therapy in western Kenya (2011-2016): a population-based cohort study. AIDS. 2019;33:2423-2430.

37. Borgdorff MW, Kwaro D, Obor D, et al. Reduction of HIV incidence in western Kenya during scale up of antiretroviral therapy and voluntary medical male circumcision, a population-based cohort analysis. Lancet HIV. 2018;5:e241-249.

38. Bailey RC, Moses S, Parker CB, et al. Male circumcision for HIV prevention in young men in Kisumu, Kenya: a randomised controlled trial. Lancet. 2007;369:643-656.

39. Auvert B, Taljaard D, Lagarde E, Sobngwi-Tambekou J, Sitta R, Puren A. Randomized, controlled intervention trial of male

circumcision for reduction of HIV infection risk: the ANRS 1265 Trial [published correct appears in PLoS Med. 2006;3:e298]. PLoS Med. 2005;2:e298.

40. Gray RH, Kigozi G, Serwadda D, Makumbi F, et al. Male circumcision for HIV prevention in men in Rakai, Uganda: a randomised trial. Lancet. 2007;369:657–666.

41. De Cock KM, Rutherford G, Akhwale W, eds. Kenya AIDS Indicator Survey 2012. J Aquir Immune Defic Syndr. 2014;66:S1–S137.

42. Cherutich P, Kim AA, Kellogg TA, et al. Detectable HIV viral load in Kenya: data from a population-based survey. PLoS One. 2016;11: e0154318.

43. Kim AA, Mukui I, Nganga L, et al. Progress in reversing the HIV epidemic through intensified access to antiretroviral therapy: results from a nationally representative population -based survey in Kenya, 2012. PLoS One. 2016;11:e0148068.

44. Kim AA, Parekh B, Umuro M, et al. Identifying risk factors for recent HIV infection in Kenya using a recent infection testing algorithm: results from a nationally representative population-based survey. PLoS One. 2016;11:e0155498.

45. Blaizot S, Kim AA, Zeh C, et al. Estimating HIV incidence using a cross-sectional survey: comparison of three approaches in a hyperendemic setting, Ndhiwa sub-county, Kenya, 2012. AIDS Res Hum Retroviruses. 2017;33:472-481.

46. Waruru A, Achia T, Muttai H, et al. Spatial-temporal trend for mother to child transmission of HIV up to infancy and during Pre-Option B+ in western Kenya, 2007-13. PeerJ. 2018;6:e4427.

47. Young PW, Zielinski-Gutierrez E, Wamicwe J, et al. Use of viral load to improve survey estimates of known HIV-positive status and antiretroviral treatment coverage. AIDS. 2020;34:631-636.

48. Young PW, Musingila P, Kingwara L, et al. HIV incidence, recent HIV infection, and associated factors, Kenya, 2007-2018. AIDS Res Hum Retroviruses. 2023;39:57-67.

49. Mutisya I, Muthoni E, Ondondo RO, et al. A national household survey on HIV prevalence and clinical cascade among children aged < 15 years in Kenya (2018). PLoS One. 2022;17:e0277613.

50. Kiplagat S. Davy Koech: Letter that won former Kemri boss freedom. Business Daily, July 30, 2023. Accessed March 23, 2025. https://www .businessdailyafrica.com/bd/lifestyle/profiles/davy-koech-letter-that -won-former-kemri-boss-freedom--4321062

51. Nairobi DusitD2 complex attack. Last edited March 19, 2025. Accessed March 23, 2025. https://en.wikipedia.org/wiki/Nairobi_DusitD2 _complex_attack

52. Joseph R, Musingila P, Miruka F, et al. Expanded eligibility for HIV testing increases HIV diagnoses—a cross-sectional study in seven facilities in western Kenya. PLoS One. 2019;14:e0225877.

53. Herman-Roloff A, Aman R, Samandari T, Kasera K, et al. Adapting longstanding public health collaborations between government of Kenya and CDC Kenya in response to the COVID-19 pandemic, 2020–2021. Emerg Infect Dis. 2022;28:S159–S167.

Chapter 13. Health Bureaucracy

1. De Cock KM, Jaffe HW, Curran JW. *Dispatches From the AIDS Pandemic: A Public Health Story.* Oxford University Press; 2023.

2. Sinek S. *Start With Why: How Great Leaders Inspire Everyone to Take Action.* Portfolio; 2009.

3. *The Economist.* Embrace crunchiness: societies are strongest when people are clear where they stand. August 27, 1988.

4. Foege WH. *The Fears of the Rich, the Needs of the Poor: My Years at the CDC.* Johns Hopkins University Press; 2018.

5. Department of Health and Human Services. Fiscal Year 2024. Centers for Disease Control and Prevention Fiscal Year 2024. Justification of Estimates for Appropriations Committees. https://www.cdc.gov /budget/documents/fy2024/FY-2024-CDC-congressional -justification.pdf

6. KPMG. Bill and Melinda Gates Foundation. Consolidated Financial Statements, December 31, 2022 and 2021. Accessed March 23, 2025. https://docs.gatesfoundation.org/documents/f_428053e-1a _billmelindagatesfoundation_fs.pdf

7. Moulds J. How is the World Health Organization funded? World Economic Forum. April 15, 2020. Accessed March 23, 2025. https:// www.weforum.org/agenda/2020/04/who-funds-world-health -organization-un-coronavirus-pandemic-covid-trump/

8. World Health Organization. Programme budget 2022–2023 approval (WHA74.3). Accessed March 23, 2025. https://www.who.int/publications /i/item/programme-budget-2020-2021-approval-(wha74.5)

9. Power S. *Chasing the Flame: Sergio Vieira de Mello and the Fight to Save the World.* Penguin Press; 2008.

10. Anan K, Mousavizadeh N. *Interventions: A Life in War and Peace.* Penguin Press; 2012.

11. Duke A. *Quit: The Power of Knowing When to Walk Away.* Portfolio; 2022.

12. Cohen J. *The Lancet* jousts with CDC's Center for Global Health. March 8, 2012. Accessed March 23, 2025. https://www.science.org /content/article/lancet-jousts-cdcs-center-global-health

13. Southwick SM, Charney DS. *Resilience: The Science of Mastering Life's Greatest Challenges.* 2nd ed. Cambridge University Press; 2018.

14. Watts G. Thomas Earl Starzl. Lancet. 2017;389:1096.

Epilogue

1. Callaway E. "It is chaos": US funding freezes are endangering global health. Nature. 2025. Accessed April 14, 2025. https://www.nature.com/articles/d41586-025-00385-9

2. Siegel J, Morehouse C, Guillén A. Trump's new goal: Revive a major climate pollutant that power markets have turned against. Politico. 2025. Accessed April 17, 2025. https://www.politico.com/news/2025/04/08/trump-launches-last-ditch-crusade-to-rescue-coal-00279245

3. Noguchi Y. Coal miners' health care hit hard in job cuts to CDC. NPR. 2025. Accessed April 17, 2025. https://www.npr.org/sections/shots-health-news/2025/04/09/nx-s1-5356067/niosh-cdc-coal-miner-black-lung-trump-doge

4. De Cock KM, Jaffe HW, Curran JW. *Dispatches from the AIDS Pandemic: A Public Health Story.* Oxford University Press; 2023.

5. The Heritage Foundation. *Mandate for Leadership: The Conservative Promise.* Project 2025, Presidential Transition Project. Accessed April 14, 2025. https://static.project2025.org/2025_MandateForLeadership_FULL.pdf

6. Miller BJ, Gowda N, Ranasinghe P, Phan P, Cullen TA, Lushniak BD. A vision for supporting and reforming the CDC. Health Affairs. June 10, 2022. Accessed March 22, 2025. https://www.healthaffairs.org/content/forefront/vision-supporting-and-reforming-cdc

7. Hartley LP. *The Go-Between.* Hamish Hamilton; 1953.

8. Koplan JP, Bond TC, Merson MH, et al. Towards a common definition of global health. Lancet. 2009;373:1993–1995.

9. De Cock KM, Lucas SB, Mabey D, Parry E. Tropical medicine for the 21st century. BMJ. 1995;311:860–862.

10. De Cock KM, Simone PM, Davison V, Slutsker L. The new global health. Emerg Infect Dis. 2013;19:1192–1197.

11. De Cock KM. Global health's evolution and search for identity. Emerg Infect Dis. 2025;31:1-7.

12. Institute for Health Metrics and Evaluation (IHME). Financing Global Health 2020: The Impact of COVID-19. IHME; 2021.

13. United Nations, Department of Economic and Social Affairs. World Population Prospects, 2022. Summary of Results. United Nations; 2022.

14. United Nations. UNHCR: A record 100 million people forcibly displaced worldwide. UN News. May 23, 2022. Accessed March 23, 2025. https://news.un.org/en/story/2022/05/1118772#:~:text=Accord-

ing%20to%20UNHCR%2C%20the%20number%20of%20forc
ibly%20displaced,Afghanistan%20and%20the%20Democratic%20
Republic%20of%20the%20Congo

15. Haines A, Ebi K. The imperative for climate action to protect health. New Engl J Med. 2019;380:263-273.

16. Binagwaho A, Ngarambe B, Mathewos K. Eliminating the white supremacy mindset from global health education. Ann Glob Health. 2022;88:32.

17. Banerjee AT, Bandara S, Senga J, González-Domínguez N, Pai M. Are we training our students to be white saviours in global health? Lancet. 2023;402:520-521.

INDEX

Browse more books from **HOPKINS PRESS**

ADVENTURES
OF A FEMALE
MEDICAL DETECTIVE
IN PURSUIT OF SMALLPOX AND AIDS
Mary Guinan, PhD, MD
with Anne D. Mather

T
H
E FEARS OF
THE RICH,
T
H
E NEEDS OF
THE POOR
MY YEARS AT THE CDC
WILLIAM H. FOEGE

The
TASK FORCE
for
CHILD
SURVIVAL
SECRETS OF
SUCCESSFUL COALITIONS
WILLIAM H. FOEGE
Foreword by PRESIDENT JIMMY CARTER

Collapse and
Resiliency
The Inside Story
of Liberia's
Unprecedented
Ebola Response
TOLBERT NYENSWAH, LLB, MPH, DrPH
with Mardia Stone, MD, MPH
foreword by
Former Liberian President Ellen Johnson Sirleaf

JOHNS HOPKINS
UNIVERSITY PRESS

PRESS.JHU.EDU

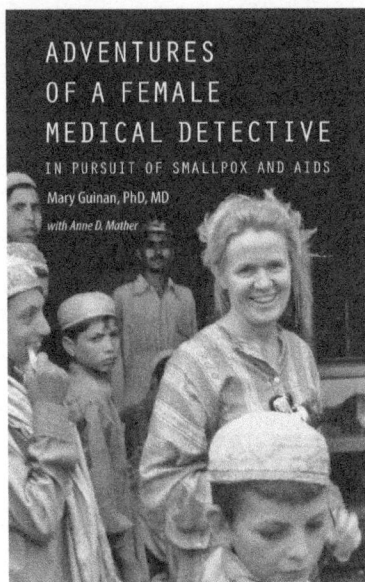

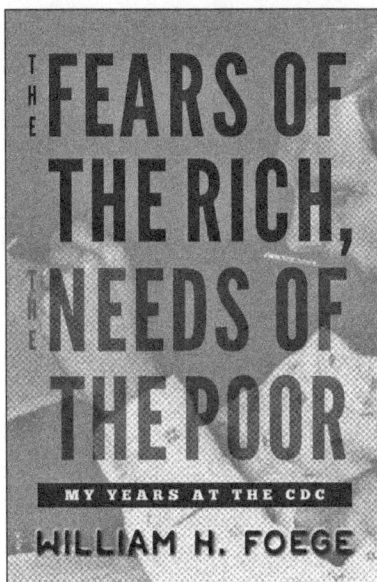

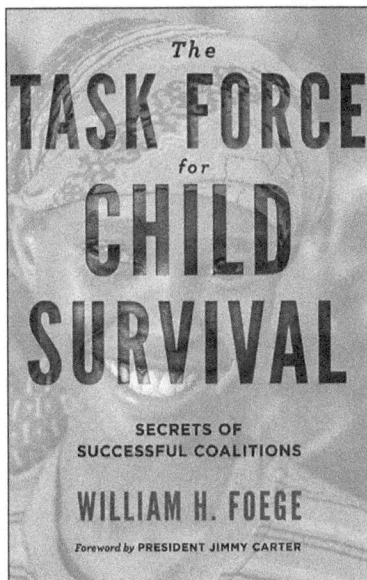

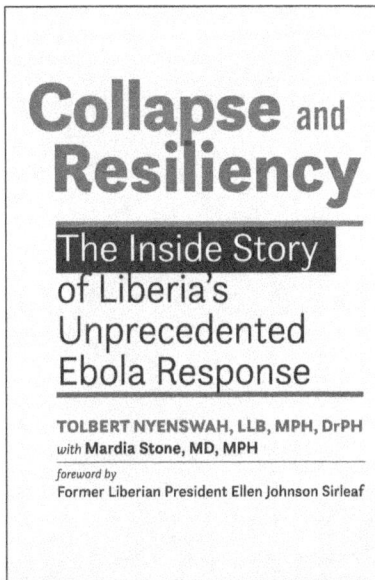